Physics, Simulation, and Treatment Planning

Principles and Practice of Radiation Therapy

Physics, Simulation, and Treatment Planning

Edited by

Charles M. Washington, BS, RT(T)

Director, Radiation Therapy Program
The University of Texas
MD Anderson Cancer Center
Houston, Texas

Dennis T. Leaver, MS, RT(R)(T)

Director, Radiation Therapy Program
Southern Maine Technical College
South Portland, Maine

with 271 illustrations

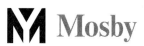 Mosby

St. Louis Baltimore Boston Carlsbad Chicago Naples New York Philadelphia Portland
London Madrid Mexico City Singapore Sydney Tokyo Toronto Wiesbaden

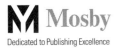
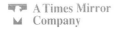

Vice President and Publisher: Don Ladig
Senior Editor: Jeanne Rowland
Senior Developmental Editor: Lisa Potts
Project Manager: John Rogers
Project Specialist: Kathleen L. Teal
Designer: Elizabeth Young
Composition Specialist: Terri Schwaegel
Manufacturing Manager: David Graybill

Printed in the United States of America

Composition by Mosby Electronic Production—St. Louis
Lithography by Top Graphics
Printing/binding by Maple Vail Book Manufacturing Group

Mosby–Year Book, Inc.
11830 Westline Industrial Drive
St. Louis, Missouri 63146

International Standard Book Number 0-8151-9136-7

98 99 00 / 9 8 7 6 5 4 3 2

To those who have run and continue to run the race against cancer.
We sincerely hope those who read this work will grow in the knowledge
and understanding necessary to provide direction and compassion to their patients.
Let us not grow tired in running our own race,
but instead encourage those around us.

Contributors

Julius Armstrong, MBA, RT(T)
Program Chairman,
Radiation Therapy Program,
Bellevue Community College,
Bellevue, Washington

E. Richard Bawiec, MS
Coordinator,
Hembree Regional Cancer Center,
Saint Edward Mercy Medical Center,
Fort Smith, Arkansas

Joseph S. Blinick, PhD
Maine Medical Center,
Radiation Physics Department,
Portland Maine

Beverly A. Buck, BS, RT, (R)(T)
Education and Development Coordinator,
Joint Center for Radiation Therapy,
Harvard Medical School,
Boston, Massachusetts

Teresa L. Bruno, BSN, RT(T), CMD
Director,
Dosimetry Training Program,
The University of Texas,
MD Anderson Cancer Center,
Houston, Texas

Joseph Buono, BS, RT(T)
Assistant Professor,
Nassau Community College,
Garden City, New York

Patton Griggs, BS
Department of Radiation Oncology,
Central Maine Medical Center,
Lewiston, Maine

Rosann Keller, MEd, RT(T)
Radiation Therapist,
Gershenson Radiation Oncology Center,
Harper Hospital,
Detroit, Michigan
and
Wayne State University,
Department of Radiation Therapy Technology,
Detroit, Michigan

Adam Kempa, MEd, RT(T)
Senior Lecturer,
Wayne State University,
Department of Radiation Therapy Technology,
Detroit, Michigan

Dennis T. Leaver, MS, RT(R)(T)
Director, Radiation Therapy Program,
Southern Maine Technical College,
South Portland, Maine

Jeremy Myles
Varian Oncology Systems,
Varian-TEM, Ltd.,
Crawley, West Sussex, UK

Sandra Nava, AS, RT(T)
Radiotherapy Program Educational Coordinator,
Division of Radiotherapy,
The University of Texas,
MD Anderson Cancer Center,
Houston, Texas

Tim Ochran, MS
Medical Physicist,
Paris Regional Cancer Center,
Paris, Texas

Elizabeth G. Quate, MS
Maine Medical Center,
Radiation Physics Department,
Portland, Maine

Judith M. Schneider, MS, RT(T)
Assistant Professor and Clinical Coordinator,
University School of Medicine,
School of Allied Health Sciences,
Radiation Therapy Program,
Indianapolis, Indiana

Thaddeus Sokolowski, MS
Medical Physicist,
Texas Oncology, PA
Sammons Cancer Center,
Dallas, Texas

Frances Taylor, BA, RT(R)(T)
Program Director,
Radiation Therapy Program,
University School of Medicine,
School of Allied Health Sciences,
Radiation Therapy Program,
University of Virginia Health Sciences Center,
Charlottesville, Virginia

Charles M. Washington, BS, RT(T)
Director, Radiation Therapy Program,
The University of Texas,
MD Anderson Cancer Center,
Houston, Texas

Reviewers

Eric Anderson, PhD
Assistant Professor of Physics,
Avila College,
Kansas City, Missouri

Sucha Asbell, MD
Chairman, Radiation Oncology,
Albert Einstein Medical Center,
Philadelphia, Pennsylvania

Joseph Baranowsky, BS
Field Service Engineer,
Dornier Medical Systems,
Kennesaw, Georgia

Cecelia Bouchard, MS, RT(R)(T)
Clinical Coordinator, Radiation Therapy Technology,
Southern Maine Technical College,
South Portland, Maine

Andrew P. Brown, MD
Radiation Oncologist,
Elliott Regional Cancer Center,
Manchester, New Hampshire

Cynthia P. Burns, AS, RT(R)(T)
Radiation Therapist,
Cynthia A. Rydholm Cancer Treatment Center,
Central Maine Medical Center,
Lewiston, Maine

Shaun T. Caldwell, BS, RT(R)(T)
Educational Director, Radiation Therapy,
College of Health Professions,
Weber State University,
Ogden, Utah

Anne T. Campbell, BHS, RT(R)(T)
Program Director, Radiation Therapy Technology Program,
Chandler Medical Center,
University of Kentucky,
Lexington, Kentucky

Sandra Bouquet Carslick, RT(R)(T)
Senior Radiation Therapist,
Costal Cancer Treatment Center,
Maine Medical Center,
Bath, Maine

Peter Y. Chen, MD
Associate Director of Education,
Department of Radiation Oncology,
William Beaumont Hospital,
Royal Oak, Michigan

Melvin C. Cheney, MS, RT(T)
Director of Patient Services,
Northwest Arkansas Radiation Therapy Institute;
Program Director, Radiation Therapist Program,
Northwest Arkansas Community College,
Springdale, Arkansas

Annette Coleman, MA, RT(T)
Educational Coordinator/Therapy,
Joint Center for Radiation Therapy,
Harvard Medical School,
Boston, Massachusetts

Joseph Digel, RT(R)(T)
Chief Therapist, Radiation Oncology,
Program Director, Radiation Therapy Program,
The Johns Hopkins Hospital,
Baltimore, Maryland

Barbara Flexner, BS, RT(T)
Educational Coordinator, Program Director,
Allied Health and Radiation Therapy Technology,
Vanderbilt University Medical Center,
Nashville, Tennessee

Diana Freeman, BS, RT(T)
Program Director, Certified Medical Dosimetrist,
Parkland College,
Decatur Memorial Hospital,
Decatur, Illinois

Tilly Gibbs, BA, RT(T)
Chief Therapist, Program Director,
Radiation Therapy Program,
University of Utah Hospital,
Salt Lake City, Utah

Patricia Giordano, MS, RT(T)
Program Director, Assistant Professor,
Gwynedd-Mercy College,
Gwynedd Valley, Pennsylvania

Charleen Gombert, BS, RT(T)
Professor, Program Director,
Radiation Therapy Technology Program,
Community College of Allegheny County,
Pittsburgh, Pennsylvania

Mark Graniero, BS, RT(T)
Chief Radiation Therapist,
Four County Radiation Medicine,
Utica, New York

Roslyn Ham, AS, RT(T)
Radiation Therapist,
Florida East Coast Cancer Center,
Ft. Pierce, Florida

Robert Holihan, BS, RT(R)
Instructor, Radiography Program,
Ferris State University,
Big Rapids, Michigan

Edna Holmes, MPA, RT(R)
Director, Radiography Program,
Lake Michigan College,
Benton Harbor, Michigan

Kathleen Kienstra, BS, RT(R)(T)
Program Director,
Barnes Hospital School of Radiation Therapy,
St. Louis, Missouri

Julianne Kinsman, MEd, RT(T)
Department Chairperson, Radiation Therapy Technology,
Springfield Technical Community College,
Springfield, Massachusetts

Druellen Kolker, BS, RT(T)
Program Director, Radiation Therapy Technology,
University of Chicago Hospitals,
Roosevelt University,
Chicago, Illinois

Sue M. Merkel, BS, RT(R)(T)
Program Director, Radiation Oncology,
University of Michigan Medical Center,
Ann Arbor, Michigan

Carmen Mesina, MS, RT(R)(T)
American Board of Radiology;
American Board of Medical Physics in Radiation
    Oncology Physics;
Clinical Radiation Therapy Physicist,
Harper Hospital,
Wayne State University,
Detroit, Michigan

Roy A. Miller, BS, RT(T)
Coordinator, Radiation Therapy Program,
Owens Community College,
Toledo, Ohio

Sharon J. Morretti, RT(T)
Supervisor, Radiation Therapy Program,
North Shore Cancer Center,
Peabody, Massachusetts

Cindy Mueller, BS, RT(R)(T)
Program Director, School of Radiation Therapy,
St. Joseph's Hospital,
Milwaukee, Wisconsin

Diane Mulkhey, AS, RT(T)
Manager, Radiation Therapy Department,
Central Maine Medical Center,
Lewiston, Maine

Joann M. Murray, BS, RT(R)(T)
Program Director, School of Radiation Therapy,
Welborn Cancer Center,
Evansville, Indiana

Larry Oliver, RT(T)
Program Director, Radiation Therapy Technology,
University of Kansas Medical Center,
Kansas City, Kansas

Brad Owen, RT(T)
Radiation Therapist,
Glen Falls Hospital,
Glen Falls, New York

Christina M. Paugh, BA, RT(R)(T)
Program Director, Educational Coordinator,
Radiation Oncology,
West Virginia University Hospital,
Morgantown, West Virginia

Joan Pierson, RT(R)(T)
Program Coordinator,
School of Radiation Therapy,
Henry Ford Hospital,
Detroit, Michigan

Nancy Quinn-Fagan, MEd, RT(R)(T)
Director of Education,
M.D. Anderson-Moncrief Cancer Center,
Ft. Worth, Texas

Marie L.A. Racine, BS, RT(R)(T)
Program Director, Radiation Therapy Technology,
Galveston College/University of Texas School of Allied
Health Sciences,
Galveston, Texas

Mary Jo Repasky, MHSA, RT(R)(T)
Program Director, Radiation Therapy Technology,
College of Health Professions,
Medical University of South Carolina,
Charleston, South Carolina

Pamela J. Ross, RT(T)
Coordinator of Technology,
Clinical Coordinator,
School of Radiation Therapy,
New York Methodist Hospital,
Brooklyn, New York

David Schatanoff, MD
Radiation Oncologist,
Radiation Oncology Department,
Mercy Regional Health System,
Altoona, Pennsylvania

Deborah Semanchik, RT(R)(T)
Radiation Therapist,
Radiation Oncology Department,
Mercy Regional Health System,
Altoona, Pennsylvania

Diane Skog, BS, RT(T)
Senior Radiation Therapist,
Maine Medical Center,
Portland, Maine

Shirley N. Smith, MPA, RT(R)(T)
Program Director, Radiation Therapy Technology,
Lansing Community College,
Lansing, Michigan

Carole A. Sullivan, PhD, RT(R)(T), FASRT
Dean, College of Allied Health,
Health Sciences Center,
University of Oklahoma,
Oklahoma City, Oklahoma

Larry Swafford, BS, RT(T)
Program Director, Radiation Therapy Technology,
Virginia Commonwealth University/Medical College of Virginia,
Richmond, Virginia

Wanda Teasley, BS, MHSA, RT(R)(T), FASRT
Chairperson, Associate Professor,
Clinical Services Department,
College of Health Professions,
Medical University of South Carolina,
Charleston, South Carolina

Giles Toole, MS, RT(R)(T)
Program Director, Radiation Therapy Technology,
Thomas Technical Institute,
Thomasville, Georgia

George M. Ushold, EdD, RT(T)
Director of Education, School of Radiation Therapy,
University of Rochester Cancer Center,
Rochester, New York

Ann Marie Vann, MEd, RT(R)(T)
Program Director, Radiation Therapy,
Medical College of Georgia,
Augusta, Georgia

David G. Ward, BS, Ed, RT(R)(T)
Program Director, Radiation Therapy Technology,
University Hospital of Cleveland,
Cleveland, Ohio

Preface

Cancer is the second leading cause of death in the United States. According to estimates of the American Cancer Society, over 1.3 million new cases of cancer will be diagnosed in 1996. The problem of controlling the disease and the important role of those involved in clinical and research activities is evident by the vast amount of money spent on cancer research each year and the immeasurable cost in compromised quality and loss of human life. Radiation therapy, a vital resource involved in cancer management, is used in well over half the diagnosed cases.

Physics, Simulation, and Treatment Planning is one of three texts in the *Principles and Practice of Radiation Therapy* series designed to contribute to a comprehensive understanding of cancer management, improve techniques involved in delivering a prescribed dose of radiation therapy, and apply knowledge and complex concepts associated with radiation therapy treatment. Each text is designed to stand on its own and at the same time provide a continuum of information in the series to the student, therapist, dosimetrist, oncologist, nurse, and others involved in radiation oncology.

This first-ever text offers a comprehensive overview of radiation therapy. Unit I explores the basic principles of physics as they relate to radiation therapy. Discussions include x-ray and gamma ray production, naturally produced radiation, teletherapy and brachytherapy, radiation safety and protection, teletherapy unit design and operation, and quality assurance. Units II and III present information on simulation, dosimetry, and treatment planning from a historical perspective as well as modern day approaches. Highlights include

the correlation between imaging studies and treatment planning, topographical and cross-sectional anatomy, and lymphatic chains and their application to patient care.

Pedagogical features designed to enhance comprehension and high-level learning are incorporated into each chapter. Elements include chapter outlines, key terms, and a complete glossary. Other notable features are the review questions and questions to ponder at the end of each chapter. The review questions reiterate the cognitive information presented in the chapter to help the reader incorporate the information into the basic understanding of radiation therapy concepts. The questions to ponder are open-ended, divergent questions intended to stimulate critical thinking and analytical judgment during information processing. Each chapter offers a reference list, thus providing the reader with additional sources. Again, the focus on each chapter is the comprehensive needs of the radiation therapy management team.

Creating a series of this magnitude has been a collaborative effort by numerous individuals. Although the idea for such a work began several years ago as one comprehensive text, the impossibility of the task was soon realized, considering the complexity and vast amount of information. Instead, three texts were proposed: *Introduction to Radiation Therapy; Physics, Simulation, and Treatment Planning;* and *Practical Applications in Radiation Therapy.* A survey of nearly all radiation therapy, dosimetry, and radiation oncology resident program directors and a smaller number of oncology nurses revealed a strong need for such a work with a notable percentage of the respondents recommending a multivolume approach. Survey results not only were encouraging, but also provided us with various individuals interested in lending their expertise as contributing authors, consultants, and reviewers. The result is a truly collaborative effort from the oncology community. This has been especially helpful because a great deal of individuality exists among treatment centers, hospitals, and universities in the techniques of irradiation.

Our hope is that the *Principles and Practice of Radiation Therapy* series will add to the body of knowledge specific to the profession. In addition, we sincerely hope the expanded knowledge and progress gained in administering a prescribed dose of radiation will ultimately enrich the quality of life of the patient and reduce suffering from cancer.

Charles M. Washington
Dennis T. Leaver

Acknowledgments

This book is the result of a tremendous team effort involving 61 contributing authors, more than 50 reviewers, our illustrators, and the dedicated professionals at Mosby–Year Book, Inc. All of us have had individuals who believed in and encouraged us when we encountered obstacles. We would like to acknowledge and thank those professionals who were instrumental in helping us build our professional foundation: Diane Chadwell and Adam Kempa from Wayne State University in Detroit, Michigan, and Dr. Banice Webber and Beverly Raymond from Radiation Oncology Associates in Providence, Rhode Island. Without their guidance and support, we could not have addressed the need for this work.

We would like to give special thanks to our students and reviewers who provided suggestions and comments that improved the manuscript. The continued support and encouragement of our colleagues at The University of Texas MD Anderson Cancer Center and Southern Maine Technical College are greatly appreciated. We are also grateful to Deborah Nickson and Jeanne Leaver for their dedicated service, secretarial assistance, and help with the glossary.

Above all, we gratefully acknowledge our families because they are the silent force behind this book. The idea for this project began at a conference in 1992. The idea was developed by many colleagues, friends, and the challenge to add to the body of knowledge in radiation oncology. We are grateful for the love, support, and encouragement from our wives, Connie Washington and Jeanne Leaver. They are also extremely important to this project. Finally, a special thanks goes to our heavenly Father, who sustains us and makes things grow.

Contents

Aspects of Radiation Therapy Physics

Applied Mathematics Review

Charles M. Washington
Thaddeus Sokolowski
E. Richard Bawiec

Outline

Key terms

Adjacent
Algebraic Equation
Base
Centigray
Cosine
Dimensional Analysis
Direct Proportionality
Exponent
Hypotenuse
Interpolation

Inverse Proportionality
Logarithm
Opposite
Proportion
Ratio
Right Triangle
Scientific Notation
Sine
Tangent

The practice of radiation therapy requires the use of exact quantitative measurements for the accurate delivery of a therapeutic dose. Patient simulation, treatment planning, and quality assurance have a strong functional dependence on mathematics. Because of this fact, the radiation therapist and the dosimetrist must have a good working knowledge of basic as well as advanced mathematical skills to accurately perform their respective duties. This chapter serves as a review of the principles of the mathematical concepts pertinent to the delivery of ionizing radiation in cancer management. The emphasis is on practical application, not on teaching theoretical principles. The chapter will review ratios and proportions, exponential functions, logarithms, basic units, uncertainty, and dimensional analysis. Practical applications are emphasized. The initial sections of the chapter are structured as a review and are not intended to "teach" mathematical concepts. The reader is presumed to have a working knowledge of basic entry-level college algebra.

REVIEW OF MATHEMATICAL CONCEPTS
Algebraic equations with one unknown

In many situations an **algebraic equation** is used to describe a physical phenomenon based on the interaction of several factors. For example, the dose to any point from a brachytherapy source requires knowledge of the source activity, source filtration, distance from the source to the point of interest, and several other factors. The ability to solve an equation for the value of an unknown variable is important. The following "rules" of algebra are helpful in remembering how do to this:

- When an unknown is multiplied by some quantity, divide both sides of an equation by that quantity to isolate the unknown.
- When a quantity is added to an unknown, subtract that quantity from both sides of the equation to isolate the unknown. When the quantity is subtracted from the unknown, add it to both sides.
- When an equation appears in fractional form, that is, the unknown is divided by some quantity, cross multiply, then solve for the unknown.[3]

Algebraic manipulation is used commonly in radiation therapy so the radiation therapist and dosimetrist should be comfortable solving these types of equations. An example of a typical algebraic manipulation scenario is shown in the practical examples at the end of this chapter.

Ratios and proportions

A **ratio** is the comparison of two numbers, values, or terms. The ratio denotes a relationship between the two components. Often these relationships allow the radiation therapist to predict trends. The notation for writing a ratio of a value or term, x, to another value or term, y, is most often written as follows:

$$\frac{x}{y} \text{ or } x{:}y$$

One important property of a ratio is that any ratio, x/y, will remain unchanged if both terms undergo operations by the same number. For example, the ratio $32/80$ can be simplified to the ratio $2/5$ by dividing both the numerator and the denominator by 16, a common factor of both numbers.

If two ratios are equal, this is known as a **proportion**. A proportion can also be looked at as an equation relating two ratios. This principle can assist in solving for an unknown factor in a proportion. For example, examine the following proportion:

$$5{:}7 = n{:}49$$

This can be rewritten in a more recognizable form as follows:

$$\frac{5}{7} = \frac{n}{49}$$

By cross multiplication, this proportion can be solved for n:

$$7 \times n = 5 \times 49$$

$$7n = 245$$

$$n = 35$$

In the clinical radiation therapy environment, inverse and direct proportions can occur in various ways. The concepts of inverse and direct proportionality are pertinent in the management of cancer with ionizing radiation, so a brief review of these concepts will be beneficial.

Inverse proportionality

Consider a hypothetical situation in which a number of aircraft must complete a trip of 1000 miles. Each aircraft travels at a different velocity. The time required for each plane to make the trip depends on that plane's velocity. Table 1-1 lists the times and velocities for each aircraft.

What simple relationship can we determine from these data? By examining the table, the following conclusions can be made:

- As velocity increases, time decreases.
- As velocity is doubled, time is halved.
- As velocity is quadrupled, time decreases by a factor of four.

This example exhibits the concept of **inverse proportionality**. Velocity (V) is inversely proportional to time (t). Mathematically, that is written as follows:

$$v \propto \frac{1}{t} \quad \text{or} \quad v = \frac{k}{t}$$

where k is a constant of proportionality. We can also relate two different aircraft's velocities and times as an inverse proportion:

$$v_1{:}v_2 = t_2{:}t_1 \quad \text{or} \quad \frac{v_1}{v_2} = \frac{t_2}{t_1}$$

Example 2 in the practical examples section demonstrates inverse proportionality while solving for an unknown.

Inverse proportionality is commonly seen in radiation therapy. For example, depth and percentage depth dose are inversely related (as depth increases, percentage depth dose decreases), as are beam energy and penumbra width (as energy increases, the width of the beam's penumbra decreases). Another good example of inverse proportionality is the inverse square law, which states that the intensity of radiation from a point source varies inversely with the square of the distance from the source.

Direct proportionality

The distance traveled by an aircraft moving at a constant velocity depends on the length of time that the aircraft is

Table 1-1	Aircraft velocities and times to complete the trip	
Aircraft	Velocity (miles/hr)	Time (hr)
A	500	2.0
B	400	2.5
C	250	4.0
D	200	5.0
E	125	8.0

aloft. Suppose we consider an aircraft traveling at a constant velocity of 400 miles per hour. The time required for this aircraft to travel 100 miles is 0.25 hour, for 200 miles the time is 0.5 hour, etc. Table 1-2 lists several distances and the time required by the aircraft to complete each distance.

Similar to the inverse proportionality example, conclusions can be reached from the data in this table, as follows:

- As time increases, distance increases.
- As time doubles, distance doubles.
- As time triples, distance triples.

Therefore we say that distance (D) is **directly proportional** to time (t). Mathematically, that is written as follows:

$$D \propto t \quad \text{or} \quad D = kt$$

where k is the constant of proportionality. We can also relate two different distances and times as a direct proportion:

$$D_1 : D_2 = t_1 : t_2$$
$$\text{or} \quad \frac{D_1}{D_2} = \frac{t_1}{t_2}$$

Example 3 in the practical examples section demonstrates direct proportionality while solving for an unknown.

Direct proportionality is also commonly seen in radiation therapy. For example, field size and percentage depth dose are directly proportional (as field size increases, percentage depth dose increases), as are beam energy and tissue air ratio (as energy increases, tissue air ratio increases). These relationships assume that all other related factors are constant.

Trigonometric ratios and the right angle triangle

Calculating angles, such as collimator and gantry angles, and depths and lengths that are related to such angles is quite common in setups during patient simulation and treatment. In many of these cases a solution is derived by using the properties of a right triangle. A **right triangle** is a three-sided polygon on which one corner measures 90°. The three most common functions associated with the right triangle are the sine, cosine, and tangent. Fig. 1-1 diagrams these quantities. There are six quantities that describe a right triangle: the three angles (α, β, and the 90° angle) and the three lengths (line segments AB, AC, and BC). The **sine, cosine,** and **tan-**

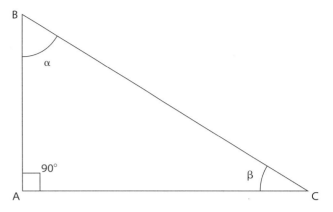

Fig. 1-1 A right triangle.

gent of an angle on a right triangle are defined mathematically (using the angle α, for example), as follows:

$$\sin(\alpha) = \frac{\text{Opposite}}{\text{Hypotenuse}} = \frac{\text{AC}}{\text{BC}}$$

$$\cos(\alpha) = \frac{\text{Adjacent}}{\text{Hypotenuse}} = \frac{\text{AB}}{\text{BC}}$$

$$\tan(\alpha) = \frac{\text{Opposite}}{\text{Adjacent}} = \frac{\text{AC}}{\text{AB}}$$

In these equations, **opposite** refers to the length of the side of the right triangle that is opposite the specified angle, **hypotenuse** refers to the length of the longest side of the triangle, and **adjacent** refers to the length of the side of the right triangle that is close, or adjacent, to the specified angle.

To solve for any unknown quantity on a right triangle, only specific combinations of two of the five remaining quantities (excluding the 90° angle) must be known. One other characteristic of the right triangle is that the angles all add up to 180°. Expressed mathematically, this is simply: $\alpha + \beta + 90 = 180$. Example 4 in the practical example section illustrates how one can determine unknown quantities in a right triangle.

Sine, cosine, and tangent are the primary trigonometric knowledge required of the radiation therapy worker and will be used frequently for specific clinical functions such as matching the divergences of two abutting treatment fields or measuring the angle or thickness of a chest wall. Values of specific trigonometric functions can be determined either by looking them up in tables or by using a hand-held scientific calculator. Because of the simplicity and common use of such calculators, this method for calculating the sine, cosine, or tangent of an angle will be used.[1]

Scientific calculators use the SIN, COS, and TAN keys. To obtain the specific trigonometric value desired, enter the known angle into the calculator in degrees and press the desired trigonometric function key. For example, to find the tangent of 30°, type in the following:

$$\boxed{3}\quad\boxed{0}\quad\boxed{\text{TAN}}\quad\boxed{=}$$

Table 1-2	Distance and time values for aircraft	
Distance		**Time (hr)**
0		0.00
100		0.25
200		0.50
300		0.75
500		1.00

The calculator should display 0.57735. This means that the ratio of the opposite side of the 30° angle to the side adjacent to the 30° is 0.57735. It is also possible to determine the measure of an angle by knowing the ratio between the two sides. If the ratio of the opposite side to the hypotenuse is 0.6, then the angle associated with this ratio can be calculated. Remember that the ratio opposite of hypotenuse defines the sine of the angle. Therefore sin ($\propto$) = 0.6. To calculate the angle, one simply needs the inverse sine of 0.6. This is obtained on most scientific calculators by pressing either the SIN⁻¹ button or the INV button followed by the SIN button. For the example, the inverse sine of 0.6 is 36.86°. Therefore $\propto$ = 36.86°.

Success in understanding trigonometric functions and identities depends, to a large degree, on the clinical application. Trigonometric functions are the most difficult type of mathematical problems for many therapy practitioners. Practice through didactic work or through experiencing these problems firsthand can aid the therapist and dosimetrist in recognizing these problems and solving them when they occur in the future.

Interpolation

To determine many of the factors that are used quite often in the practice of radiation therapy, one must be able to interpolate from tables that contain these factors. Field-size dependence factors, tissue-air ratios (TARs), tissue-maximum ratios (TMRs), percentage-depth doses, etc. are conveniently listed in easy-to-read tables. For example, a dosimetrist/therapist can easily look up the TAR for a 10 × 10 cm field size at a 10 cm depth. However, the tables only list the factors in incremental values. What happens if the exact depth of calculation and/or field size is not listed in the table or lies between two table values? In this case the dosimetrist/therapist can use an approximate evaluation for the intermediate point. This procedure is called **interpolation**. In most tables used in radiation therapy dose calculations, algebraic ratios can be employed to assist the therapist in finding the intermediate number. Interpolation is more precise when the table values listed are close together. If a desired point is directly between two known points, a simple average of the two factors for the two respective points is all that is required to determine the new value. Example 5 in the practical example section demonstrates how factors are interpolated from a table when the known values lie "above" and "below" the intermediate value. Relationships are established between the known values, and these relationships must be maintained through the computation to arrive at the correct factor.

Working with exponents

An exponent, or "power," is a shorthand notation that represents the multiplication of a number by itself a given number of times. For example, $4^3 = 4 \times 4 \times 4 = 64$. In this case the superscript 3 represents the **exponent**, while the 4 represents the **base**. The 3 is also said to be the "power." One could ver-

bally express 4^3 as "four raised to the third power." The following simple rules are important to remember when working with exponents:

1. $x^0 = 1$
2. $x^a \times x^b = x^{a+b}$
3. $(x^a)^b = x^{ab}$
4. $(xy)^a = x^a y^a$
5. $(x/y)^a = x^a/y^a$
6. $x^{-a} = 1/x^a$ and $1/x^{-a} = x^a$
7. $\sqrt[n]{x^n} = x^3$

Scientific notation is a special use of exponents that uses base 10 notation. It is used to represent either very large or very small numbers.[2] Numbers written in scientific notation are written in the following form:

$$n.nnn \times 10^p$$

where *n.nnn* indicates the first four numerical values of the specified number. The power to which the base of 10 is raised (*p*) depends on the size of the specified number. For example, 2657.89 can be written in scientific notation as 2.65789×10^3; it can also be written as 26.5789×10^2_3. However, in the scientific community, placing only one number to the left of the decimal point is the preferred style. Example 6 illustrates the use of exponents.

Natural logarithms and the exponential function

A **logarithm** operates as the reverse of exponential notation. Whereas the example 4^3 is considered "four raised to the third power" in exponential notation and equals 64, the logarithm base 4 of 64 equals 3. In mathematical notation the logarithm is written as follows:

$$\log_b(N) = x$$

where *b* is the base, *N* is the desired product, and *x* is the power. In exponential notation, this is written as follows:

$$b^x = N$$

Certain physical processes have been discovered in nature that obey a special type of logarithmic, and thus exponential, behavior. A radioactive substance is said to decay exponentially.[1,3,4,5] This simply means that the physical process that occurs can be described by exponential notation. However, rather than the base being an integer, the base is a special number that was discovered by Euler, a mathematician. This special number is represented by the letter *e* and is called Euler's constant or the "base of the natural logarithms." Numerically, *e* is equal to 2.718272.... Logarithms based on *e* are called "natural logarithms." Exponential function is the terminology used to describe *e* raised to a power and is written as follows:

$$e^x = N$$

A special notation is also given to the natural logarithm. The symbol ln is shorthand for "(natural) logarithm base *e*" and can be written as follows:

$$\ln(N) = x$$

These two equations can be combined to yield an important identity:

$$\ln(e^x) = x$$

In other words the natural logarithm and the exponential functions are inverses of each other. The exponential function has a few important properties that can be beneficial to the radiation therapy practitioner:

- If the power (x) is greater than 0 (meaning the power is positive), then the value of e^x will be greater than 1.
- If the power is less than 0 (meaning the power is negative), then the value of e^x will be a number greater than 0 and less than 1.
- If the power is exactly 0, then the value of e^x will be exactly equal to 1.

To summarize:

$$e^x > 1 \text{ if } x > 0$$

$$0 < e^x < 1 \text{ if } x < 0$$

$$e^x = 1 \text{ if } x = 0$$

Example 7 demonstrates how to use the exponential function.

Basic units

The system of basic units used most commonly in radiation therapy clinics is the metric or SI system. This system is the world standard for scientific and technical work. The metric system is based on fundamental units of time, distance, mass, and electrical current and several derived units that are combinations of the four fundamental units. Additionally, prefixes may be added to the four fundamental units to represent large or small quantities of the fundamental units.[2-5]

The four fundamental units in the metric system are the second (time), the meter (distance), the kilogram (mass), and the ampere (electrical current). These units are defined internationally by standards kept at a laboratory near Paris, France. However, secondary standards are kept in national laboratories in most countries. In the United States the National Institute of Standards and Technology (NIST) maintains the secondary standards.[2] Commonly used prefixes and their meanings are listed in Table 1-3.

Special units have been defined for the radiological sciences. The roentgen (r) is the unit of radiation exposure that represents a measure of the amount of ionization created by radiation in the air. A derived unit for exposure is the coulomb/kilogram (C/kg). Thus the relationship between these two quantities is 1 roentgen = 2.58×10^{-4} C/kg.

The accepted unit of absorbed dose is the Gray. Absorbed dose, which will be discussed in more detail in further chapters, describes the amount of radiation energy absorbed by a medium. The Gray can be expressed in units as joule/kilo-

Table 1-3	Numerical prefixes used with SI units	
Prefix	**Symbol**	**Multiplier**
pico	p	10^{-12}
nano	n	10^{-9}
micro	μ	10^{-6}
milli	m	10^{-3}
centi	c	10^{-2}
deci	d	10^{-1}
kilo	k	10^3
mega	M	10^6
giga	G	10^9

gram (J/kg). An outdated unit that was replaced by the Gray is the rad. A rad is equal to 0.01 Gray, or, restated, 100 rads equals 1 Gray. Therefore, 1 rad equals one **centigray** (cGy).[3]

The accepted unit of energy is the joule (J), which is equal to 1 kilogram-meter^2 per second^2 (1 kgm^2/s^2). A joule of energy is a rather large amount of energy, relative to the energies associated with radiation therapy. Therefore another special "derived" unit is the electron volt (eV). The relationship between the electron volt and the joule is as follows:

$$1 \text{ eV} = 1.602 \times 10^{-19} \text{ J}$$

The kilo-electron volt (keV = 10^3 eV) and the mega-electron volt (MeV = 10 eV) are the most common energy units used in the radiation therapy clinic.[3]

Measurements and experimental uncertainty

During the course of a program in radiation therapy a student eventually becomes familiar with certain quantities such as source-to-axis distance (SAD) and source-to-skin distance (SSD) measurements as well as certain units such as absorbed dose (cGy), exposure (roentgen), and activity (millicurie).[2-5] Various instruments can be used to measure these and various other quantities. The process of taking a measurement is basically an attempt to determine a value or magnitude of known quantity.

For example, the quantity SSD is a physical measurement of distance. Suppose an SSD of 73.5 centimeters was measured from the source of radiation to the chest wall of a patient during the treatment simulation process. This indicates that the centimeter was used as a unit of length and that the distance to the skin surface was 73.5 times larger than this unit. Stated differently, a measurement is a comparison of the magnitude (how large or small) of a quantity to that of an accepted standard. In this measurement and in other measurements such as determining the temperature using a thermometer, the barometric pressure using a barometer, or the exposure rate using an exposure rate meter, an amount of uncertainty is inherent. Therefore the measuring process requires that the person taking the measurement must have the knowledge that this uncertainty exists. Referring to the

SSD measurement, the distance of 73.5 centimeters will contain error that is introduced not only by the measuring device but also by the fact that the patient will most probably be moving as a result of inhalation and exhalation. This inherent or built-in uncertainty in making a measurement is a characteristic of almost all of science. Uncertainties can be grouped into three categories: systematic errors, random errors, and blunders.

Systematic errors. A systematic error is an error or uncertainty inherent within the measuring device. A systematic error will always affect the measurement in the same way: the measurement will either be too large or too small, depending on the device. These errors are commonly obtained, for example, from one or more of the following: human biases such as vision inaccuracies; imperfect techniques that may occur, for example, during experimental setup; and unacceptable instrument calibrations. Stem leakage of an ionization chamber and the inaccuracy of reading an analog temperature meter on an annealing oven are examples of systematic errors.

Random errors. Random errors, as the name implies, are a result of variations attributed to chance that are unavoidable. Random errors can either increase or decrease the result of a measurement. To correct for this type of error, a common practice is to take several measurements and average them. Random errors can also be reduced by making improvements in the measuring device and/or technique. An uncontrolled rapid change in temperature or barometric pressure, accidental movement of a patient during setup, and electronic noise are all examples of random errors.

Blunders. Blunders during measurement are those errors that occur as a result of human error in algebraic or arithmetic calculations or from improper use of a measuring device. Errors such as these can be avoided by properly educating the individuals who will be making the measurements. They can also be avoided by comparing the measurements being made to previous measurements that are known to be correct or even comparing them to theoretical values. If large discrepancies exist between the correct values and the values that the individual is obtaining, then something must have been done incorrectly, and retracing the setup and procedure can be an easy way to remedy the error.

Accuracy and precision of measurements. Another facet of measurements that must be discussed is the importance of and also the difference between the accuracy and precision of a measurement. When measurements are made, the individual must be concerned with how close the measurements are to the "true" value. Although the "true" value cannot be known exactly, theoretical calculations can define a value that is accepted as a "true" value. How close a measurement comes to this "true" value is referred to as accuracy. The precision of a measurement indicates how reproducible a particular measurement is or how consistent the measurement is.

Fig. 1-2 illustrates the difference between accuracy and precision. The bull's eye represents the "true value." The

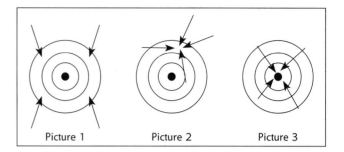

Fig. 1-2 Representation of the contrast between accuracy and precision. The *first picture* is neither accurate nor precise. *Picture 2* demonstrates precision but not accuracy. *Picture 3* illustrates both precision and accuracy.

arrows represent measurements. In the first picture the measurements are neither precise nor accurate. The arrows (measurements) did not hit the bull's eye, nor did they land close to each other. In the second picture the arrows were precise but inaccurate. They all hit close to the same location, but were not close to the bull's eye. In the third picture the arrows were precise and accurate because they were grouped together close to the bull's eye.

As another example, consider the output measurement of a linear accelerator as performed by three therapists as part of the daily quality assurance program. After setting up the necessary apparatus and following the policy and procedure outline, the following data were gathered. Each therapist made four measurements with the ionization chamber to obtain an average value for the output and thereby eliminate random errors.

	Therapist A	Therapist B	Therapist C
	2.702	2.650	2.738
	2.701	2.660	2.578
	2.702	2.655	2.737
	2.702	2.651	2.579
Average:	2.702	2.654	2.657

The accepted value for the output for that accelerator was 2.658. So a number of questions could be asked about the values obtained by the therapists. Which therapist had the most accurate values? Which therapist had the most precise values? Which therapist had the best overall results? The measurements made by Therapist A were more consistent and more precise because values do not differ by more than 0.001 from each other. However, the average results obtained by Therapists B and C were closer to the accepted value. Apparently, Therapists B and C were more accurate than Therapist A, even though Therapist A was the most precise. By comparing the individual values that were obtained by Therapists B and C, one can see that Therapist C's values had a large range. Therefore, although Therapist C's average value was the closest to the accepted value, it was obtained through imprecise readings. Therefore the values obtained by

Therapist B are deemed the most acceptable because they were precise and accurate.

From this example, it is apparent that a measurement can be precise without being accurate and vice versa. Radiation therapy practitioners should be concerned not only with accuracy, but also with precision. Discerning between the two is a function of analytical judgment and critical thinking skills, both very important in the practice of radiation therapy.

Experimental uncertainty. Because it is impossible to eliminate all systematic errors, random errors, and blunders, an absolutely accurate and precise measurement cannot be achieved. Although this seems disheartening to the scientist, there is a method that is accepted by the scientific community to handle this experimental uncertainty. It is common practice to measure the percent relative error in a measurement in order to discover the degree of accuracy. The percent relative error can be thought of as the percentage of error in a measurement relative to the accepted value. It is calculated by using the following equation:

$$\% \text{ Relative} \atop \text{certainty} = \frac{\text{Experimental value} - \text{Accepted value}}{\text{Accepted value}} \times 100\%$$

Consider the measurement result of Therapist A. The percent relative error in that result can be calculated as follows using the above equation:

$$\% \text{ Relative error} = \frac{2.702 - 2.658}{2.658} \times 100\% = 1.65\%$$

The percent relative error in the result obtained by Therapist A was +1.65%. This means that the result was 1.65% higher than the accepted value. The percent relative errors in the results obtained by Therapists B and C can be calculated by the reader and are −0.15% and −0.04%, respectively. Both of these values were low.

Dimensional analysis

A technique that can be very useful in radiation therapy (as well as in many other branches of science) is dimensional analysis. **Dimensional analysis** is a process that involves the careful assessment of the units of measurement used in calculating a specific quantity. This technique involves canceling common units that appear in the numerator and denominator of an equation. When one or more quantities are manipulated to obtain a specified quantity, the units of the known quantities when combined must be equivalent to the unit of measurement of that specified quantity. For example, to obtain the specific quantity of velocity, one must divide distance by time. In other words, velocity is measured in meters per second, distance is measured in meters, and time is measured in seconds.[3]

When using an equation, it is important to ensure that all of the units when combined equate to the units desired. There are a few "rules of thumb" that can be used when analyzing the dimensions of an equation. First, any quantity divided by 1 is equal to the quantity itself. Next, any quantity divided by

itself is equal to 1. Also, the process of division is equivalent to multiplying the numerator by the inverse of the denominator.[2,3] Using these facts, one can cancel units in any equation until no cancellation possibility remains. The units that remain should be equivalent to the desired units. If this is not true, then an error must have occurred.

PRACTICAL EXAMPLES OF MATHEMATICS IN RADIATION THERAPY

Mathematical theories must be put into practice. Several examples have been used throughout this chapter to help focus the content into useful information. This section of the chapter provides more in-depth analysis of practical application examples of mathematical principles as seen in radiation therapy.

Example 1—algebraic equations: To determine the value of an unknown, it is necessary to use the rules of algebra. For example, if a therapist knows the total dose that a patient is to receive and the dose per fraction, then the number of treatments can be determined. Assume that the total dose is 5000 cGy and the daily dose is 200 cGy. The number of fractions can be determined from the following equation:

$$200 \text{ cGy/fraction} \times N \text{ (fractions)} = 5000 \text{ cGy}$$

where N represents the number of fractions. To isolate the unknown (N), the value of 200 can be divided out of both sides of the equation without disturbing the equality:

$$\frac{200 \text{ cGy / fraction}}{200 \text{ cGy / fraction}} \times N = \frac{5000 \text{ cGy}}{200 \text{ cGy / fraction}}$$

The first term in this equation is equal to 1, and any value multiplied by 1 equals that number. Also, because the unit cGy appears in both the numerator and the denominator of the fraction on the right side of the equation, it can be canceled. The resulting equation is thus:

$$N = \frac{5000}{200} \cdot \frac{1}{1 / \text{Fraction}}$$

At this point, one other algebraic rule can be applied. Any fraction that appears in the denominator of a fraction can be written as the reciprocal of that fraction. Therefore our final answer becomes the following:

$$N = \frac{5000}{200} \text{ fractions} = 25 \text{ fractions}$$

So the therapist knows that the patient will be treated for 25 fractions.

As already stated, one can also abstract values from both sides of an equation to find an answer. Suppose that a therapist knows that the physician wants to deliver 200 cGy on a particular day and knows that on the previous day the patient received 250 cGy. Therefore the unknown can be determined from the following equation:

$$250 \text{ cGy} - X = 200 \text{ cGy}$$

Obviously, this is a simple problem, but it is used to illustrate a principle. From this point, one can subtract 250 cGy from both sides of the equation, as follows:

$$250 \text{ cGy} - X - 250 \text{ cGy} = 200 \text{ cGy} - 250 \text{ cGy}$$

Subtracting 250 from itself equals 0, and 0 added to any value simply equals that value. Also, one can multiply both sides of an equation by the same value without disturbing the equality. Therefore, if we multiply both sides of the equation by -1, the following results:

$$^{-}X = 200 \text{ cGy} - 250 \text{ cGy} = {}^{-}50 \text{ cGy}$$

$$(^{-}1) \times {}^{-}X = (^{-}1) \times {}^{-}50 \text{cGy}$$

$$X = 50 \text{ cGy}$$

So the therapist knows that the daily dose was reduced by 50 cGy.

Example 2—inverse proportionality: A therapist had just learned from a physicist that the therapy unit would be running at a dose rate of 400 cGy/min on a given day. The therapist knows that the normal dose rate is 300 cGy/min. Therefore the therapist wonders how this new dose rate will affect the patient's treatment times. This example illustrates inverse proportionality. If a particular patient's treatments took 1.2 minutes with the normal dose rate of 300 cGy/min, then what would it be with the new dose rate? This can be solved by the following equation:

$$300 \text{ cGy/min} \times 1.2 \text{ min} = 360 \text{ cGy}$$

$$\frac{360 \text{ cGy}}{400 \text{ cGy / min}} = 0.9 \text{ minutes}$$

Therefore as the dose rate increases, the treatment times decrease, thus demonstrating inverse proportionality.

Example 3—direct proportionality: A radiation oncologist wants to increase the dose that a patient receives per fraction but does not want to change the total number of fractions. Assume that, originally, the physician had planned to give 200 cGy per fraction for 25 fractions, then decided that 230 cGy would achieve better results. Initially, the total dose would have been:

$$200 \text{ cGy/fraction} \times 25 \text{ fractions} = 5000 \text{ cGy}$$

But, since the dose per fraction was changed to 230 cGy, the total dose would also change:

$$230 \text{ cGy/fraction} \times 25 \text{ fractions} = 5750 \text{ cGy}$$

Therefore note that as the dose per fraction increases, the total dose increases. This is an example of direct proportionality.

Example 4—unknown quantities and the right triangle: A radiation physicist wants to know at what angle a wall-mounted laser is directed at the floor. Assume that she also wants to know the distance from the laser to its intersection point on the floor. First, she measures the distance from the wall to the intersection point on the floor (segment AC measures 12 feet). Then she measures how far up the wall the laser is mounted (segment AB measures 8 feet).

From the trigonometric identities outlined in the text, the physicist knows that the tangent of the angle is equal to the

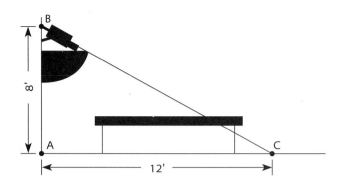

length of the opposite side divided by the length of the adjacent side. That can be stated in mathematical form as follows:

$$\tan \beta = \frac{\text{Opposite side}}{\text{Adjacent side}}$$

$$\tan \beta = \frac{\text{Segment AC}}{\text{Segment AB}} = \frac{12 \text{ feet}}{8 \text{ feet}}$$

$$\tan \beta = 1.5$$

$$\beta = \tan^{-1}(1.5)$$

$$\beta = 56°$$

Therefore angle β is equal to 56°. Also, the physicist knows that the sine of β is equal to the length of the opposite side divided by the hypotenuse. This can be written as follows:

$$\sin \beta = \frac{\text{Opposite}}{\text{Hypotenuse}} = \frac{\text{Segment AC}}{\text{Segment BC}}$$

Because the length of segment BC is desired, the equation can be rewritten and solved for that length:

$$\text{Segment BC} = \frac{\text{Opposite}}{\sin \beta} = \frac{12}{\sin(56°)} = \frac{12}{0.829} = 14.5 \text{ feet}$$

Therefore the distance from the laser's position on the beam wall to the point where the beam intersects the floor is 14.5 feet.

Example 5—interpolation: A radiation dosimetrist wants to determine the output of a cobalt machine for two different field sizes for one specific date from the following output table. The field sizes are 12 cm × 12 cm and 19 × 19 cm². The desired date is March 30. Assume that this date is exactly halfway between March 15 and April 15.

Output (cGy/min) for Theratron 780 @ 80 cm in AIR (SAD treatment) 1994 (15th of month)

Field size	Jan 15	Feb 15	Mar 15	Apr 15	May 15
5 cm× 5 cm	210.71	208.41	206.13	203.88	201.66
10 cm×10 cm	218.58	216.19	213.83	211.50	209.19
12 cm×12 cm	220.98	218.57	216.18	213.82	211.49
15 cm×15 cm	224.48	222.03	219.60	217.21	214.83
20 cm×20 cm	228.19	225.70	223.24	220.80	218.39

Because the 12 cm × 12 cm field size is listed on the table, the only step required to determine the output for that field size is to determine the intermediate value between the March 15 and April 15 outputs for that field size. The outputs for a 12 × 12 field size for March 15 and April 15 are 216.18 and 213.82 cGy/min, respectively. Therefore the output for the 12 × 12 field size for March 30 will be the simple average of the two outputs:

$$\frac{216.18 + 213.82}{2} = \frac{430.0}{2} = 215.00 \text{ cGy/min}$$

The first step in determining the desired output for the 19 × 19 field size is to determine the intermediate values of the output for March 30 for the field sizes nearest to 19 × 19. These would be the 15 × 15 and 20 × 20 field sizes. The outputs for March 15 and April 15 for the 15 × 15 field size are 219.60 and 217.21 cGy/min, respectively, whereas the outputs for March 15 and April 15 for the 20 × 20 field size are 223.24 and 220.80 cGy/min, respectively. To determine the intermediate values, the simple averages are calculated and can be shown to be 214.81 cGy/min for the 15 × 15 field size and 222.02 cGy/min for the 20 × 20 field size. The next step is to determine the ratio of how "far" the 19 × 19 field size is from either the smaller or the larger field size. For this example, we will choose the smaller field size. The 19 × 19 field size is 4 cm greater than the 15 × 15 field size. Therefore the 19 × 19 field size is four fifths of the "distance" between the two known values. Therefore the output must also be four fifths of the "distance" between the two intermediate outputs in the same direction on the table. To calculate the desired output, one must know the "distance" between the two intermediate values and then multiply that "distance" by the field size "distances" ratio. This will give the desired output of 221.30 cGy/min:

$$222.02 \text{ cGy/min} - 218.41 \text{ cGy/min} = 3.61 \text{ cGy}$$

$$3.61 \text{ cGy/min} \times 4/5 = 2.89 \text{ cGy/min}$$

$$218.41 \text{ cGy/min} + 2.89 \text{ cGy/min} = 221.30 \text{ cGy/min}$$

Therefore, the output for March 15 for the 19 × 19 field size was 221.30 cGy/min.

Example 6—exponents: A brief example of the use of exponents is all that will be demonstrated here. The primary use of exponents in the field of radiation therapy is in scientific notation. If one must calculate the product of two numbers that are represented in scientific notation, some of the rules outlined in this chapter can be useful. For example, assume that a radiation physicist desires to determine the total amount of exposure produced by ionizing radiation in a specified mass of air. She knows that 1 roentgen is equal to 2.58×10^{-4} coulombs of charge liberated per kilogram of air

present. She measured 3.23×10^{-2} coulombs in 1 kilogram of air mass. Mathematically, this is written:

Exposure (x) =

$$\frac{3.23 \times 10^{-2} \text{ coulombs}}{1 \text{ kilogram of air}} \times \frac{1 \text{ roentgen}}{2.58 \times 10^{-4} \text{ coulombs} / 1 \text{ kg air}}$$

Exposure (x) =

$$\frac{3.23 \times 10^{-2} \text{ coulombs} / 1 \text{ kilogram of air}}{1 \text{ kilogram of air} / 1 \text{ kilogram of air}} \times 1 \text{ roentgen}$$

$$\text{Exposure } (x) = 1.25 \times \frac{10^{-2}}{10^{-4}} \text{ roentgens}$$

If a number with a negative exponent is in the denominator of a fraction, then that is the same as the same number with the equal positive exponent moved to the numerator of the equation.

$$\text{Exposure } (x) = 1.25 \times 10^{-2} \times 10^{4} \text{ roentgens}$$

$$\text{Exposure } (x) = 1.25 \times 10^{(-2+4)} \text{ roentgens}$$

$$\text{Exposure } (x) = 1.25 \times 10^{2} \text{ roentgens} = 125 \text{ roentgens}$$

Example 7—exponential functions: The decay of a radioactive substance behaves in an exponential manner. Therefore if one wishes to calculate the amount of activity of a particular substance that remains after a specific amount of time, the following equation can be used:

$$A_t = A_0 \times e^{-\lambda t}$$

where A_t is the activity after time t, A_0 is the initial activity, and λ is the decay constant that is specific to the particular radioactive substance being used. As an example, assume that the activity of a sample of iridium 131 is known exactly 2 days after it was received from a manufacturer. Assume that we would like to know what the activity was when it arrived. The activity at the present time is 5 curies (Ci). Therefore we know that $t = 2$ days and $A_t = 5$ Ci. Also, the decay constant for iridium 131 is 8.6×10^{-2}/day. So plugging these values into the decay equation gives the following:

$$5 \text{ Ci} = A_0 \times e^{-(8.6 \times 10^{-2}/\text{day}) \times (2 \text{ days})}$$

$$5 \text{ Ci} = A_0 \times e^{-0.172}$$

$$A_0 = \frac{5 \text{ Ci}}{e^{-0.172}} = \frac{5 \text{ Ci}}{0.842}$$

$$A_0 = 5.938 \text{ Ci}$$

Therefore the activity on arrival 2 days earlier was 5.938 Ci. One can also determine the activity of the substance 2 days after the present date using the same equation. The reader can calculate this independently.

Review Questions

Multiple Choice

1. $(10^3)^5$ equals:
   a. 10^8
   b. 10^2
   c. 10^{15}

2. Convert the following to scientific notation: 910,000,000.
   a. 9.1×10^8
   b. 9.01×10^7
   c. 91.0×10^8
   d. 9×10^7

3. If an instrument positioned 1 meter from a point source is moved 50 centimeters closer to the source, the radiation intensity will be:
   a. Increased by a factor of 4
   b. Increased by a factor of 2
   c. Decreased by a factor of 4
   d. Decreased by a factor of 2

4. As the depth in tissue increases, the percentage depth dose values decreases. This is an example of:
   a. Inverse proportionality
   b. Direct proportionality
   c. Interpolation
   d. None of the above

5. What is the ratio of 100 cGy to 500 cGy?
   a. 5:1
   b. 1:5
   c. Both A and B
   d. Neither A nor B

True or False

6. $\ln(e^x) = x$.
   True _____ False _____

7. $\dfrac{10^x}{10^y} = 10^{x+y}$.
   True _____ False _____

REFERENCES

1. Bernier D et al: *Nuclear medicine technology and techniques*, ed 3. St. Louis, 1994, Mosby.
2. Bushong S: *Radiologic science for technologists: physics, biology, and protection*, ed 5. St. Louis, 1993, Mosby.
3. Harris M: *Radiation therapy physics handbook*, The University of Texas MD Anderson Cancer Center, 1992.
4. Khan FM: *The physics of radiation therapy*, ed 2. Baltimore, 1994, Williams & Wilkins.
5. Stanton R, Stinson D: *An introduction to radiation oncology*. Madison, WI, 1992, Medical Physics Publishing Corp.

Introduction to Radiation Therapy Physics

Timothy Ochran

Outline

Key terms

Atom
Atomic mass unit
Binding energy per nucleon
Bohr atom model
Bremsstrahlung
Electrical charge
Electron binding energy
Frequency of the wave
Ground state
Half value layer

Mass equivalence
Neutron activation
Nuclear binding energy
Nuclear energy level
Nuclear force
Photon
Radioactivity
Rest mass
Wave-particle duality
Wavelength of the wave

Shortly after Roentgen's discovery of x-rays at the University of Wurzberg in Germany, medical applications of x-rays were used worldwide. At that time, x-rays were such a news item that they were discussed in the press. Many physicists began the task of understanding the principles critical to the use and production of x-rays.

Over the past century, great strides have been taken in the area of radiation physics to define the interaction of radiation and matter. Without a basic understanding of this relationship, radiation therapy practitioners would not be able to cure and palliate the multitude of cancer patients treated each year. To that end, this chapter will describe the basic principles of radiation therapy physics.

QUANTITIES AND UNITS

Four major quantities that one must know to be versed in radiation physics are as follows: (1) radioactivity, (2) radiation exposure, (3) radiation absorbed dose, and (4) radiation dose equivalent. The original units for each of these quantities can be found in Table 2-1, as well as the new Système Internationale d'Unités (SI units) and conversion factors. These conversion factors compare original units to the SI units that were developed in 1977 to help simplify things worldwide. These quantities will be discussed in more detail in following sections.

Table 2-1	Radiation activity, exposure, and dose units of measurement		
Measured property	**Old unit**	**New SI unit**	**Conversion factor**
Radioactivity	curie (Ci) = 3.7×10^{10} dps	becquerel (Bq) = 1 dps	1 Ci = 3.7×10^{10} Bq 1 Bq = 2.7×10^{-11} Ci
Radiation exposure	roentgen (R) = 2.58×10^{-4} C/kg	coulomb/kg (C/kg)	1 R = 2.58×10^{-4} C/kg 1 C/kg = 3.88×10^{3} R
Radiation absorbed dose	rad = 100 erg/g	gray (Gy) = 1 J/kg	1 rad = 0.01 Gy 1 Gy = 100 rad
Radiation dose equivalent	rem = QF $\times$ rad	sievert (Sv) = QF $\times$ Gy	1 rem = 0.01 Sv Sv = 100 rem

From Bernier DR, Christian PE, Langan JK, editors: *Nuclear medicine: technology and techniques*, ed 3. St Louis, 1994, Mosby.
QF, Quality factor.

Units are agreed upon standard quantities of measurements such as meters, seconds, and grams, to name just a few. From these fundamental units we can derive the units such as meters per second or even 1 erg ($1g \times cm^2/sec^2$). There are two different measurement systems: (1) the foot-pound-second and (2) the meter-kilogram-second systems.[1]

It will often be necessary to convert between various systems and magnitudes of units.

1. *How many minutes are in 2 hours and 14 minutes?*

$$2 \text{ hours} \times \frac{60 \text{ minutes}}{1 \text{ hour}} + 14 \text{ min} = 134 \text{ min}$$

2. *How many meters are in 5.5 miles?*

$$5.5 \text{ miles} \times \frac{5280 \text{ feet}}{1 \text{ mile}} \times \frac{12 \text{ inches}}{1 \text{ foot}} \times \frac{2.54 \text{ cm}}{1 \text{ inch}} \times$$

$$\frac{1 \text{ meter}}{100 \text{ cm}} \cong 8851.4 \text{ m}$$

The "trick," as you can see, is to always multiply by 1. Throughout this chapter and this text you will find the opportunity to convert many types of units.

ATOMIC PHYSICS
Subatomic particles

The smallest unit of an element that retains the properties of that element is known as an **atom**. Atoms are made up of smaller units called subatomic particles.[1-3] There are many types of subatomic particles that have been discovered or postulated. J.J. Thomson postulated in 1897 that the atom must consist of a tiny cloud of positive charge, with the electrons floating in it.[2] Lenard in 1903 proposed that atoms were made up of "clumps" of positive charge, electrons floating around them, and a relatively large empty space between them. Twentieth century physicists working with "atom smashers" have been able to break the atom not only into its component parts but also into smaller units, thus discovering the six quarks.

Radiation therapy physics deals with the most basic of the subatomic particles: electrons, neutrons, and protons. Rest mass and electrical charge are the properties of these parti-cles with which we will be concerned. The **rest mass** refers to the mass (weight) of the particle when it is not moving. Einstein's theory of special relativity states that subatomic particles moving at high speeds will have increased mass. At this point we will not need to concern ourselves with this theory, other than to know of it.

The mass of subatomic particles can be measured in terms of the standard metric system mass unit, the kilogram. For those more familiar with US units of measure, 1 kg is equivalent to about 2.2 pounds. Because of the very small masses of these particles, expressing them in kilograms would make these values very cumbersome to handle; therefore a quantity called the atomic mass unit (amu) was defined. The **atomic mass unit** is defined such that the mass of an atom of carbon 12 is exactly 12.000 amu. From this it was determined that the following is true:

$$1 \text{ amu} = 1.66 \times 10^{-27} \text{ kg}$$

This relationship can be used to convert from one mass unit to another.[2]

The mass of a proton is equal to 1.00727 amu. Express this mass in terms of kilograms.

$$(1.00727 \text{ amu}) \times \frac{(1.66 \times 10^{-27} \text{ kg})}{(1 \text{ amu})} = 1.672 \times 10^{-27} \text{ kg}$$

The **electrical charge** is a measure of how strongly the particle is attracted to an electrical field, and can be either positive or negative. A positively charged particle will be attracted to a negative electrical field, and a negatively charged particle will be attracted to a positive electrical field. The electron and the proton have the same amount of electrical charge, 1.6×10^{-19} coulombs (the coulomb is the metric unit of electrical charge), but they differ in that the electron's charge is negative and the proton's is positive. The neutron, as the name implies, carries no electrical charge.

The Bohr atom

In 1913 Neils Bohr attempted to explain the spectral phenomena of atoms by combining Rutherford's atomic model with

tum theories of Einstein and Planck.
Bohr atom, has since been replaced
echanical models of the atom; how-
way to derive a mental picture of the
hr atom model stated that the elec-
cleus existed only in certain energy
r stated that when an electron moved
r it needed to gain or lose energy. The
s the spectra that had been observed
d by adding energy to them.
in Fig. 2-1 consists of a central core,
d the electron cloud or orbits. The
nucleus consists protons and neutrons tightly bound
together by a force known as the strong nuclear force. This
force is strong enough at the extremely small distances found
within the nucleus that it can hold together the positive
charged protons that are trying to repel each other. Outside
the nucleus the strong nuclear force quickly becomes ineffective. The number of protons and neutrons within the
nucleus defines the physical and chemical properties of the
atom. Elements are substances made up entirely of atoms of
a single kind. Some familiar substances that are elements
include oxygen, carbon, helium, aluminum, and cobalt. All
other substances are called compounds and are made up of
various combinations of elements. As previously stated, each
element contains a unique number of protons in its nucleus:

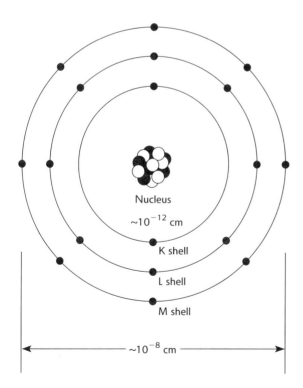

Fig. 2-1 The Bohr atomic model with central nucleus surrounded by
the electron orbits. (From Bernier DR, Christian PE, Langan JK,
editors: *Nuclear medicine: technology and techniques*, ed 3. St
Louis, 1994, Mosby.)

carbon has six, oxygen has eight, etc. If a nucleus gains or
loses protons, its elemental identity changes. For example, if
a carbon atom gains a proton, it becomes an atom of nitrogen
(which has seven protons). The number of protons in the
nucleus is known as the atomic number of the atom.

Atomic nomenclature

The symbolism used to identify an atom (X), its atomic number (Z), and atomic mass number (A) is as follows:

$$^A_Z X$$

The periodic table in Fig. 2-2 is a listing of the elements and
their symbols.

Nuclear stability and isotopes

The total amount of energy that it takes to hold a nucleus
together is called the **nuclear binding energy** and is measured in MeV (10^6 electron volts). To compare the binding
energy of one atom to another, one must calculate the binding energy per nucleon. The **binding energy per nucleon** is
the binding energy divided by the atomic mass number. It
should be noted that a peak at an atomic mass number of
about 56 represents the most stable state of iron (Fe). A
nucleus can have more energy than is required for stability;
to illustrate this, one can think of a staircase. The bottom step
represents the binding energy of the atom and is called the
ground state. The **ground state** is the minimum amount of
energy needed to keep the atom together. Higher and higher
steps of the staircase represent higher and higher energy
states of the atom. As in a staircase, the steps have finite levels. The energy levels of an atom do not have transition zones
between the steps, so the atom's energy level must be one
step or the other, not between. Each of the higher steps is
called a **nuclear energy level**. Unstable atoms are those that
are not at their ground state. An atom at an energy level different from its ground state tends to try to lose the energy and
return to its ground state. This can be achieved in a number
of ways, including radioactivity. **Radioactivity** in this case is
the emission of energy in the form of electromagnetic radiation or energetic particles.[4] As you can see, any element can
have different nuclear configurations. Atoms with the same
atomic number but different atomic mass numbers are called
isotopes of that atom.[2,4] Other nuclear configurations, related
to the various combinations of atomic number and number of
neutrons, are summarized in Table 2-2. An easy way to
remember this table is to recall the next to last letter of the
configuration—isoto*p*e, isob*a*r, isoto*n*e, and isom*e*r—which
tells the value that remains constant (one must assume that *e*
stands for everything).

Atomic energy levels

The Bohr atom's other major component, besides the
nucleus, consists of the electron orbits or shells that surround it. These are not actually orbits, but this term gives
us a way to imagine the atom. The **electron binding**

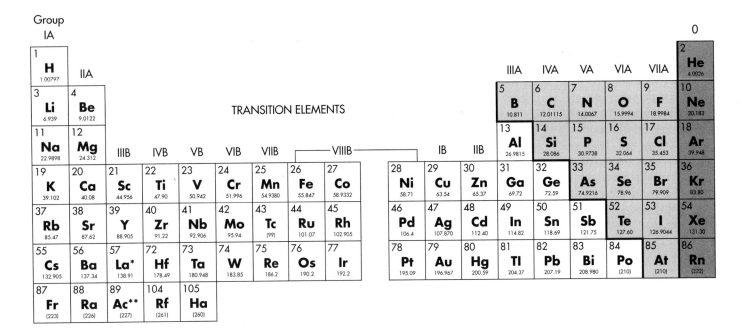

Fig. 2-2 Periodic table of elements. (From Bernier DR, Christian PE, Langan JK, editors: *Nuclear medicine: technology and techniques*, ed 3. St Louis, 1994, Mosby.)

Table 2-2	Nuclear configurations		
Name	**Z**	**A**	**N**
Isotope	Same	Different	Different
Isobar	Different	Same	Different
Isotone	Different	Different	Same
Isomer	Same	Same	Same

Z, Atomic number; *A*, Atomic mass number; *N*, number of neutrons.

energy is the amount of energy required to remove that electron from the atom. The binding energy is different for each shell and depends on the makeup of the nucleus. The larger the number of positive charges in the nucleus, the greater the attraction of the electrons toward it, and thus the higher the binding energy.

The electron binding energy has a negative value and is usually measured in kiloelectron volts. It represents the amount of energy that must be added to the electron's total energy before the electron can begin to move away from the atom.

As previously seen in Fig. 2-1, electron shells are numbered and given letter names that represent, in increasing order, their distance from the nucleus. The maximum number of electrons in any shell is determined by the formula $2n^2$, where n is the shell number. As the atomic number increases, the number of electrons needed to keep the atom electrically neutral also increases. The rules by which the electrons fill the shells are as follows:

1. No shell can contain more than its maximum number of electrons.
2. The outermost shell can contain no more than eight electrons.

Describe the electron shell configuration of an atom of stable nitrogen (Z = 7).

The first two electrons will fill the K shell. The five remaining electrons will fill five of the eight electron positions in the L shell.

What is the electron configuration of an atom of electrically neutral cobalt (Z = 27)?

The K and L shells contain 10 electrons. The remaining 17 electrons would be spread between the M and N shells, even though the M shell can hold 18 electrons. This results from the second rule, which states that only 8 electrons can be in the outermost shell. Predicting the exact configuration of the electrons will involve using chemical principles, which we are not concerned with here. The important fact is that the electrons will be in four shells.

Nuclear forces

To hold a nucleus together, a force must be present. This force must be strong enough to overcome the electrostatic force that is attempting to break up the nucleus. This particular binding force is called the **nuclear force**. The nuclear force comes into play only over very short distances (~10^{-14} m). The nature of this force and others within the nucleus to hold it together is complex. We will not discuss this in detail, but the major force that holds the nucleus of an atom together is the nuclear force.

Nuclear energy levels

The nucleus possess energy levels similar to the atomic energy levels. The nucleus attempts to remain at a stable or ground state, that is, if the nucleus absorbs energy through rising energy level to an excited state, it will attempt to return to the stable state by giving up the excess energy. This process will be discussed later.

Particle radiation

In 1925 deBroglie hypothesized that photons (EM wave) sometimes act as particles. They exhibit momentum, and particles exhibit wavelike properties. This is important to the definition of particle radiation, since it is the propagated energy that has a definite rest mass, definite momentum (within limits), and a position at any time. This hypothesis will be discussed in more detail later.

ELECTROMAGNETIC RADIATION

Radiation is defined as energy that is emitted by an atom and travels through space. This energy can take the form of electromagnetic radiation or can be transferred to subatomic particles such as electrons and cause the particles to move away from the atom. This section will cover the phenomenon of electromagnetic radiation.

Photons

A **photon** is any "packet" of energy traveling through space at the speed of light, 3×10^8 m/s (in a vacuum). Although a photon can be envisioned as a particle, it has no mass of its own nor does it have an electrical charge. It has only its energy, which is a fixed quantity for that particular photon. Thus high energy photons can pass through miles of dense material unscathed, since they have no mass to "bump" into atoms with and no electrical charges to attract or repel other particles that might interfere with their travels.

The nature of photons puzzled physicists until early in the twentieth century, when a new branch of physics called quantum mechanics burst into prominence. This field of study was an attempt to explain atomic and nuclear phenomena on their own level rather than trying to make the physics of these extremely small and special bits of matter correspond to the physics of large objects like automobiles or planets. One of the discoveries of the new science was that photons can be viewed in one of two ways, depending on the situation: either as massless particles, as described previously, or, alternatively, as waves, like the movements of a violin string or the human voice. Photons are a special case of a type of wave called an electromagnetic (EM) wave, which consists of an electrical field and a magnetic field traveling through space at right angles to each other (see Fig. 2-3).[1] Thus photons exhibit the characteristics of a particle at times and the characteristics of a wave at other times. This phenomenon is known as **wave-particle duality**. In the following sections, we will look at both of these

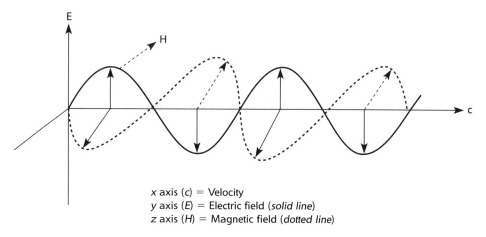

x axis (*c*) = Velocity
y axis (*E*) = Electric field (*solid line*)
z axis (*H*) = Magnetic field (*dotted line*)

Fig. 2-3 Electromagnetic wave component energy fields. (From Bernier DR, Christian PE, Langan JK, editors: *Nuclear medicine: technology and techniques*, ed 3. St Louis, 1994, Mosby.)

manifestations of the photon and see how they can be related to each other in a single equation.

Physical characteristics of an EM wave

An electromagnetic wave has three major distinguishing physical characteristics, which are closely interrelated. They are as follows:

- The **frequency of the wave**, which is represented by the Greek letter nu (υ) is the number of times the wave oscillates per second and is measured in units of waves per second. Since the term "waves" is not really a unit, but simply a number, the unit for frequency turns out to be 1/sec, called the hertz (Hz).
- The **wavelength of the wave** is the physical distance between peaks of the wave. Wavelength is represented by the Greek letter lambda (λ) and is measured in meters (m). Usually the waves we will be working with have wavelengths of about one billionth of a meter, so, to avoid having to constantly write very small numbers, we will express wavelengths in terms of the nanometer (nm), which is equal to 10^9 meters. Another unit of wavelength seen frequently is the angstrom (Å), equal to 10^{-10} m, or 0.1 nm.
- The final important wave characteristic is the velocity of the wave as it travels through space. For our purposes, we will assume that all EM waves travel at the same speed, which is the "speed of light in a vacuum," represented by the letter c and equal to 3×10^8 m/s.

The relationship between these three quantities is as follows:

$$c = \upsilon\lambda$$

Note that if you rearrange the variables, there are two other forms of this equation:

$$\upsilon = \frac{c}{\lambda}$$

$$\lambda = \frac{c}{\upsilon}$$

Looking closely at these equations, you can see that the frequency υ and wavelength λ of an electromagnetic wave are inversely related. As one gets larger, the other gets smaller. Table 2-3 lists some of the frequencies and wavelengths present in the range of known electromagnetic waves.

Calculate the wavelength of an EM wave that has a frequency of 4.5×10^{14} Hz.

To calculate wavelength from frequency, we can use the equation $\lambda = \frac{c}{\upsilon}$.

$$\lambda = \frac{c}{\upsilon} = \frac{3 \times 10^8 \text{ m/s}}{4.5 \times 10^{14} \text{ Hz}} = 6.67 \times 10^{-7} \text{ m}$$

This answer could also be expressed in nanometers and angstroms:

$$(6.67 \times 10^{-7} \text{ m}) (1 \text{ nm}/10^{-9} \text{ m}) = 667 \text{ nm, or } 6670 \text{ Å}$$

An FM radio station broadcasts at a wavelength of 3.125 m. At what frequency will you find this station on your radio dial?

Table 2-3	The electromagnetic spectrum	
Radiation	**Average λ (m)**	**Average υ (Hz)**
Gamma rays	10^{-12}	10^{20}
Ultraviolet light	10^{-8}	10^{17}
Visible light	10^{-6}	10^{14}
Infrared light	10^{-5}	10^{13}
Microwaves	10^{-2}	10^{10}
Radio and television	10^{2}	10^{6}

From Bernier DR, Christian PE, Langan JK, editors: *Nuclear medicine: technology and techniques*, ed 3. St Louis, 1994, Mosby.

$$\upsilon = \frac{c}{\lambda} = \frac{3 \times 10^8 \text{ m/s}}{3.125 \text{ m}} = 96,000,000 \text{ Hz, or } 96 \times 10^6 \text{ Hz}$$

This station broadcasts at 96 megahertz (MHz).

Photon energy

As stated previously, the energy of a photon is its major characteristic, especially from the viewpoint of radiation therapy physics. Fortunately, there are ways to calculate the energy of the wave when its other properties are known. The energy can, for example, be calculated when the frequency (υ) of the wave is known, using the following equation:

$$E = h\upsilon$$

where E is the energy of the wave, and h is a constant called Planck's constant, which has the value 6.626×10^{-34} J·s; this is equivalent to 4.15×10^{-15} eV·s. Either value can be used, depending on whether you want the resultant energy in joules or electron volts.

A joule (J) is the "metric system," or SI, unit of energy and is equivalent to 1 kg m²/s². This unit is typically used for applications involving "real world" objects, such as billiard balls, cans of light beer, and space shuttles. However, the energies of EM waves are usually much smaller than the energies involved in these situations (with the possible exception of light beer), so another smaller unit is used. This unit is the electron volt and represents the amount of energy that one electron would pick up as it passed through an electrical field whose potential difference was 1 V. This unit will be the standard unit for photon energy in this text and is related to the joule as follows:

$$1 \text{ eV} = 1.6 \times 10^{-19} \text{ J, or } 1 \text{ J} = 6.25 \times 10^{18} \text{ eV}$$

If an EM wave has a frequency of 1.8×10^{20} Hz, what are its wavelength and energy (in eV)?

$$\lambda = \frac{c}{\upsilon} = \frac{3 \times 10^8 \text{ m/s}}{1.8 \times 10^{20} \text{ Hz}} = 1.667 \times 10^{-12} \text{ m}$$

$$E = h\upsilon = (4.15 \times 10^{-15} \text{ eV} \cdot \text{s}) (1.8 \times 10^{20} \text{ Hz}) = 747,000 \text{ eV} = 0.747 \text{ MeV}$$

The photon emitted from the decay of the radioisotope ^{99m}Tc has an energy of about 142 keV. What are the frequency and wavelength of this photon?

Since we know that E = 142 keV = 142,000 eV, we can find υ by the following:

$$\upsilon = \frac{E}{h} = \frac{142,000 \text{ eV}}{4.15 \times 10^{-15} \text{ eVs}} = 3.422 \times 10^{19} \text{ Hz}$$

Now λ can be found:

$$\lambda = \frac{c}{\upsilon} = \frac{3 \times 10^8 \text{ m/s}}{3.422 \times 10^{-19} \text{ Hz}} = 8.77 \times 10^{-12} \text{ m}$$

Another interesting fact about photons can be discovered using Einstein's theories of relativity, in which he postulated the famous equation for relating the mass of any object to the amount of energy that it can be converted into:

$$E = mc^2$$

where E is the energy, m is the mass of the object, and c is the speed of light. Note that, since c^2 will have units of m^2/s^2, it is necessary to express the mass of the object in kilograms so that we obtain an answer in joules whenever using this equation.

This equation gave the first indication to the scientific world that matter and energy are really different aspects of the same thing and that one can be directly converted into the other. This discovery has drastically changed the world we live in by increasing our understanding of the universe as well as giving us the ability to harness the power of the stars in nuclear fusion reactions, which convert a small amount of matter directly into a huge amount of energy. Unfortunately, the only current use of this knowledge in any viable sense is the stockpile of "hydrogen bombs" present in our defense arsenals.

If you set this equation for E equal to the Planck equation and solve, you find that:

$$m = \frac{h\upsilon}{c^2}$$

With this equation, it is possible to calculate the **mass equivalence** of a photon. Although the photon has no actual mass, the equation allows you to treat the photon as if it actually had mass of its own—the more energy, the greater the mass equivalence. Thus, the above equation neatly combines the particle and wave natures of the photon into a single, tidy equation.

Calculate the mass equivalence of a photon of green light, with a nominal wavelength of 520 nm.

First, calculate the energy of this wave, letting $\upsilon = \frac{c}{\lambda}$:

$$E = \frac{hc}{\lambda} = \frac{(6.626 \times 10^{-34} \text{ Js})(3 \times 10^8 \text{ m/s})}{520 \times 10^{-9} \text{ m}}$$
$$= 3.823 \times 10^{-19} \text{ J}$$

Notice that to keep the units consistent, we have used the value for Planck's constant that includes joules, so that the SI unit of meters present in the photon wavelength will cancel out.

Having found the energy, we can now calculate the mass equivalence by solving Einstein's equation for the mass:

$$m = \frac{E}{c^2} = \frac{(3.823 \times 10^{-19} \text{ J})}{3 \times 10^8 \text{ m/s}} = 4.248 \times 10^{-36} \text{ kg}$$

RADIOACTIVITY

Unstable atomic nuclei tend to seek their ground state, meaning that they tend to give off their excess energy until they reach a point at which the energy in the nucleus is just enough to maintain nuclear stability. The process by which they lose this energy is called radioactivity. Radioactivity may involve the emission of particles, electromagnetic radiation (photons), or a combination of the two. In this section we will study the processes by which atoms rid themselves of this excess nuclear energy, and the mathematical methods used to describe them.

The nuclear stability curve

The nuclear stability curve is shown in Fig. 2-4. The vertical axis represents the atomic number (Z) of the atom, that is, the number of protons in the nucleus. The horizontal axis represents the number of neutrons (N) in the nucleus. The solid line represents the condition $^N/z = 1$, that is, atoms with the same number of neutrons and protons in the nucleus. The curved line shows the "line of stability"; atoms whose proton/neutron combinations place them on this line are stable and will not undergo radioactive decay, since they have no excess energy. The two curves are coincident at low values of Z, for example, Z < 20, indicating that these atoms have identical numbers of protons and neutrons. As Z increases, however, you can see that the curve begins to diverge from the "ideal" line, curving to the right. This indicates that, as the number of protons grows larger, more neutrons than protons are required to maintain stability and the required neutron/proton ratio increases as Z increases. Atoms that do not

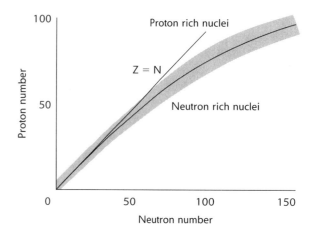

Fig. 2-4 Nuclear stability curve. (From Bernier DR, Christian PE, Langan JK, editors: *Nuclear medicine: technology and techniques,* ed 3. St Louis, 1994, Mosby.)

meet this criterion appear at other positions on the graph, away from the stability curve; these represent unstable atoms. As these atoms lose energy, they will move closer to the stability curve, finally reaching a stable state.

You may recall that the combinations called isotope, isobar, and isotone refer to different arrangements of nuclear particles. Similarly, the terms *isotopic*, *isobaric*, and *isotonic* refer to types of transformations that change the atom to an isotope, isobar, or isotone of itself. For example, an isotopic transition is one in which the Z of the atom remains constant, but the atomic mass number (A) increases or decreases. Similarly, during an isobaric transition the A of the atom remains the same, while the Z and N change appropriately; during an isotonic transition, the N remains constant while Z (and therefore A) changes. By undergoing as many of these transitions as necessary, atoms can move from an unstable to a stable state.

Types of radioactive decay

Alpha decay. An alpha particle, symbolized by the Greek letter α, consists of two neutrons and two protons bound together; this is equivalent to a helium atom (Z = 2) that has been stripped of its two electrons.[1-4] Large, unstable atoms that have a large amount of excess energy tend to undergo radioactive decay by the emission of α particles, which eliminates four nuclear particles and therefore a substantial amount (in nuclear terms) of excess energy. The equation for α decay is as follows:

$$^{A}_{Z}X \rightarrow {}^{A-4}_{Z-2}Y + {}^{4}_{2}\alpha + Q$$

where Q represents the excess energy shed by the nucleus. This energy frequently appears in the form of photons, which, because of their nuclear origin, are called gamma rays (γ-rays).

Examine this equation carefully. "Reading" it, it says that a nucleus X with a known A and Z decays by α decay to a new atom with atomic mass number A-4 and atomic number Z-2; the two missing protons and two missing neutrons appear as an α particle emitted from the nucleus. In addition, a certain amount of energy is given off, either in the form of kinetic energy (i.e., speed of the α particle) or as γ-rays or, more commonly, as a combination of the two. A key feature of this equation is that the numbers of protons, neutrons, and electrical charges on both sides of the arrow are equal. This is a critical feature of all radioactive decay equations: the two sides of the arrow must balance exactly in terms of number of particles, electrical charges, and energy. The most important thing to note, however, is that the original atom has now changed into a new element by the loss of two nuclear protons.

An atom of uranium, $^{238}_{92}U$, undergoes α decay. What is the result?

$$^{238}_{92}U \quad {}^{234}_{90}Th + {}^{4}_{2}\alpha + \gamma$$

The atom of uranium has been transformed into an atom of thorium.

Alpha decay occurs when the N/z ratio is too low, that is, when the atom falls "underneath" the stability curve on the N/z graph. By eliminating two neutrons and two protons, plus the associated energy, this transition increases the N/z ratio, attempting to correct for the too low N/z ratio that existed before the transition.

The energies of the α particles emitted by a given isotope are fixed and discrete. Even though an isotope may emit more than one α particle energy as the atoms in the sample decay, each α will have one of a selection of fixed energies. This contrasts with ß decay, described in the next two sections, in which essentially infinite numbers of particle energies are possible.

Beta minus decay. Recall that a beta minus (ß⁻) particle is the same as an electron, the difference in name arising because of the difference in place of origin. An electron is found orbiting in the electron shells, whereas a ß⁻ particle is emitted as the result of a nuclear decay. To understand ß⁻ decay, think of a neutron as a "mixture" of a proton plus an electron:

$$n^{\circ} \rightarrow p^{+} + e^{-}$$

What essentially happens during a ß⁻ decay is that a neutron in the nucleus "decays" into a proton plus an electron, as shown. The proton remains in the nucleus, and the electron is ejected and leaves the atom; this ejected electron is called the ß⁻ particle. The equation for ß⁻ decay is as follows:

$$^{A}_{Z}X \rightarrow {}^{A}_{Z+1}Y + {}^{0}_{-1}\beta + \upsilon$$

where the symbol υ stands for the emission of a tiny particle called the antineutrino. This particle carries away the energy that is left over when the ß⁻ does not carry away all of the atom's excess energy. You can see that when undergoing ß⁻ decay, the atom increases its Z by one, while maintaining the same A (having lost a neutron but gained a proton), making this an isobaric transition. Since the number of protons increases while the number of neutrons decreases constant, the N/z ratio of this atom will decrease. (The ß⁻ particle has an "atomic number" of $^{-}1$, representing its electrical charge relative to the proton.) Usually the daughter nucleus of a ß⁻ decay is itself radioactive and can undergo radioactive decay in many ways, typically by giving off its excess energy as γ-rays. In fact, there are very few isotopes that emit only ß⁻ particles; the majority are accompanied by γ-ray emission from the daughter nucleus.[1-4]

Cobalt 60 decays by β⁻ decay to an excited state of ^{60}Ni, which then decays by the emission of two high energy γ-rays, as follows:

$$^{60}_{27}Co \rightarrow {}^{60}_{28}Ni + {}^{0}_{-1}\beta + \upsilon \rightarrow {}^{60}_{28}Ni + 2\gamma$$

Beta-emitting isotopes do not give off ß particles of fixed energy, as do α emitters. Instead the emitted ß⁻ particles possess energies between 0 and a given maximum (E_{max}), creating what is called a beta spectrum (see Fig. 2-5). The average energy of the beta particle in the spectrum is about one third

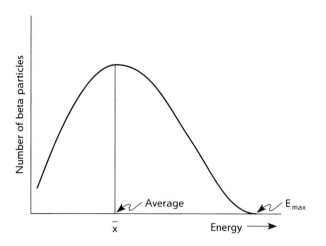

Fig. 2-5 Beta particle energy spectrum. (From Bernier DR, Christian PE, Langan JK, editors: *Nuclear medicine: technology and techniques*, ed 3. St Louis, 1994, Mosby.)

of E_{max}. The extra energy between E_{max} and the actual energy of the ß- particle is carried away by the antineutrino (υ).

Beta plus decay. There is a subatomic particle that has exactly the same characteristics as an electron, except that it possesses a positive electrical charge rather than a negative charge. This particle is called a positron and has the symbol ß+. Also, like an electron, it can be ejected from an atomic nucleus; in this case, a nuclear proton "decays" into a neutron and a positron:

$$p^+ \rightarrow n^0 + ß^+$$

So the equation for ß+ decay is

$$_Z^A X \rightarrow _{Z-1}^A Y + _{+1}^0 ß + υ$$

Because of the loss of a proton but the gain of a neutron, the atom retains the same A but the Z of the atoms decreases and the N/z ratio of the atom increases, making this an isobaric transition.[1]

Sodium 22 ($_{11}^{22} Na$) is a common radioactive isotope of natural sodium. It decays by ß+ decay to a stable isotope of the gas neon, with the emission of a ß+ particle and a γ-ray, as follows:

$$_{11}^{22} Na \rightarrow _{10}^{22} Ne^* + _{+1}^0 ß \rightarrow _{10}^{22} Ne + γ$$

As with ß+ decay, a spectrum of energies is emitted, with an average energy of one third E_{max}; the remainder of the energy is carried off by the neutrino (υ), as in ß- decay.

Electron capture. Although the Bohr model of the atom depicts the electrons as being in fixed orbits outside of the nucleus, the discoveries of quantum mechanics tell us that it is possible that the electrons may, at some time, come very close to the nucleus. An electron that strays too close to the nucleus may be captured and combined with a proton, reversing the process for ß- decay:

$$p^+ + e^- \rightarrow n^0 + υ$$

This process is known as electron capture, and has the same result as ß+ decay; in other words, the Z of the parent nucleus decreases by 1, and the N/z ratio of the atom increases.

Because of the proximity of the K shell to the nucleus, it is most likely that the captured electron will be taken from this shell, although it is possible to capture an electron from the L or M shells. When an electron is taken from one of the electron shells, it leaves a "hole" in the shell; this will place the atom in an unstable configuration in terms of energy, since an inner shell electron has lower energy than an electron from an outer shell. As a result, one of the electrons from an outer shell will "fall" toward the nucleus, moving from a higher energy state to a lower one, and this excess energy, no longer needed to maintain stability, will be given off in the form of an x-ray. This type of radiation is called characteristic radiation and is an important part of many radioactive decay schemes and radiation/matter interactions.

Isomeric transition. An isomer is an atom whose Z and A are identical to another atom's but that is currently in what is called a metastable state. This represents a daughter product of some other kind of decay that is itself in an excited state, but, instead of instantly decaying by γ emission (see the example for ß- decay), it remains in this excited state for a given period of time, then decays. Such a nucleus is represented by a small "m" next to its atomic mass number, as in ^{99m}Tc. A nucleus that has no metastable state but decays instantly has a star to the right of its chemical symbol (^{60}Ni*). Metastable isotopes, or isomers, usually decay by emitting the excess energy as a γ-ray.

^{99m}Tc is an isotope used daily in nuclear medicine procedures. It is a daughter product of ^{99}Mo, and the decay equation looks like this:

$$_{42}^{99} Mo \rightarrow _{43}^{99m} Tc^* + _{-1}^0 ß \rightarrow _{43}^{99} Tc + γ$$

Specification of radioactivity

To quantify the amount of radioactivity present in a given sample, in the early 20th century the curie was defined as the activity of 1 g of ^{226}Ra, the most well-known isotope in use at that time. Unfortunately, as measurement techniques improved, disputes arose as to exactly what the activity of 1 g of ^{226}Ra meant in terms of the number of radioactive atoms present. So eventually the unit of radioactivity, the curie, was defined as follows:

$$1 \text{ Ci} = 3.7 \times 10^{10} \text{ dis/sec}$$

where dis/sec stands for "nuclear disintegrations per second," that is, the number of atoms that undergo some kind of radioactive decay every second. Since "disintegrations" is not really a unit but merely a quantity, the curie is numerically equal to 1/s or s^{-1}. In fact, the new proposed unit of radioactivity, the becquerel (Bq), is equal to 1 dis/sec; this unit, however, is rarely used because of the large number of dis/sec present in even a small sample of radioactive material.

For various amounts of radioactive material, multiples of the curie such as the millicurie (mCi, 10^{-3} Ci) and the microcurie (μCi, 10^{-6} Ci) are used. A typical nuclear medicine procedure employs amounts of radioactivity in the range of hundreds of millicuries, whereas a cobalt teletherapy machine uses a source of ^{60}Co of an activity in the range of 5000 to 6000 Ci.

Exponential decay of radioactivity. The amount of radioactivity present in a given sample is never a constant quantity, but rather is being reduced continuously by the decay of the radioactive atoms in the sample.[2,4] This decay process follows a mathematical pattern known as exponential behavior. Any value that increases or decreases exponentially will double or halve its value within a certain amount of time; when that time interval passes again, the value will have further reduced by half or increased by two times. Although it is impossible to say exactly which atoms in a radioactive sample will decay at any given time, it is reasonably straightforward to determine what percentage of the atoms will remain after a given amount of time.

The equation of exponential decay of radioactivity is as follows:

$$A_t = A_o e^{-\lambda t}$$

where A_t is the activity at time t, A_0 is the activity at time "zero" (when the activity was measured), and λ is a value known as the exponential decay constant, which will be discussed in more detail below. The symbol e represents the base of the natural logarithms, which governs exponential behavior; it has the value e = 2.718282... .

According to the rules of logarithms, e to any negative power will always be less than 1.000; e to a very small negative number will be very close to 1.000; and many hand calculators will give the value of 1.000 in this case. However, the number should never be greater than 1.000; if this is the case, you have made a mathematical error because radioactive decay will always result in a decrease in the amount of radioactivity present.

To make this point absolutely clear, we will use a little algebra to rearrange the previous equation:

$$\frac{A_t}{A_o} = e^{-\lambda t}$$

This says that the final amount of radioactivity divided by the initial amount is equal to the exponential side of the equation, which will always be between 0 and 1.

Another important principle in working with natural logarithms is that the "inverse" of the exponential function e is the natural logarithm ln. This means that

$$\ln (e^{\text{anything}}) = \text{Anything}$$

or, in our case,

$$\ln(e^{-\lambda t}) = -\lambda t$$

A radioactive sample is measured to contain 100 mCi of radioactivity. If the decay constant of this isotope is 0.115 hr^{-1}, how much activity will remain after 24 hours?

$$A_t = A_o e^{-\lambda t} = (100 \text{ mCi})e^{(-0.115)(24)} = 6.329 \text{ mCi}$$

Note the units on λ, which are time^{-1}. Since the units of t are in time and the units of λ are time^{-1}, these must cancel out, leaving the exponent of e with no units. To accomplish this, λ and t must be in the same unit of time, that is, minutes, hours, days, years, etc.

λ is a constant for a given isotope, that is, all atoms of a given isotope will decay with the same λ, which will not change no matter what environmental conditions persist— you cannot change the λ of an isotope with heat, pressure, or any other known factors.

How can we use the exponential decay equation to derive the useful quantity, known as the half-life of an isotope? The half-life is the time required for the activity of any sample of a particular radioisotope to decay to half of its initial value. So the quantity we seek to solve for is t, the time, which we will give the special symbol t_h to represent half-life.

How do we solve the equation for half-life? We know that the activity after 1 half-life will be half of the initial activity, by definition. So we can say that:

$$\frac{A_t}{A_o} = 0.5$$

Knowing this, solve for t_h:

$$\frac{A_t}{A_o} = e^{-\lambda t}$$

$$0.5 = e^{-\lambda t_h}$$

$$\ln (0.5) = -\lambda t_h$$

$$-0.693 = -\lambda t_h$$

We now divide and cancel the minus signs to get the final solution:

$$t_h = \frac{0.693}{\lambda}$$

We can, if needed, also rearrange this equation to give:

$$\lambda = \frac{0.693}{t_h}$$

You should go through this derivation several times and try it yourself, so that the method is clear. These equations will be used frequently in our calculations involving radioactive isotopes.

A sample of an isotope with a half-life of 8.0 days is measured to have an activity of 25.0 mCi on Monday at noon. What would the activity be on Friday of that week, at noon?

Find λ using the above equations with 4.0 days as the value for t:

$$\lambda = \frac{0.693}{t_h} = \frac{0.693}{8.0\text{d}} = 0.087\text{d}^{-1}$$

$$A_t = (25.0 \text{ mCi})e^{(-0.087\text{d}^{-1})(4.0\text{d})} = 17.679 \text{ mCi}$$

The exponential decay equation is quite powerful, since it can be solved algebraically in a number of ways, depending on the results required. For example, if you take two activity readings from an isotope sample, you can call these A_o and A_t, and the elapsed time between the two readings will be t. You can now find the decay constant and half-life of this isotope by rearranging the exponential decay equation into a new form:

$$\frac{A_t}{A_o} = e^{-\lambda t}$$

$$\ln \frac{A_t}{A_o} = e^{-\lambda t}$$

$$\ln \frac{A_t}{A_o} \times \frac{-1}{t} = \lambda$$

Note that we have made use of the relationship between ln and e, that is, that the natural log function and the exponential function are inverse functions—one will "cancel" the effect of the other. This allows us to find any unknown quantities that may exist in the exponent of the exponential function, such as λ or t. The previous equation can be used to find λ and, therefore, the half-life of the isotope.

Two readings of the activity of a radioactive sample are taken 40 hours apart. The first reading is 125.0 mCi, the second one is 1.232 mCi. Calculate the half-life of this isotope.

Find λ, then find t_h:

$$\ln \frac{A_t}{A_o} \times \frac{-1}{t} = \lambda$$

$$\ln \frac{1.232 \text{ mCi}}{125.0 \text{ mCi}} \times \frac{-1}{40.0 \text{ hrs}} = \lambda$$

$$(-4.620)(-0.025) = 0.116 \text{ hr}^{-1} = \lambda$$

$$t_h = \frac{0.693}{0.116 \text{ hr}^{-1}} = 6.0 \text{ hr}$$

An isotope with a decay constant $\lambda = 0.043$ hr^{-1} is allowed to decay for 24 hours. The activity at the end of this period is measured as 17.8 mCi. What was the initial activity?

$$A_t = A_0 e^{-\lambda t}$$

$$17.8 = A_0 e^{(-0.043)(24)}$$

$$17.8 = A_0 (0.356)$$

$$A_0 = 50 \text{ mCi}$$

A quantity called the mean life (t) of the isotope is sometimes used in brachytherapy calculations involving short-lived isotopes (i.e., isotopes with short half-lives). The mean life t is related to the half-life and decay constant of the isotope as follows:

$$t = 1.44 t_h = \frac{1}{\lambda}$$

Radioactive equilibrium

It is quite common for some radioisotopes, especially high Z isotopes, to decay to daughter products that are themselves radioactive. An example of this process is ^{226}Ra, which is one of a number of isotopes along a "chain" of daughter products created when ^{238}U, found in nature, decays to ^{206}Pb over the course of millions of years. When parent and daughter isotopes exist in this manner, it is possible that a condition of equilibrium (i.e., balance) will be established in this system—the daughter and parent isotopes will begin to appear to decay with nearly the same half-lives and to have the same activities.

To illustrate this, consider the case of the decay of ^{226}Ra to ^{222}Rn via α-decay:

$$^{226}_{88}\text{Ra} \rightarrow\ ^{222}_{86}\text{Rn} + ^{4}_{2}\alpha + Q$$

^{226}Ra has a half-life of over 1600 years, while the half-life of the daughter ^{222}Rn is only about 3.8 days. A sample that starts out as pure radium begins to decay to radon, causing a buildup of radon. But the radon decays with a shorter half-life and so will have a higher activity (number of disintegrations per second). Eventually the daughter product is so active that it essentially equals the activity of the parent. This condition is called secular equilibrium and can occur only when the half-life of the parent is much greater than the half-life of the daughter isotope, that is, when:

$$t_{hparent} >> t_{hdaughter}$$

If the differences in parent and daughter half-life are not as dramatic but the parent is still longer lived than the daughter, the daughter activity will actually grow slightly larger than the parent activity and then appear to decay at the same rate (with the same half-life). This condition is called transient equilibrium and occurs when:

$$t_{hparent} > t_{hdaughter}$$

In the case $t_{hparent} < t_{hdaughter}$, no equilibrium can exist.

Radioactive equilibrium conditions can be exploited to provide a steady source of some radioisotopes used in nuclear medicine procedures. An excellent example of this is the use of "generators" that contain a source of $^{99}_{42}$Mo, which decays by ß- decay to the metastable isotope $^{99}_{43}$Tc. The parent half-life of 67 hours is greater than the daughter half-life of 6 hours, so that transient equilibrium is reached. Each week a fresh generator is delivered to the nuclear medicine department. At the beginning of each day the technologist adds a solvent to the generator, which chemically separates the ^{99m}Tc from the ^{99}Mo, and the ^{99m}Tc is drawn off. It can then be used as a radioactive injection in a number of diagnostic studies. Of course, since the ^{99}Mo is decaying away, at the beginning of each day less ^{99m}Tc is available than the day before. So at the end of the week the generator is stored for further decay, then returned to the manufacturer when radiation levels reach acceptable levels.

PHOTON INTERACTIONS

When a beam of radiation from any source strikes some material, a number of processes can occur that serve to transfer energy from the radiation to the medium; this energy can then affect the medium in many ways. Biological tissue, for example, may suffer damage to the nucleic acid structures (DNA) and lose its ability to reproduce itself, thereby damaging the organism as a whole. Other materials may undergo physical or chemical changes as a result of the energy transfer, such as heating or disruption of crystal structures. In this section, we will look at the ways in which photons (x-rays or γ-rays) interact with matter.

The inverse square law

The intensity of flux of a radiation beam is defined as the number of photons in the beam per square centimeter. Note that this definition does not take into account the energy of the radiation in the beam, only the number of photons present in the beam at a given instant per square centimeter. So a beam can be called "low intensity" if it has just a few photons per square centimeter, even if the photons are very high energy; similarly, a "high intensity" beam may consist entirely of a large number of very low energy photons. For practical purposes the intensity of a radiation beam is usually measured in terms of the exposure rate (X, mR/hr) or dose rate (D, cGy/min) of the beam at that point, rather than the number of photons present.

Frequently in radiation therapy physics, we are interested in describing the intensity from a point source of radiation. A point source is a source that is so small (from the viewpoint of the observer) that it appears to have no area, and all photons coming from it appear to originate at the same point. In reality, most radiation sources have some finite area; however, if the distance from the source is large it will appear to be a point. For example, a coin viewed from a distance of 3 meters will appear to be a "point". So, if the distance from the source to the "point of interest" is at least five times the physical size of the source, the source can be treated as a point source. This assumption greatly simplifies most radiation therapy calculations; since the distance from a radiation therapy source to the point of interest is rarely shorter than five times the source size, most sources can be considered point sources for our purposes. This is not always true in the case of internally implanted radioisotopes.

Given that we are working with a point source, the intensity of the radiation beam coming from this source can be determined first by assuming that the radiation is emitted isotropically from the source—that is, it is emitted evenly in all directions from the point source. If this is the case, the intensity of the beam at any distance from the source is calculated by dividing the number of photons coming from the source by the area of the sphere surrounding the source at that distance. If we let Δp represent the number of photons emitted by the point source in any instant, we can say that the intensity of the beam at distance d_1 from the point source is equal to:

$$I_1 = \frac{\text{Number of photons}}{\text{Area of sphere}} = \frac{\Delta p}{4\pi d_1^2}$$

where $4\pi d_1^2$ is the area of the sphere of radius d_1.

How does the intensity change as we move closer to or farther away from our point source? If we assume that none of the photons are attenuated (taken out of the beam), then Δp will remain the same; only d, the distance from the point source, will change. If we call the new distance d_2, then the intensity at this point is equal to:

$$I_2 = \frac{\Delta p}{4\pi d_2^2}$$

So the change in intensity moving from distance d_1 to distance d_2 is the ratio of I_1 to I_2:

$$\frac{I_1}{I_2} = \left(\frac{\Delta p / 4\pi d_1^2}{\Delta p / 4\pi d_2^2}\right) = \left(\frac{d_2^2}{d_1^2}\right) = \left(\frac{d_2}{d_1}\right)^2$$

When we solve this equation for I_2, we get:

$$I_2 = I_1\left(\frac{d_1}{d_2}\right)^2$$

This is one statement of the inverse square law, an important principle in radiation therapy physics. The basic idea of the inverse square law is that the intensity of a radiation beam decreases or increases as the inverse of the square of the distance.[1] A few examples should clarify the use of this principle.

The intensity of a radiation beam is measured at 10.0 mR/hr at a distance of 10 cm. What will be the intensity of this beam at 20.0 cm?

Let I_1 = 10 mR/hr, d_1 = 10.0 cm, and d_2 = 20.0 cm. The intensity at d_2 will be:

$$I_2 = (10.0 \text{ mR/hr})\left(\frac{10.0 \text{ cm}}{20.0 \text{ cm}}\right)^2 = 2.5 \text{ mR/hr}$$

The intensity at twice the distance is one fourth of the original intensity.

If, in the preceding example, d_2 is equal to 5 cm (i.e., the new distance is closer to the source than the original), what will be the change in beam intensity?

With d_2 now equal to 5 cm, the solution becomes:

$$I_2 = (10.0 \text{ mR/hr})\left(\frac{10.0 \text{ cm}}{5.0 \text{ cm}}\right)^2 = 40.0 \text{ mR/hr}$$

Since the distance change was in the opposite direction to the previous example, the intensity increased by four times.

The inverse square law, as indicated earlier, is an important factor in radiation therapy patient calculations.

Exponential attenuation

The inverse square law is strictly correct only when certain conditions are met. For example, the source of the radiation must be small enough to be treated as a point source. In addition, we have assumed that none of the radiation emitted from the source is removed from the beam, but rather continues outward from the source, unmolested. When working with photons in air, this condition is met well enough that the inverse square law can be said to apply in most of these cases. For high energy medical accelerators the inverse square law applies to a limited degree when the photons are traveling in some material such as water or a patient. In most cases of photon interactions with material, however, the photons will indeed interact with the atoms of the material, giving up their energy and being removed from the beam. This process is called attenuation.

Earlier we saw that the decay of a radioactive source is an exponential function, described by the following equation:

$$A_t = A_o e^{-\lambda t}$$

where λ is a constant for a given radioisotope and t is the time between measurements A_o and A_t. This represents a statistical view of the problem; it is impossible to say exactly when each individual atom will decay, but large numbers of atoms can be described with high precision. The attenuation of radiation by a medium can also be described in this way. To do this, we define a value called the linear attenuation coefficient with the symbol μ. This describes the probability that each photon in the beam will interact with the medium and lose its energy, per centimeter of material that the photons pass through, and has units of cm^{-1}. It is not a constant like λ, but instead depends greatly on the energy of the photon beam and the medium in which the interaction is taking place.

The degree of attenuation of a photon beam by a medium is then calculated by the following:

$$I_x = I_o e^{-\mu x}$$

where I_o is the intensity of the beam before striking the medium, I_x is the intensity after passing through the medium, μ is the linear attenuation coefficient for this beam energy and medium, and x is the thickness of the medium (in cm). Note that this equation is in exactly the same form as the equation for radioactive decay, indicating that the two processes are similar to each other in being statistical in nature, rather than exact.

As with the radioactive decay equation, the equation of attenuation can be used in may ways.

A beam of ^{60}Co photons is incident on a lead sheet 1.0 cm thick. If the initial dose rate of the cobalt beam (I_o) was 50 cGy/min, what will the dose rate be after passing through the lead sheet if the value of μ for this beam in lead is 0.533 cm^{-1}?

$$I_x = I_o e^{-\mu x}$$

$$I_x = (50)e^{(-0.533)(1.0)}$$

$$I_x = (50)(0.587)$$

$$I_x = 29.34 \text{ cGy/min}$$

Using the data from the previous example, calculate the initial dose rate if the dose rate after passing through the lead sheet was measured to be 15.0 cGy/min.

From the previous example, $\mu = 0.533$ cm^{-1} and x = 1.0 cm:

$$I_x = I_o e^{-\mu x}$$

$$15.0 = I_o e^{(-0.533)(1.0)}$$

$$15.0 = I_o(0.587)$$

$$I_o = 25.52 \text{ cGy/min}$$

A table of μ values for materials and photon energies important in radiation therapy is provided in Table 2-4.

Table 2-4	Linear attenuation coeffecients (μ) (cm^{-1})				
Energy (MeV)	**Water**	**Tissue**	**Aluminum**	**Copper**	**Lead**
0.010	5.0660	5.360	71.1187	1964.0300	1507.4720
0.050	0.2245	0.2330	0.9803	22.9466	88.7330
0.100	0.1706	0.1760	0.4604	4.0759	62.0370
0.200	0.1370	0.1412	0.3306	1.4067	11.2612
0.500	0.0969	0.0998	0.2281	0.7500	1.8040
0.662	0.0857	0.0883	0.2013	0.6496	1.2314
0.800	0.0787	0.0810	0.1846	0.5914	0.9906
1.000	0.0707	0.0729	0.1660	0.5277	0.7963
1.250	0.0632	0.0651	0.1482	0.4704	0.6600
1.500	0.0575	0.0593	0.1352	0.4301	0.5873
2.000	0.0494	0.0510	0.1169	0.3763	0.5146
3.000	0.0397	0.0409	0.0955	0.3226	0.4737
4.000	0.0340	0.0350	0.0839	0.2975	0.4714
5.000	0.0303	0.0312	0.0767	0.2840	0.4805
8.000	0.0242	0.0249	0.0713	0.2715	0.5157
10.00	0.0222	0.0229	0.0626	0.2778	0.5544
20.00	0.0182	0.0186	0.0586	0.3055	0.6952
30.00	0.0171	0.0176	0.0594	0.3324	0.7952
50.00	0.0167	0.0172	0.0623	0.3692	0.9168
80.00	0.0169	0.0173	0.0656	0.4005	1.0122
100.0	0.0172	0.0177	0.0677	0.4184	1.0544

The exponential decay equation may be used to derive a special quantity, the half-life, that describes the amount of time required for the isotope to decay to half of its original activity. In the same manner, we can define a quantity, called the **half value layer** (HVL), that is the thickness of some added material required to reduce the beam intensity to half of its original value:

$$HVL = \frac{0.693}{\mu}$$

Since μ depends on the energy of the beam and the material with which the radiation is interacting, HVL values must be defined by both energy and attenuating material. This procedure is fairly straightforward if the photon beam is monoenergetic, that is, if it consists of only a single photon energy. Unfortunately, this is not the case with photon beams produced by most modern radiation therapy equipment, which produce polyenergetic beams consisting of a wide spectrum of photon energies. So, usually, the HVL is simply measured for a given machine and beam energy and, in the case of low energy x-ray units, is used to describe the characteristics of the treatment beam.

We know that exponential decay data plotted on a similar graph yields a straight line. This technique can also be applied to exponential attenuation by plotting the percentage of radiation passing through a material as a function of the material thickness. By plotting data such as these, and drawing in the straight line formed by the data, the HVL of the beam can be determined experimentally. Once the graph is done, the thickness of material required to reduce the beam intensity to one fraction of its initial value can be found simply by reading the graph. If a large number of attenuation readings are taken, the curve may not actually display a single line but a series of line segments of decreasing slope. This effect results from the "hardening" of the beam, explained in the next section.

X-ray beam quality

The HVL is an important quantity for photon beams and can be used as a description of "beam quality." Photon beams can be classified as "hard" or "soft" beams, depending on their HVL.[4] Although there are no hard and fast rules for determining the hardness or softness of a radiation beam, a "hard" beam will have a higher HVL and higher penetrating ability than a "soft" beam.

This concept of beam hardness becomes more important when one considers the various factors involved. Softer beams have less penetrating ability and will therefore tend to deposit their energy in a medium fairly quickly. If the medium in question is actually a radiation therapy patient, this means that the skin dose to that patient will be increased. In some situations this is desirable; in many situations, however, it is not. Consider, for example, a radiation therapy simulator (or any diagnostic x-ray device). A soft beam will not penetrate adequately through the patient to the film, but will instead leave a large amount of dose inside the patient without contributing any quality to the final film. In this setting, one should attempt to reduce the softness of the beam (and therefore the patient dose) without requiring a large increase in radiation exposure to take the film.

To understand one solution to these problems, consider a polyenergetic beam of radiation striking a medium such as lead. The beam consists of a large variety of x-ray energies—some low, some more energetic. As it passes through the lead, the "softer" x-rays (those with the lower energy) tend to be absorbed by the lead, while the "harder" x-rays, whose μ value is lower, are not as likely to be absorbed and may pass through the lead untouched. So if you examine the various energies in the beam before and after it passes through the lead, you can see that the beam exiting from the lead will have a higher average energy (i.e., fewer low energy x-rays) and a larger HVL than the initial beam. By passing the beam through this lead attenuator, we have actually increased the overall HVL of the beam, although the intensity of the beam has probably been decreased. This effect is called beam hardening and is very important in the design and use of diagnostic and radiation therapy equipment.[2-4]

Low energy x-ray units (diagnostic and superficial therapy) usually have a certain amount of "inherent filtration," that is, there is some filtration material built into the machine. Usually this consists of the metal window where the radiation beam exits the inside chamber of the tube, where it is produced, together with a small amount of added filtration (usually aluminum) to harden the beam for use in patient diagnosis and treatment. High energy x-ray units (linear accelerators and betatrons) have several devices in the treatment head that harden the beam, as well as change the distribution of the radiation within the field so that the dose across the patient is uniform. These devices assist in improving the uniformity of dose within the treatment volume while eliminating excessive dose in areas where tissue sparing is desirable.

Types of photon interactions

The exact mechanisms of the interactions of photons with the atoms of the irradiated medium are known to a large extent from the work done in the late 19th and early 20th centuries by Thomson, Einstein, Compton, Rutherford, and many others. There are five basic mechanisms that occur in the energy range of concern in radiation therapy:

- Thomson (coherent) scattering
- Photoelectric scattering
- Compton (incoherent) scattering
- Pair production
- Photodisintegration

Thomson (coherent) scattering. In Thompson scattering the incident photon is of very low energy, not quite energetic enough to ionize the atom. The photon, coming into the region close to the atom, is absorbed, but since not enough energy is present to cause the release of any electrons, the atom re-emits a second photon of exactly the same energy as the incident photon, but headed in a new direction. So, from the outside, it appears that the photon bounced off of the atom into another direction. In this case, no damage is done to the atom, so this interaction has no biological effect. The interaction is called "coherent" because the wavelength and energy of the emitted photon are identical to those of the incident photon, a condition known in physics as "coherency."

Photoelectric scattering. The photoelectric effect was first described in detail by Einstein, who was awarded the Nobel Prize in physics for the discovery—his other theories were believed to be too controversial and far-out for serious consideration (at the time). This interaction occurs exclusively at low photon energies (≤ 1 MeV) and so is more common in diagnostic radiology than in radiation therapy.

In a photoelectric interaction (see Fig. 2-6), the incident photon interacts with an electron in the inner shells of the atom—usually the K or L shell. By adding energy to this shell, the electron binding energy is overcome, and an electron from the involved shell is ejected from the atom with an energy equal to:

$$E_{electron} = E_{photon} - E_{binding}$$

where $E_{electron}$ is the kinetic energy of the electron leaving the atom (related to its mass and speed), E_{photon} is the energy of the incident photon, and $E_{binding}$ is binding energy of the involved electron shell. After ejection of the electron, there is a "hole" in the electron shell, which is then filled by outer shell electrons "falling" into it, losing energy in the process. The energy lost by these outer shell electrons usually appears as low energy x-rays, called characteristic radiation.[1-4]

Whenever characteristic radiation is produced, there is a possibility that the characteristic x-ray photon may be absorbed by an orbital electron rather than leaving the atom. The electron, now having an excess of energy, will be ejected from the atom in place of the photon. An electron that leaves the atom in this manner is called an Auger electron (pronounced "O-zhey") and is capable of causing biological damage on its own.

Compton (incoherent) scattering. Compton scattering is the most common photon interaction that occurs in the energy range used in radiation therapy.[4] In a Compton interaction, as shown in Fig. 2-7, the incident photon interacts with an outer shell electron, that is, one very loosely bound to the atom (sometimes called a "free" electron). The atom absorbs all of the photon's energy, and the electron is ejected from the outer shell. But the electron does not carry away all of the remaining energy; instead, a second photon is emitted, which carries off a portion of the leftover energy. This secondary photon has a different energy and wavelength than the incident photon, and this interaction is called "incoherent."

The secondary electron and secondary photon travel away from the atom at different angles, which can be calculated using several complex equations relating the angles and energies of the particles involved both before and after the interaction takes place. Although the mathematics of this situation are complex, a few examples can show the effect of angle on the results of a Compton interaction.

- *Direct hit on the target atom.* If the incident photon makes a "direct hit" on the atom, the electron will go straight forward (in the same direction the incident photon was traveling) and carry away most of the energy, whereas the secondary photon will travel backward from the atom and carry away a minimum of energy. This effect is called backscatter. At high photon energies (like those from a typical therapy accelerator), the energy of the secondary photon approaches a maximum value of 0.255 MeV, and the number of photons that scatter directly back is very small.

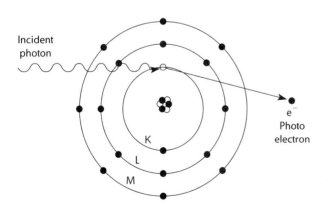

Fig. 2-6 In the photoelectric effect, the incident photon is totally absorbed and transfers all of its energy to the resultant photoelectron. (From Bernier DR, Christian PE, Langan JK, editors: *Nuclear medicine: technology and techniques*, ed 3. St Louis, 1994, Mosby.)

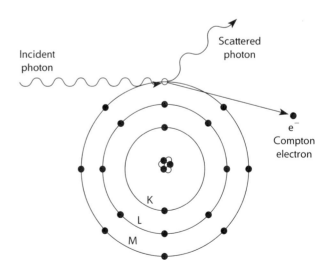

Fig. 2-7 Compton scattering occurs in outer electron shells. The atom is left ionized. (From Bernier DR, Christian PE, Langan JK, editors: *Nuclear medicine: technology and techniques*, ed 3. St Louis, 1994, Mosby.)

- *Grazing hit on the target atom.* A "grazing" hit on the atom by the incident photon will cause very little energy loss; most of the energy will be carried away by the secondary photon, which as a result will have nearly the same energy as the incident photon.
- *90-degree scatter.* It is important for radiation protection purposes to look at what takes place when the secondary photon emerges at an angle 90° to the incident photon. It turns out that the energy of this photon reaches a maximum value of 0.511 MeV and is essentially independent of the energy of the incident photon, even at very high photon energies.

Pair production. Pair production interactions occur at high energies; in fact, they are physically impossible below an energy of 1.022 MeV for the incoming photon.[1-4] In the pair production interaction (shown in Fig. 2-8) the incident photon passes close to the nucleus of the atom. When the photon interacts with the electromagnetic field of the nucleus, it is absorbed, and instantly the energy is re-emitted as an electron/positron pair (ß⁻, ß⁺), which then is ejected from the atom. If you use Einstein's equation $E = mc^2$, letting m equal the mass of an electron, you can calculate that the rest energy of an electron or positron, that is, the energy needed to "create" one during an interaction, is equal to 0.511 MeV. Since two such particles are created, this explains why you must have at least two times that energy, or 1.022 MeV, for pair production interaction to occur. Whatever energy is left over after the 1.022 MeV has been used is divided between the electron and positron.

The electron created usually begins to interact with other atoms outside of the original atom, until it loses its excess energy and is absorbed. The positron, however, suffers a more interesting fate. When it has undergone several interactions and is moving somewhat more slowly than when it left the atom where the pair production interaction took place, it

will collide with a free electron, creating an annihilation reaction. The positron is called an "antimatter" version of the electron, and when the two meet, both are destroyed, with the energy of the two being emitted as two photons of 0.511 MeV each, traveling at 180° to each other (i.e., in opposite directions). Thus, following a pair production interaction, two photons as well as the electron/positron pair will be available for further interactions.

Photodisintegration. A photodisintegration reaction is one in which the photon strikes the nucleus of the target atom directly and is absorbed. The sudden absorption of this energy causes the nucleus to emit both neutrons and γ-rays in an attempt to maintain stability. This interaction occurs mainly in high Z materials and at usually higher energies ($\approx$ 7 MeV), depending on the material. Thus it is a very unimportant interaction in tissue, where the Z_{eff} is approximately 7.42 (in other words, very low Z). However, it is extremely important when working with high energy medical accelerators, those with photon or electron beam energies of 10 MeV or greater. Because of the high energies of these beams, combined with the massive amounts of high Z materials like lead and tungsten in the beam production systems of these accelerators, a substantial neutron hazard to patients or personnel can occur. If you look at the inside of the treatment head of a high energy linear accelerator, you will probably see some neutron shielding in the form of a borated plastic that slows down ("moderates") the neutrons so that they can be captured.

Effects of combined interactions. When a radiation beam interacts with a medium, no single type of photon interaction occurs; instead, the result is usually a combination of two or more of the previous interactions. The factor μ, discussed earlier, actually represents the combined effects of all of the previous interactions for a given energy and material:

$$\mu = \sigma_{coh} + \tau + \sigma_{inc} + \pi + \Pi$$

where σ_{coh} represents Thomson ("coherent") scattering; τ, photoelectric interactions; σ_{inc} the Compton ("incoherent") interactions; π, the pair production interactions; and Π, the photodisintegration and other high energy reactions that we did not study here. Each of these symbols represents a probability that the photon, when it interacts with the medium, will undergo that type of reaction; μ describes the total probability of an interaction. Table 2-5 shows the relative importance of the three interactions of greatest concern in radiation therapy physics: the photoelectric, Compton, and pair production interactions.

As you can see from the table, at low energies the majority of the photon interactions taking place are photoelectric (τ) interactions. But as energy increases, the Compton (σ_{inc}) interaction quickly takes precedence and is itself slowly replaced by the pair production (π) and other interactions as the energy continues to increase. Most radiation therapy energies fall into the range of 1 to 5 MeV, where Compton predominates. You can also see this trend in Table 2-4, especially for lead; the values of μ start at extremely high values,

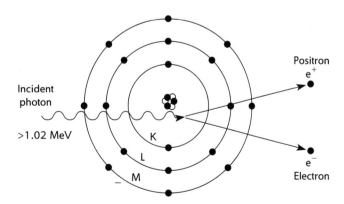

Fig. 2-8 In the pair production interaction the incident photon passes close to the nucleus of the atom and creates a positron/electron pair. The positron will undergo annihilation with another electron. (From Bernier DR, Christian PE, Langan JK, editors: *Nuclear medicine: technology and techniques*, ed 3. St Louis, 1994, Mosby.)

Table 2-5	Relative importance of photon interactions in water (the number of each type that occurs out of 100 photons)		
Photon Energy (MeV)	τ	σ_{inc}	π
0.010	95	5	0
0.026	50	50	0
0.060	7	93	0
0.150	0	100	0
4.000	0	94	6
10.00	0	77	23
24.00	0	50	50
100.0	0	16	84

drop to a minimum at energies around 4.0 MeV, then begin to climb again as the pair production interactions begin to produce more and more interactions as energy increases. You should keep this behavior of μ in mind when thinking about exponential attenuation problems.

PARTICLE INTERACTIONS

The interactions of particulate radiation with matter differ considerably from those of photons because of the different nature of particulate radiation. While photons have no mass and no electrical charge, particles do have mass, and most have some type of electrical charge as well. As a result, interactions between particles and atoms tend to resemble "billiard ball" interactions, familiar to us on an everyday level. In this section we will examine some of the interactions that take place in the cases of two major particle radiations used in radiation therapy: electrons and neutrons.

Elastic and inelastic collisions

The collisions of particle radiations can be likened to the collisions between large scale objects such as billiard balls. Each ball can be described as possessing kinetic energy, that is, energy caused by its motion through space. When the balls collide, their directions and speeds will change depending on the conditions of the collision, and thus each ball may lose or gain kinetic energy; the total kinetic energy, however, may or may not remain the same before and after the collision. If no kinetic energy is lost to the system in the collision, the collision is elastic; if energy is lost from the system, the collision is inelastic.

Two balls with kinetic energies equal to 10 joules each collide. After the collision, one ball has a kinetic energy of 15 joules, while the other has a kinetic energy of 5 joules. Since the total energy in the system has not changed (20 joules = 20 joules), the collision was elastic.

If, in the same example, the energies of the two balls after the collision had been measured as 12 joules and 6 joules, this would have been an inelastic collision, since energy was lost during the collision (20 joules > 18 joules). The remaining two joules of energy were converted into other forms of energy, such as vibrational energy or heat.

Note that, whether or not kinetic energy is conserved, the total energy of the system (which includes all other forms of energy such as heat) must remain the same. In the second example, the two joules of kinetic energy lost to the billiard balls did not "disappear" but rather were converted into another form of energy. This concept is called the principle of conservation of energy and is one of the basic concepts of physics and chemistry.

The interactions between atoms and particle radiations can be classified in the same manner. If the total kinetic energies of the particle and atom are the same after the interaction, then an elastic collision has taken place; if not, the collision was inelastic. We will look at how these definitions apply in the cases of electron and neutron radiations.

Electron interactions

Electron-electron interactions. When electrons in a medium interact with the electrons in the electron shells of the atoms in the medium, they give up energy to those electrons and are then deflected away from the atom in a new direction. Since they have given up energy to the atomic electron, the original electron is now moving more slowly (and therefore has less kinetic energy). The target electron, in the atomic orbit, may be "kicked up" to a shell farther from the nucleus (call excitation) or may be ejected completely from the atom (ionization) if the energy gained from the incident electron is high enough. Remember that a "collision" between two particles does not necessarily mean that actual physical contact between the particles has occurred; a collision can also result if the electromagnetic fields of the two particles come close enough to interact with each other, a distance that may be several times larger than the physical size of the particle itself.

Recall from our study of the Compton interaction that outer shell electrons are considered "free" electrons because their binding energies are very low compared to the energy of the incoming photons. If one of these "free" electrons is involved in the electron-electron interaction just described, the binding energy of the target electron is so small that it may be ignored; therefore the energy before the collision (incident electron plus target electron), in this case, can be considered elastic. If, however, the interaction involved an electron in a shell close to the nucleus, the binding energy must be taken into account. In this case, because of the principle of conservation of energy already discussed, some of the energy of the original electron will be "lost" to overcome the binding energy of the target electron before the target electron can change shell or leave the atom, making this an inelastic collision.

When the electron's energy is finally depleted by a series of collisions, it is captured by an atom in the vicinity, exhausted but satisfied.

Elastic electron-nuclei collisions. In materials heavier than hydrogen (Z = 1), electrons with certain energies are more likely to undergo elastic scattering with the nuclei of atoms than with the atomic electrons. Like an electron-electron elastic collision (already described), the incident electrons lose a small amount of energy to the nucleus of the atom and bounce away with reduced energy. Since the nuclei are so much larger than electrons, the electron will retain a larger percentage of its energy than if it had collided with an electron and is more likely to bounce straight backward from the atom after the collision. This effect diminishes quickly as the energy of the incident electrons is increased, and, at energies in the range usually used in radiation therapy (4 to 25 MeV), the electrons interact mainly by electron-electron scattering (above) or inelastic nuclear scattering (below).

Inelastic electron-nuclei collisions. High energy electrons can pass close to the nucleus of a target atom, as seen in Fig. 2-9, and be so strongly attracted by the charges in the nucleus that they will slow down, losing some of their kinetic energy; this energy will be emitted from the atom as a photon with energy (hυ) equal to the energy lost by the electron when it slowed down.[1] This process is called **bremsstrahlung** (German, "braking radiation") and is the most important method of producing x-ray beams in therapy units.

The photon created in the bremsstrahlung process can be of any energy from 0 up to the energy of the incident electron and can emerge from the atom in any direction. Thus, like ß decay, bremsstrahlung produces not a single energy x-ray but rather a spectrum of x-ray energies ranging from 0 to the energy of the incident electron beam. The average energy of the bremsstrahlung spectrum will be about a third of the maximum possible energy (E^{max}).

When the electron beam is in the lower energy range used in therapy (50 to 300 keV), the photons are emitted in a wide range of angles. As the electron beam energy increases, the photons tend to be emitted closer to the direction of the incident electron, a phenomenon known as forward peaking of the photon beam. This effect is very important in the design and use of high energy photon machines such as linear accelerators and betatrons, since at the high energies used in these machines, the bremsstrahlung photon beam is highly forward peaked.

Bremsstrahlung production is more likely in high Z materials such as lead or tungsten than in a low Z material like water or tissue. For this reason, high Z materials can be bombarded with a beam of high energy electrons to produce high energy photon beams in radiation therapy machines.

Neutron interactions

Basic mechanisms of neutron interactions. Neutrons are being studied as an alternative modality in some types of radiation therapy treatments. They can be obtained by bombarding some types of materials ($^3_1$H or Be) with heavy particles such as protons (p+) or deuterons ($^2_1$H) or from an isotope of the high Z element californium (^{252}Cf), which emits neutrons spontaneously when it undergoes radioactive decay.

For neutron energies below about 20 MeV, neutron interactions are primarily of the elastic type discussed previously; since neutrons have no electrical charge, they will not interact by electrical repulsion or attraction. In this type of elastic interaction the maximum energy transfer from the incident particles to the target nucleus occurs if they have identical masses. Neutrons and protons have nearly the same mass, therefore, if the incident atom has one proton in its nucleus (i.e., hydrogen), this interaction will transfer nearly the maximum possible amount of energy from the neutron to the medium. Since there is a large amount of hydrogen in tissue (in water and organic molecules), this interaction accounts for the bulk of energy transfer in tissue for therapeutic energy neutrons. Like electrons, if the neutron has energy remaining after this collision, it will bounce off of the atom into a new direction and interact again, finally being absorbed by the medium. This process of continual slowing down that takes place in a neutron beam is called moderation of the beam; so you may have materials that have a high hydrogen content are referred to as "moderators." The final absorption of the neutron usually excites the nucleus of the atom that absorbed the neutron, frequently causing it to emit energy in the form of gamma rays.

For higher energy neutrons, or neutrons incident on a high Z material, inelastic scattering is more likely. The colliding neutron gives up its energy to the nucleus, then bounces away. The excited nucleus will frequently give off protons or perhaps even heavier particles such as α particles, which possess very high linear energy transfers (LETs).

Neutrons, since they have no electrical charge of their own, are called indirectly ionizing radiations; they themselves do not create ionizations, but their interactions release particles that cause ionizations. Photons ionize in the same fashion—by the release of electrons or heavier particles and not by their own direct action. Charged particles, such as electrons, α particles, protons, or heavier nuclei that have been stripped of their orbital electrons, do the actual work of ionization and tissue damage.

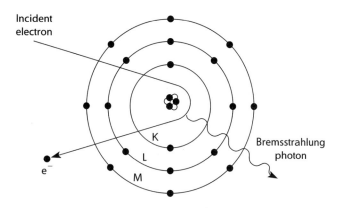

Fig. 2-9 Deceleration of charged particle passing near nucleus results in release of energy in the form of bremsstrahlung radiation. (From Bernier DR, Christian PE, Langan JK, editors: *Nuclear medicine: technology and techniques*, ed 3. St Louis, 1994, Mosby.)

As we saw earlier, a large number of unstable, radioactive atoms exist in nature. In the late 1940s and 1950s, after the development of nuclear reactors, another source of radioactive isotopes became available—the production of artificial isotopes by a process called **neutron activation**. Using this process, normally stable atoms can be converted into radioactive isotopes, some of which have found use in medicine and industry.[2-4]

Neutron activation can occur when a neutron is absorbed by the nucleus of a stable atom. By adding this additional neutron to its nucleus, the A of the atom increases by 1. This moves it from its previous position on the nuclear stability curve and adds more energy to the nucleus because of the increase in mass. Frequently the new isotope is radioactive; in some cases, two or more neutrons must be absorbed before a radioisotope is produced.

Not all stable nuclei can be readily activated by exposure to a neutron beam. If you imagine the neutron-nucleus interaction as a bullet hitting a target, then the probability of this interaction occurring can be related to the "size" of the target presented to the neutron. The larger the target size, the more likely it is that a neutron will hit the target and be absorbed by the nucleus. In fact, this is exactly how nuclear physicists describe the probability of a neutron activation—by expressing the "target size" of an atom as seen by the neutron. This quantity, called a neutron cross section, is measured in terms of square centimeters. However, given the size of atoms, you can see that the cross section will be a very small area. (The cross section is not the same thing as the physical area of the atom—the neutron does not actually have to touch the nucleus to be absorbed but must come close to the vicinity of the nucleus before the nuclear forces can capture the neutron.) To express this small area more conveniently, cross sections are expressed in units of barns, where:

$$1 \text{ barn} = 10^{-24} \text{ cm}^2$$

The name of the unit, of course, is a reference to the expression "hit the broad side of a barn." Subunits of the barn continue this whimsical nomenclature (humor is relatively rare in nuclear physics), with names like "shed" (1 millibarn) and "outhouse" (1 microbarn).

The cross section of an atom for neutron activation depends on the A of the atom as well as on the energy of the neutrons. Very low energy neutrons, like thermal neutrons (energy 0.025 eV), may be more easily captured than fast neutrons (energy above 1 MeV). The activity that can be produced by placing a sample into a neutron beam can be calculated by:

$$\text{Activity} = \Delta A = \lambda N \sigma \phi \Delta \tau$$

where λ is the decay constant of the new radioactive isotope, N is the number of nonradioactive target atoms originally present in the sample, σ is the cross section of the target atoms for that neutron energy, ϕ is the intensity of the neutron beam (neutrons per square centimeter per second), and $\Delta \tau$ is the time the sample is left in the neutron beam. Although we will not be using this equation for problem solving purposes, you should note that the amount of radiation produced in a neutron beam depends on all of the above factors, so it is necessary to ensure, when making radioisotopes, that all of these factors are optimized for the activation in question.

The activation of ^{60}Co from natural cobalt metal can be accomplished using a thermal neutron flux:

$$^{59}_{27}\text{Co} + ^{1}_{0}\text{n} \rightarrow ^{60}_{27}\text{Co} + \lambda$$

A number of other radioisotopes used in radiation therapy are obtained from neutron activation of other atomic species, including ^{198}Au, ^{192}Ir, and ^{125}I. Whereas ^{60}Co is normally used in external beam therapy, these other isotopes are used in brachytherapy (implant) applications.

SUMMARY

To understand the discipline of radiation physics, one must be familiar with the developments, theories, and technological advances that have taken place since Roentgen discovered the x-ray in 1895. From the Curies who defined the activity of 1 g of radium (^{226}Ra), to Bohr's attempt to explain the atom, to Einstein's Nobel Prize, the area of physics has grown and developed. Using the work of those who have come before us, we are able to understand why an x-ray image taken with photons in the kilovoltage range is superior to one taken with photons in the megavoltage range. The knowledge of the interactions of subatomic particles is critical to understanding these issues.

The inverse square law, linear attenuation, half-life, and exponential decay are a few of the concepts, terms, and tools needed to begin understanding the discipline of radiation physics. It has been the objective of this chapter to provide an understanding of these issues and concepts. It is our hope that after review and study, you will have a solid foundation on which to build.

Review Questions

Multiple Choice

1. How many seconds are there in 2.54 minutes?
   a. 174.0
   b. 114.0
   c. 152.4
   d. 92.4
   e. 254

2. Calculate the wavelength of an electromagnetic wave that has a frequency of 3.95×1014 Hz.
   a. 1.32×10^6 m
   b. 13.2×10^6 m
   c. 7.59×10^{-8} m
   d. 7.59×10^{-7} m
   e. 7.59×10^{-6} m

3. An FM radio station broadcasts at 102.0 MHz on your radio dial. What is the wavelength of the station's signal?
   a. 34.0 m
   b. 3.40 m
   c. 2.941 m
   d. 2.941×10^6 m
   e. 29.41 m

4. An electromagnetic wave has a frequency of 2.1×10^{21} Hz. What is the energy of the wave?
   a. 3.355×10^{54} eV
   b. 1.39×10^{12} eV
   c. 5.060×10^{35} eV
   d. 8.250 MeV
   e. 8.715 MeV

5. If an electromagnetic wave has an energy of 6 MeV, what would its wavelength be?
   a. 50 m
   b. 3.313×10^{-32} m
   c. 2.075×10^{-13} m
   d. 2.075×10^{-12} m
   e. 2.075×10^{-7} m

6. A sample of an isotope has a half-life of 74 days and is measured to have an activity of 8.675 Ci at noon of that day. What will the activity of the isotope be 94 days later at 6 PM?
   a. 4.338 Ci
   b. 3.588 Ci
   c. 3.596 Ci
   d. 5.034 Ci
   e. 2.37 Ci

7. The intensity of a radioactive beam is measured at a distance of 100 cm and found to be 250 mR/min. What will the intensity of this beam be at 105 cm?
   a. 226.8 mR/min
   b. 238.1 mR/min
   c. 205.7 mR/min
   d. 275.6 mR/min
   e. 262.5 mR/min

8. A 6 MV photon beam is incident on a lead sheet 1.5 cm thick. If the initial dose rate of the beam is 300 cGy/min, what will the dose rate be after passing through the lead sheet if the linear attenuation coefficient for this beam in lead is 0.4911 cm^{-1}?
   a. 79.0 cGy/min
   b. 183.6 cGy/min
   c. 147.33 cGy/min
   d. 143.6 cGy/min
   e. 221.0 cGy/min

9. What is the HVL of the beam in the previous question?
   a. 2.72 cm
   b. 4.07 cm
   c. 0.941 cm
   d. 1.386 cm
   e. 1.411 cm

10. In the problem given in question 8, what minimal thickness of lead is needed to reduce the dose rate to less than 9 cGy/min?
    a. 2 cm
    b. 10 cm
    c. 100 cm
    d. 7.0 cm
    e. 7.5 cm

Questions to Ponder

1. A shielding concern for a high energy linear accelerator, one whose energy is greater than 10 MV, is the presence of neutrons. Where do these neutrons come from and by what process or interaction are they formed?
2. A portal radiograph (port film) is taken with a high energy photon beam (MV range). Why is the radiograph inferior in diagnostic quality when compared to a radiograph taken on a simulator (keV range)?
3. Explain the difference between the tenth value layer (TVL) of a material and its linear attenuation coefficient.
4. Explain the reason for using lead as a shielding material for x-ray rooms and/or vaults.
5. Explain the concept of the exponential decay constant and how it relates to half-life.

REFERENCES

1. Bernier DR, Christian PE, Langan JK, editors: *Nuclear medicine: technology and techniques*, ed 3. St Louis, 1994, Mosby.
2. Hendee WR, Ritenour R: *Medical imaging physics*, ed 3. St Louis, 1992, Mosby.
3. Johns HE, Cunningham JR: *The physics of radiology*, ed 4. Springfield, IL, 1983, Charles C Thomas.
4. Khan FM: *The physics of radiation therapy*, ed 2. Baltimore, 1992, Williams & Wilkins.

Aspects of Brachytherapy

Charles M. Washington

Outline

Key terms

HISTORICAL OVERVIEW AND PERSPECTIVE

The discovery of x-rays by Roentgen in the late 19th century has proved, more than any other innovation, to have a dramatic impact on modern medicine. Shortly after the discovery of x-rays, Henri Becquerel and Pierre Curie began investigating the existence of similar rays produced by known fluorescent materials. Curie, in his experimentation, deliberately produced an ulcer on his arm and described in detail the various phases of a moist epidermitis and his recovery from it.[1] At that point he gave a small radium tube to a colleague and suggested he insert it into a tumor. Subsequently, several physicians began investigating the effects of these rays on malignant tumors, and the therapeutic use of ionizing radiation began.

The term **brachytherapy** refers to radiation therapy that involves the application of radioactive material directly into or immediately adjacent to the tumor, rather than through external beams. *Brachy*, meaning short, implies therapy at a short distance. Today, brachytherapy is a standard technique in the treatment of a large number of malignancies, including uterus and uterine cervix, prostate, and breast. Brachytherapy use in cancer therapy is increasing and is paralleled by the increasing desire for organ preservation and acceptable cosmetic results. In current oncologic practice there are many opportunities for dosimetrist and radiation therapist involvement in the practical application of brachytherapy. The scopes of practice for the dosimetrist and radiation therapist identify the need for critical thinking skills that involve the application of radiation through these means.

The major advantage of brachytherapy is that very high doses of radiation can be delivered locally to the tumor in a relatively short time, while very low doses are delivered in the surrounding tissue.[1] As the distance around the source of radiation increases, there is a dramatic reduction of dose absorbed in tissue. This adheres directly to the premise that in radiation therapy, homogeneous tumoricidal doses must be deposited in the tumor while sparing as much normal tissue as possible. Brachytherapy is commonly used to supplement the dose administered by external beam irradiation; this allows additional doses to be delivered to a well-defined volume of tumor tissue. Since the radiation administered in this way does not penetrate through overlying tissues to reach this volume, surrounding tissues are spared from increased doses of radiation.

Brachytherapy can be administered through several types of applications. **Interstitial brachytherapy** is characterized by the placement of radioactive sources directly into a tumor or tumor bed. Rigid needles or flexible tubes may be used in the actual placement of the sources (Fig. 3-1). Interstitial brachytherapy is commonly used in the treatment of neck, breast, soft tissue sarcomas, and skin tumors. Intracavitary brachytherapy places radioactive sources within a body cavity for treatment. This type of brachytherapy has been the mainstay in the treatment of cervical cancer for over 50 years.[3] Closely associated with interstitial brachytherapy, **intraluminal brachytherapy** places sources of radiation within body tubes such as the esophagus, uterus, trachea, bronchus, and rectum. **Topical brachytherapy** places the radioactive sources on top of the area to be treated. Molds of the body part treated may be taken and prepared to place the sources in definite arrangements to deliver the prescribed dose.

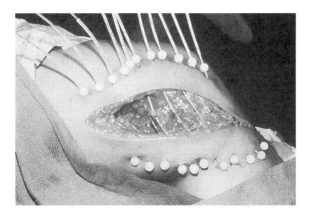

Fig. 3-1 Example of interstitial catheters placed along a tumor bed of an extremity. Sources placed inside of the catheters will deliver a high dose of radiation to the tumor bed and immediate surrounding area.

SPECIFICATION OF SOURCE STRENGTH

Source strength specification plays three roles in brachytherapy. The first is to provide a commonly accepted standard means of describing quantities of emitted radiation. The second allows practitioners to form a basis for *computational dosimetry*, which is the calculation of dose with the aid of a computerized system. Third, source strength specification serves as a prescription parameter in brachytherapy.

The historical term used to describe activity in terms of number of disintegrations per unit time is the curie (Ci). The curie is 3.7×10^{10} disintegrations per second from 1 gram of radium. The Système Internationale (SI) unit of activity is the becquerel (Bq). One becquerel equals one disintegration per second. Although the becquerel is the unit recommended for use, the curie is still commonly used in practice. Table 3-1 reviews the conversions commonly used.

Radioactive decay

The key relationship in understanding radioactivity, which is a statistical process, is as follows:

$$\frac{\Delta N}{\Delta t} \propto N$$

where N is the number of atoms and t is the time. The change in the number of atoms per change in unit time is proportional to the number of atoms present. This proportion can be made into an equation by the addition of a constant, λ, called the **decay constant**.

$$\frac{\Delta N}{\Delta t} = {}^-\lambda N$$

The negative sign is added because there are fewer atoms present after a given amount of time. The equation can be rearranged to solve for the gamma constant, as follows:

$$\lambda = {}^- \frac{\frac{\Delta N}{N}}{\Delta t}$$

Therefore the decay constant can be expressed as the total number of atoms that decay per unit time. From this are developed the definition of activity and the formula for exponential decay.

Table 3-1	Commonly used conversions relating curies to becquerels
Unit	**Definition**
1 curie (Ci)	3.7×10^{10} disintegrations/sec
1 millicurie (mCi)	3.7×10^{7} disintegrations/sec
1 microcurie (µCi)	3.7×10^{4} disintegrations/sec
1 becquerel (Bq)	1 disintegration/sec
1 megabecquerel (MBq)	1×10^{6} disintegrations/sec
1 mCi	37 MBq
1 gigabecquerel (GBq)	1×10^{9} disintegrations/sec
1 Ci	37 GBq

Activity. Activity (A) is the rate of decay of a radioactive material or the change in the number of atoms in a certain amount of time and can be written as follows:

$$A = \frac{\Delta N}{\Delta t} = {}^-\lambda N$$

The activity is directly proportional to the decay constant. So, as the decay constant increases, the activity increases.

The preceding equation can also be rearranged and integrated to yield the exponential decay equation, as follows:

$$N = N_0 e^{-\lambda t}$$

A (activity) can be substituted for N (the number of atoms) to yield the following:

$$A = A_0 e^{-\lambda t}$$

This formula, as presented in Chapter 2, is commonly used to calculate activity of a radioisotope after some length of time has passed.

Half-life. The concept used to deal with the isotope disintegration is half-life. The **half-life** is the time period in which the activity decays to one half the original value. It is the essential value to employ the decay formula for a particular isotope. Half-life ($T_{1/2}$) is related to the decay constant by the following formula:

$$T_{1/2} = \frac{0.693}{\lambda}$$

The relationship between activity and half-life is given by the following formula:

$$A = \lambda N = \frac{0.693}{T_{1/2}}$$

The relationship between half-life and activity is inversely proportional. In other words, as half-life increases, overall activity decreases.

Decay formula. These mathematical expressions can be grouped together and allow the radiation therapist and dosimetrist to derive a formula that will predict radionuclide decay. This is called the *decay formula*, which is expressed by the following:

$$A = A_0 e^{-\left(\frac{0.693}{T_{1/2}}\right)t}$$

The originally known activity is denoted by A_0, A is the current activity, $T_{1/2}$ is the half-life, and t is the length of time passed since time of originally known activity. Table 3-2 lists isotopes commonly used in radiation therapy with their half-lives. The half-life will vary somewhat from different literature sources and from past to present, but these are fairly representative of what is in common use today. A good way to remember these concepts is to put them into practical use. It is important to make sure that the units used throughout the problem are consistent.

Example 1: Every year a new decayed value must be determined for clinical use of the cesium 137 tubes. The decay is always calculated from the original assayed value obtained when the source was received. One source was

Table 3-2	Commonly used isotopes
Isotope	**$T_{1/2}$**
Radium 226	1622 years
Cobalt 60	5.26 years
Cesium137	30.0 years
Iridium 192	74.1 days
Iodine 125	60.2 days
Gold 198	2.7 days
Radon 222	3.82 days
Copper 64	12.8 hours

received on September 3, 1995; that value was determined to be 69.5 mCi. What would be the activity for this source 365 days later?

$$A = A_0 \times e^{-\left(\frac{0.693}{T_{1/2}}\right) \times t}$$

$$A = A_0 \times e^{-\left(\frac{0.693}{30\ yr}\right) \times 1\ yr}$$

$$A = 67.91\ mCi$$

Mean life. Another concept related to half-life is mean life, which is complicated in explanation, but useful and easy in calculation. **Mean life** is the average lifetime for the decay of radioactive atoms. It is the time period for a hypothetical source that decays at a constant rate equal to its initial activity to produce the same number of disintegrations as the exponentially decaying source that decays for an infinite period of time. It is primarily applicable to dose calculations in permanent implants, typically gold 198 and iodine 125. Theoretically, all the dose is delivered over a very long time period because all the activity is not decayed away until the last unstable atom disintegrates. The treatment planning team needs a practical means of calculating a final dose. The relationship between mean life and half-life is as follows:

$$\text{Mean life} = T_{1/2} \times 1.44$$

Example 2: 106 mCi of gold 198 is implanted into a pelvic mass. Determine the emitted radiation.

$$\text{Mean life of gold 198} = 1.44 \times (2.7\ days) = 3.89\ days$$

$$\text{Emitted radiation} = 106\ mCi \times 3.89\ days = 412.34\ mCi\text{-days}$$

Average energy (E_{ave}). Another property of interest in isotope usage is the average energy of the emitted photons. This is derived from the decay schemes of each isotope. Any beta emission has already been eliminated by filtrating encapsulations, since radiation treatment is not accomplished with beta particles. Table 3-3 illustrates a list of the average energy for isotopes commonly used in brachytherapy.

Table 3-3	Average energy of isotopes used in brachytherapy	
Isotope	**E_{ave} (MeV)**	
Radium 226	0.83	
Cobalt 60	1.25	
Cesium 137	0.662	
Iridium 192	0.38	
Iodine 125	0.03	
Gold 198	0.41	
Radon 222	0.83	

RADIOACTIVE SOURCES USED IN BRACHYTHERAPY

Brachytherapy most commonly uses sealed radioactive sources within or adjacent to a tumor volume. A sealed source is one in which the radioactive material is encapsulated by welded ends. Typically the isotope is encased within metal casings that serve two main functions: preventing escape of radioactivity and absorption of beta particles. Fig. 3-2 demonstrates a sealed source. The International Organization of Standardization (ISO) classifies sealed sources based on safety requirements. They also specify leak test methods, such as wipe tests, for sealed sources to be carried out at both the manufacturer and user levels.[12]

Most brachytherapy procedures were developed using radium 226, the first radioisotope to be isolated and identified.[9] Other isotopes came into use when nuclear reactor–produced isotopes became readily available. Most of the isotopes used in radiation therapy today have their dosimetry based on the original radium work and are referred to as radium substitutes. These substitutes offer several advantages over radium. Both radium and radium substitutes will be described later in the chapter.

Radium

Radium ($^{226}_{88}$Ra) decays mainly by alpha emission and is part of a long decay chain that begins with natural uranium ($^{238}_{92}$U) and concludes in an isotope of stable lead ($^{206}_{82}$Pb). The half-life for radium is about 1622 years. As part of the process, radium decays to form radon, a heavy inert gas that further decays down to the stable lead atom. Radon gas has caused concern during home construction from the Midwest to the Eastern Seaboard. As ore deposits decay, the radioactive gas seeps up into the basements of the homes, causing serious health concerns.

Use of radium is very practical because it has a very high specific activity. **Specific activity** is defined as the activity per unit mass of a radioactive material (Ci/g). The specific activity dictates the total activity that a small source can have. Even though some radionuclides might have some particular advantage for implantation, they may not be suitable because a small size and high activity may not be possible for

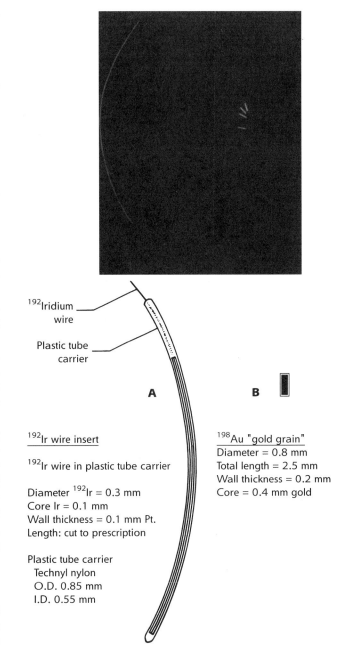

Fig. 3-2 Two isotopes used for interstitial irradiation. **A**, ^{192}Ir wire is thin, flexible, and can be tailored to any length. Its cross-section is excellent (750 barns). The half-life is acceptable for treatment times of 2 to 8 days. ^{192}Ir is the most practical isotope for afterloading removable implants. For safe and easier manipulation, iridium wire is mounted inside a nylon or Teflon tube carrier. (Iridium seed chains in Teflon may also be used, but intensity per seed is higher.) *O.D.*, outer diameter. *I.D.*, inner diameter. **B**, ^{198}Au seeds ("gold grains") are small and, therefore, can be inserted in thin mucosa overlying bone and narrow spaces. Although they are used for permanent implants, short half-life of gold allows it to deliver the most of the dose in the first 5 to 10 days. (From Levitt SH, Khan FM, and Potish RA: *Levitt and Tapley's technological basis of radiation therapy: practical clinical applications*, Baltimore, 1992, Williams and Wilkins.)

that particular isotope. The disadvantage of radium concerns itself mainly with radiation hazards.[9,12] Radiation is produced by alpha emission and produces a daughter, radon 222, a gas that can possibly leak from the encapsulated sources.

A typical radium source consists of a hollow needle or tube made of a metal such as platinum or stainless steel. Inside the tube, small capsules of radium salt are placed, giving the source a known activity. This activity, together with the thickness of the source capsule (known as the filtration), determines the dosimetric properties of the source and how it can be used in brachytherapy. Note that the area in which the radioactivity is packed is shorter than the total length of the source; the length of the area in which the radioactivity lies in the source is called the **active length** of the source and must be differentiated from the physical length, which is the total length of the source, end to end.[9,12]

The gamma (Γ) factor for radium 226 is 8.25 R · cm^2/mCi · hr, assuming a filtration of 0.5 mm of platinum. The filtration (shell thickness) of the radium source is very important, since the decay processes of radium 226 result in a large number of low energy x-rays, which are easily filtered by any additional filtration. In other words, as you increase the filtration of the radium 226 source, the Γ factor will decrease as you eliminate more and more low energy x-rays. If you have a radium 226 source with more or less than 0.5 mm platinum (Pt) filtration, the Γ factor from this source will change as follows: increase of 2% for each additional 0.1 mm of platinum added to 0.5 mm, and decrease of 2% for each 0.1 mm of platinum less than 0.5 mm.

Radium sources. The amount of radioactivity in a radium source is expressed in milligrams of radium. In the definition of a curie, it was initially the amount of activity of 1 gram of radium. Later, however, the definition of the curie was changed to exactly 3.7×10^{10} disintegrations/second, whereas $^{226}_{88}$Ra decays with about 3.66×10^{10} disintegrations/second. Despite this small discrepancy, in clinical situations it is assumed that 1 mg of radium has an activity of 1 mCi.

When brachytherapy was becoming a popular treatment method, the manufacturers of radium sources decided on a standard for specifying the ways in which radium can be distributed inside a needle source. A full strength source is defined as one that has 0.66 mg/cm of activity, and a half strength source has 0.33 mg/cm of activity.

Example 3: A full strength radium source has an active length of 3 cm. What is the activity of this source in milligrams?

$$A = (0.66 \text{ mg/cm}) (3.0 \text{ cm}) = 2.0 \text{ mg}$$

Sources that have the same concentration of radioactivity throughout their active length are called *uniform sources*. However, physicians have found that it is convenient to have available some sources with a nonuniform distribution of activity in them. Two other types of source have been developed: the *Indian club source*, which is heavily loaded with activity at one end, and the *dumbbell source*, which has heavy

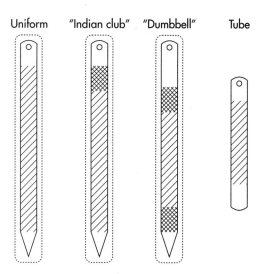

Fig. 3-3 Typical radium sources. Note the depiction of the active length and the physical length. (Redrawn with permission from Khan F: *The physics of radiation therapy*, ed. 2, Baltimore, 1992, Williams and Wilkins.)

loading at both ends, with lighter activity concentration in the middle.[9] These types of sources are all *needles*; that is, they are sharply pointed at one end and can be inserted directly into tumor tissue; the other end holds an eyelet to allow the source to be secured with sutures and easily removed (Fig. 3-3).

The use of needle sources presents several problems from medical and radiation safety viewpoints. Since they are stiff, they must be inserted into areas of the body thick enough to accept them without bending them. The possibility of breakage is always present. Also, the personnel loading the sources are continually exposed to radiation while performing the procedure, which is not in line with the recommended national policy of keeping medical radiation exposure to a minimum for both patients and staff. To avoid these problems, systems were developed to allow devices known as applicators to be inserted into the treatment area first, then loaded with radioactivity quickly and safely when the patient is back in his or her room. This technique, known as **afterloading**, led to the development of tube sources. These are small sources that are rounded on each end and contain larger amounts of activity than needle sources (up to 50 mg in a single source).

Some isotopes, such as radon 222 and gold 198, have very short half-lives and are implanted permanently rather than temporarily. Such sources are packaged in tiny versions of tube sources called seeds, which are usually about 3 to 5 mm long and the diameter of a pencil lead. These sources are implanted with a gunlike applicator that uses long needles to accurately position the seeds within the tumor during surgery. This type of therapy is used frequently in the case of prostate cancer, as well as other types of solid, localized tumors that can be reached surgically.

Radium substitutes

The term **radium substitute** is used to indicate any isotope used for brachytherapy whose dosimetry is based on the original radium work. These include but are not limited to the following: cesium 137, iridium 192, gold 198, and iodine 125. The activities of these isotopes are expressed in millicuries. However, when these isotopes were first introduced, an attempt to correlate the effect of these isotopes with that of radium was made, since all clinical experience up to that time involved the use of radium. A unit was developed, called *radium equivalence*, which is defined as follows:

$$mg\ Ra\ eq = \left(A_{isotope},\ mCi\right)\left(\frac{\Gamma_{isotope}}{\Gamma_{Ra}}\right)$$

where $A_{isotope}$ is the activity of the source in millicuries.

Example 4: What is the radium equivalence of a 25.0 mCi source of $^{137}_{55}Cs$?

$$mg\ Ra\ eq = (25.0\ mCi)\left(\frac{3.226}{8.25}\right) = 9.776\ mg\ Ra\ eq$$

Cesium 137. Cesium 137 ($^{137}_{55}Cs$) is one of the most widely used radium substitutes and has largely replaced radium as the primary isotope for brachytherapy of the uterus and cervix. It has a primary photon energy of 662 keV, which is comparable to the average photon energy of radium (830 keV). This means that the cesium photon penetrates tissue in about the same manner as radium. This makes the conversion from using radium to using cesium easier for radiation therapy practitioners.

Cesium has some positive advantages over radium. Although the average energy of radium is 830 keV, radium emits a spectrum of photon energies (0.047 to 2.45 MeV). Photon energies above 2 MeV result in a radiation safety hazard. The lower energy of cesium and the fact that it has no higher photon energy reduces the radiation safety hazard when using this isotope. This same fact makes storing the isotope less of a problem than with radium. Cesium has a half-life of 30.0 years, so sources can be used for a long time; they decay about 2% per year. Since cesium is produced in nuclear reactor fuel as a natural by-product of nuclear fission, it can be chemically separated from spent nuclear fuel and is therefore widely available. Several manufacturers can provide cesium sources in a wide variety of needle or tube configurations. These facts, plus the wide use of cesium in educational institutions, make $^{137}_{55}Cs$ very popular with hospital-based and privately owned radiation therapy practices.

Iridium 192. Iridium 192 ($^{192}_{77}Ir$) is supplied in the form of wires of iridium-platinum alloy or as small seeds of this alloy attached to nylon ribbons with a spacing of 1 cm between seeds. This radioisotope undergoes beta-decay and has an average energy of 370 keV. The wire form combines flexibility with strength along with filtration characteristics that absorb the beta particles released. The half-life of 74.2 days is shorter than that of cesium and so iridium is used for temporary implants of easily reached tumor sites such as the breast and tongue.[12]

The usual technique for iridium wire implants is to insert needles in the tissue that penetrate through the tumor area; alternatively, flexible plastic catheters can be looped through or around a tumor. Then the iridium wire or seed carrier is threaded into the catheter and left in place for a calculated amount of time. If needed, the wire or seed carrier can be cut to the proper length for insertion into the needles, an operation that requires great care to avoid spreading radioactivity around the work area or patient room. $^{192}_{77}Ir$ is ordered in batches every 2 months or so, and iridium whose activity is too low to use for treatment can be kept until it decays to a very low activity level, then returned to the manufacturer. Since $^{192}_{77}Ir$ is produced in a nuclear reactor, like cobalt, it can be reactivated for future use.

Cobalt 60. Cobalt 60 is a radionuclide that is not commonly used in brachytherapy applications. It undergoes a two-tiered beta decay after its neutron activation that produces 1.17 and 1.33 MeV gamma rays, averaging out to the commonly accepted 1.25 MeV. This radionuclide has a half-life of 5.26 years. Cobalt 60 has been typically used as an external beam radiation therapy source, but it has been used for ophthalmic applicators and, in some countries, in needles and tubes. It has also seen some application in high dose rate applications. The external beam design and use of cobalt are reviewed and described in Chapter 14 in volume I of this series.

Gold 198. Gold $^{198}_{79}Au$ is a popular replacement for $^{222}_{86}Rn$ in permanent implants. It has a very short half-life of 2.7 days and a monoenergetic (only one energy produced) energy of 412 keV. It is normally supplied in the form of cylindrical grains or seeds encapsulated in platinum.[6,12] Like cesium, the lower photon energy makes radiation safety much less of a problem with gold than with radon, and more of the dose is absorbed locally. Because of the short half-life, gold seeds are shipped with very high activities, and by the time they are ready to be used they have an activity in the range of 5 mCi/seed. Because of this, gold gives the tissue a very high dose in a short time, a method called high dose rate therapy. The prostate can benefit from interstitial implants with permanent gold seeds because other isotopes would require surgical procedures for both insertion and removal of sources.[12]

Iodine 125. The use of iodine 125 ($^{125}_{53}I$) is becoming more popular in interstitial seed implants. This radioisotope is produced as a daughter product from the neutron activation of xenon 124 to xenon 125. The activated xenon 125 decays by electron capture to produce the daughter, iodine 125. This isotope decays by electron capture to produce useful 35.5 keV gamma rays. Because of the low energy of the isotope, whose half-life is 60.2 days, shielding requirements are minimal. The dose is deposited very close to the seeds, reducing the dose to structures next to the tumor. In addition, the dose from $^{125}_{53}I$ is deposited over a longer period of time than the dose from $^{198}_{79}Au$, making iodine therapy a type of *low dose rate therapy*, which may cause a different biological reaction than the same dose from gold.[4,5,11] Education in the use of iodine 125 is an important part of any brachytherapy program using this isotope.

These last two isotopes mentioned are used as replacements for radon ($^{222}_{86}Rn$) in seed sources. $^{222}_{86}Rn$ is a radioactive gas, making its use very dangerous. If a seed breaks, the radioactivity becomes airborne and can be inhaled, doing great damage to the sensitive tissues of the lung. Because of this very real problem, radon seeds are no longer used.

EXPOSURE RATE FROM A RADIOACTIVE SOURCE

Calculation of absorbed dose from radioactive sources can be performed using any one of a number of methods, all of which are based on either calculation techniques or tables of measured data. A central component of the calculation techniques is the gamma factor (Γ factor), which can be defined as the exposure rate at 1 m from a radioactive source of known activity. The units of the Γ factor are as follows:

$$\frac{roentgen \cdot cm^2}{mCi \cdot hr}$$

The actual value of the Γ factor is different for each radioisotope; values for the radioisotopes most commonly used in radiation therapy are given in Table 3-4.

While the units of the Γ factor may seem complex, they actually make the Γ factor a very useful and easily manipulated quantity. For example, to calculate the exposure rate (roentgen/hr) at some distance from a radioactive source, the Γ factor can be used in the following equation:

$$\dot{X} = (\Gamma_{isotope})(A)(1/d)^2$$

where $\dot{X}$ is the exposure rate (recall that the dot over the X means "rate" in physics notation), d is the distance from the source to the point of calculation, and A is the activity of the source. Notice that if d is in centimeters and A is in millicuries, the units cancel neatly, leaving roentgens per hour, which is the exposure rate. An example should clarify this process.

Example 5: Calculate the exposure rate at 10 cm from a cesium 137 source with an activity of 10 mCi.

Given that the Γ factor of cesium = 3.226 roentgen $\cdot$ cm²/mCi $\cdot$ hr, d = 10 cm, and A = 10 mCi,

$$\dot{X} = (3.226 \text{ R} \cdot cm^2/mCi \cdot hr)(10 \text{ mCi})(1/10 \text{ cm})^2$$

$$\dot{X} = 0.3226 \text{ roentgen/hr} = 322.6 \text{ mR/hr}$$

Table 3-4	Gamma factors for radiation therapy isotopes	

Isotope	Γ factor $\left(\dfrac{roentgen \cdot cm^2}{mCi \cdot hr}\right)$
Radium 226	8.25
Radon 222	8.25
Cobalt 60	13.07
Cesium 137	3.226
Iridium 192	4.57
Iodine 125	1.089
Gold 198	2.327

By arranging the equation, you can find any of the four quantities included in the Γ factor if the other three are known. For example, if you know the total exposure, the distance from the source, and the activity of the source, the total time of exposure in hours can easily be calculated. Another typical use is to find the activity of a source by measuring the exposure rate at some distance and solving for the activity, as in Example 6.

Example 6: At 15 cm from an iridium 192 source, the exposure rate is 305 mR/hr (0.305 roentgen/hr). What is the activity of this source?

With a value of 4.57 roentgens $\cdot$ cm²/mCi $\cdot$ hr for Γ_{Ir}, solve for A.

$$0.305 \text{ roentgen/hr} = (4.57 \text{ roentgens} \cdot cm^2/mCi \cdot hr)(A)(1/15 \text{ cm})^2$$

$$A = \frac{(0.305 \text{ roentgen/hr})}{(4.57 \text{ roentgens} \cdot cm^2/mCi \cdot hr)(1/15 \text{ cm})^2}$$

$$A = 15.02 \text{ mCi}$$

An important limitation to the use of the Γ factor is that it is applicable only to a point source of radiation. A radioactive source can be considered a point source if the distance from the source to the calculation point is at least five times the length of the source. Therefore the size of the source will place a limitation on the distances at which the Γ factor can be applied.

BRACHYTHERAPY APPLICATORS AND INSTRUMENTS

Just as there are various sources of radioisotope that are used in radiation therapy, there are numerous methods of applying them in clinical practice. It has been apparent since the first uses of brachytherapy that applicator design is important in the maintenance of source positioning and radiation safety. As stated earlier, there are several generalized methods of brachytherapy application: external or mold, interstitial, and intracavitary.[9]

External applicators or molds

When a patient has a well-circumscribed surface lesion that requires a high localized dose, surface molds are commonly used.[1] External applicators usually are molded to fit snugly on the surface of the affected area, with areas specified for radioisotope placement. These molds can be designed to incorporate shielding for adjacent sensitive structures so that they do not receive as high a dose as the lesion. These molds can be designed to fit any shape. Sometimes impressions are made of the body part so that a detailed anatomical template with custom isotope pathways can be designed.

Eye plaques are also a means of using radioisotopes with external application. Iodine 125 is used in the management of uveal melanoma of the eye. Brachytherapy is employed in the management of this disease because of its ability to effectively treat tumors near the optic nerve and macula without causing loss of vision secondary to radiation-induced changes. The plaque carrier arranges the sources in appropriate positions so that adequate dose distributions are obtained (Fig. 3-4).

Areas commonly treated with external applicators include any areas on the skin, oral cavity, nasal cavity, hard palate, and orbital cavity, just to name a few. Ingenuity and creative thinking are typically used in creating applicators for treatment of these superficial lesions.

Interstitial applicators

Interstitial brachytherapy places the radioactive sources directly into or adjacent to the tumor or tumor bed. There are both permanent and temporary applications of interstitial implants used in radiation therapy.

Permanent implants. Permanent implants are performed when the tumor to be treated is inaccessible, making the removal of the radioisotope impossible or impractical. Iodine 125 and gold 198 are ideally suited for permanent implants because of their short half-lives. The patient who receives these types of implants does not have to have a second surgical procedure to remove the isotopes. The volumes treated commonly require placement of many sources; this requires a rapid and accurate means of application. To accomplish this, a gun-type applicator with a long hollow insertion needle is used. The needle is pushed through the skin into the deep tumor, and the sources are inserted into the tumor. The needle is withdrawn 5 to 10 mm, and the next source is inserted. This is repeated until the desired length and number of sources are applied. Permanent implants using iodine 125 and gold 198 are ideally suited for deep-seated lesions in the pelvis, abdomen, and lung. Fig. 3-5 shows a radiograph of a gold 198 pelvic implant.

Temporary implants. Temporary, removable implants are used in anatomical areas where there is no body cavity or orifice to accept radioactive sources.[1,6] The sources are placed directly into the tumor and tumor bed for a short period of time to deliver a high dose to the area. Radiation therapy boost fields can make use of this brachytherapy technique.

Hollow stainless steel needles can be pushed through the tissues to accommodate catheters holding radioisotopes. Iridium 192 afterloading is used in most applications. The tubes are spaced 1 cm apart; several planes may be used,

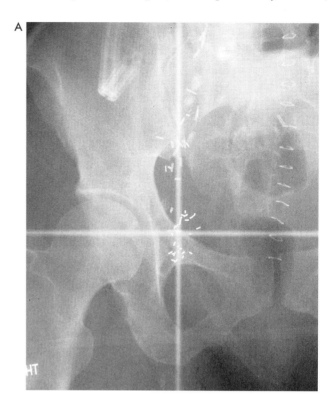

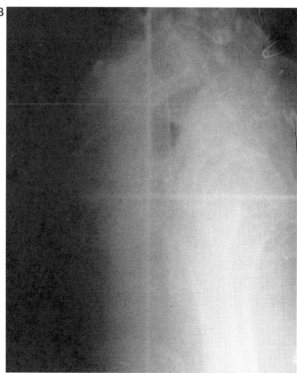

Fig. 3-5 Gold 198 seed permanent implant. Note the small size and clustering of source placement. **A,** Anterior. **B,** Lateral.

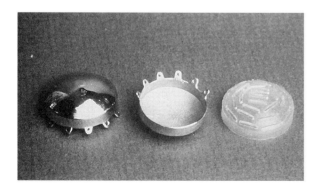

Fig. 3-4 Typical plaque used in topical brachytherapy of the eye. The thin gold shielding is sufficient to block neighboring dose-limiting structures from the damaging effects of the low energy isotope.

A

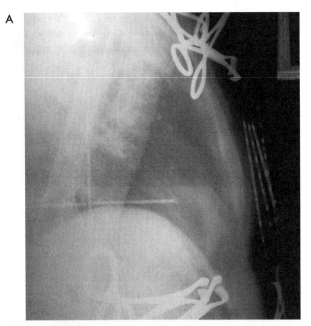

B

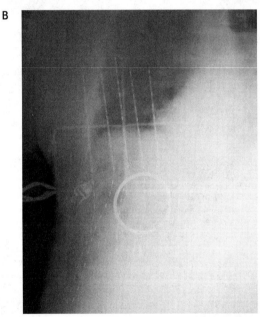

Fig. 3-6 Iridium 192 breast implant. Note how the dummy sources can be seen and used for dose calculation. Magnification ring allows for accurate size perspective to be realized. **A**, Anterior. **B**, Lateral.

depending on the tumor size. Catheters are placed in the tubes before removal. When the stainless steel tubes are removed, the catheters are left in place, ready to accommodate dummy sources. Dummy sources are nonradioactive radiopaque seeds that can be visualized on a radiograph. The sources are aligned and spaced just as the radioactive seeds would be. This is done to enable visualization of source placement, to ensure that the implants are positioned correctly, and for treatment planning and dose calculation without unnecessary radiation exposure to the patient and personnel. This is the basic principle of remote afterloading. Table 3-5 outlines the advantages and disadvantages of remote afterloaders.

Once the placement is confirmed, the dummy sources can be replaced with the radioactive sources and left in place for the desired time. This technique is commonly used in, but not limited to, breast and chest wall irradiation.[1,6,10] Fig. 3-6 demonstrates an iridium 192 breast implant radiograph. Anterior, lateral, and posterior walls of the vagina are also treated with interstitial afterloading techniques (Fig. 3-7).

To improve the accuracy of needle placement and to maintain position during treatment, stabilizers and guides can be used. These are popular in transperineal implants. In these applications, ultrasound as well as radiographs can be employed to confirm location and placement of sources. Fig. 3-8 demonstrates a Syed-Neblett template radiograph. Cancers of the rectum, prostate, vagina, and urethra are commonly treated with this applicator.

Intracavitary applicators

Insertion of radioactive sources into body cavities has been a viable component of radiation therapy for many years.[1,3,6] Several applicators have been designed and used, most for the treatment of gynecological tumors. The designs used in the newer applicators allow for customized, intricate dose distributions, maximizing dose to the tumor and sparing dose to adjacent, sensitive structures (such as the rectum and urinary bladder). Extensive knowledge of physics and anatomy is required to be effective in the dose delivery using this brachytherapy application.

Tandem and ovoids. Gynecological malignancies are usually treated using standard apparatus; however, standardized applicators typically have room in their design for cus-

Table 3-5	Advantages and disadvantages of remote afterloading systems	
Advantages		**Disadvantages**
Reduction or elimination of exposure to medical personnel		Remote afterloaders are expensive
Treatment techniques more consistent		More cost because of increased maintenance
In HDR, allows outpatient treatment, lowering cost		In HDR, increased room shielding is necessary
In LDR, sources can be retracted in case of emergency		

HDR, High dose rate; LDR, low dose rate.

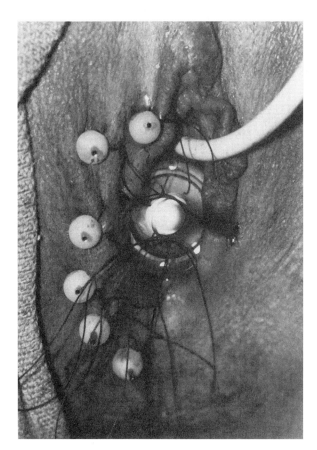

Fig. 3-7 Delco stainless steel needles for afterloading. Iridium implant of the lateral vaginal wall. Note Foley catheter and empty vaginal cylinder. (Courtesy Dr. L. Delclos.)

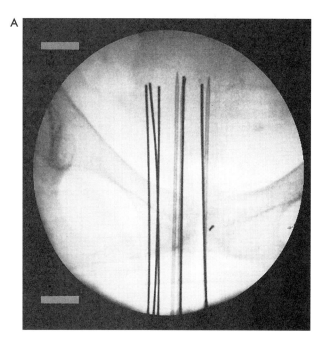

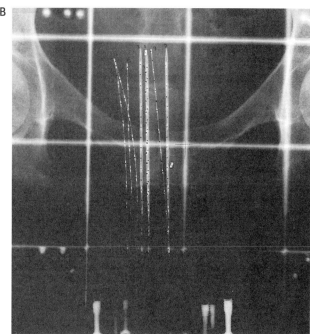

Fig. 3-8 Radiographs of a Syed-Neblett template technique for a vaginal carcinoma. **A**, Radiograph of needle placement during surgery. **B**, Radiograph of stylets loaded with dummy iridium 192 sources.

tomized modifications. Gynecological insertions are done with both low dose rate (LDR) and high dose rate (HDR) applications today. There is much debate on the merits of high dose rate applications, both pro and con. The jury is still out on high dose rate; however, its increased usage and reports of comparable complication rates have high dose rate protagonists optimistic.[7-9,11]

A central tandem and a pair of lateral ovoids are commonly used in brachytherapy applications involving the cervix (Fig. 3-9). The **tandem** is a long narrow tube that inserts into the opening of the cervix (cervical os) into the uterus. **Ovoids**, or colpostats, are oval shaped and insert into the lateral fornices of the vagina. Both components are hollow and can accommodate several radioactive sources. The ovoids come in various sizes to accommodate the variances in anatomical structures (wide or narrow vaginas) These ovoids can have shielding that customizes the dose distributions in such a way that dose to the urinary bladder and rectum is minimized. Tandems and ovoids are placed into the female anatomy and stabilized with packing. This packing (sterile gauze) not only stabilizes the apparatus during its 2- to 3-day placement in the vagina, but also serves to displace the rectum and bladder from the sources. Remember that

radioisotopes adhere to the inverse square law. The farther critical structures are from the sources, the less dose they will receive.

Location of the applicator is verified with radiographs, and dose calculations can be performed (Fig. 3-10). Once loaded with sources, the tandem and ovoids typically demonstrate a pear-shaped isodose distribution (Fig. 3-11).

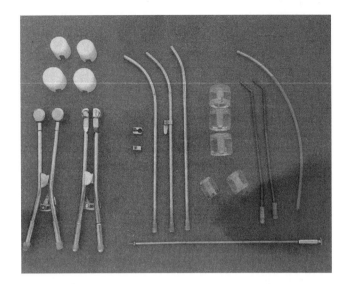

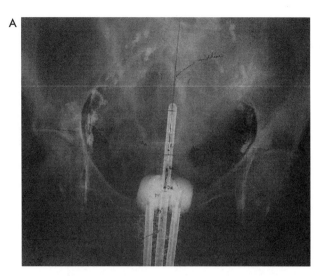

Fig. 3-9 Fletcher suit, Delclos Manual Afterloading System. *From left to right*: small colpostats with additional caps for conversion to medium and large; minicolpostats; intrauterine "tandems"; Delclos and cylindrical colpostats (selected); colpostat carriers; tandem carrier; *Bottom (horizontal)* dead-seed implanter and seeds. (From Fletcher GH: *Textbook of radiotherapy*, Baltimore, 1980, Williams and Wilkins.)

Currently the standard unit is the centigray to a specific anatomical point or isodose line. The anatomical points used historically for cervical and uterine treatment are points A and B. Point A is located 2 cm superior and 2 cm lateral to the center of the cervical canal (at the cervical os) in the plane of the uterus. Point B was originally 3 cm lateral to point A, but it is currently noted as being 1 cm lateral to the medial aspect of the pelvic side wall (Fig. 3-12). The dose at point B is typically about one third that at point A. While these points of dose specification have been used for years, their location is not standard in all patients. Anatomical differences can cause variances. Each case must be considered individually.

Heyman capsules. Heyman capsules allow the uterus to be packed with stainless steel capsules that house cesium sources to treat uterine cancers that are inoperable (Fig. 3-13). Metal wires are attached to the capsule (which now can be remote afterloaded) for removal; they protrude through the vagina. Localization of the sources for dose calculation can be done just as in the other applications.

Vaginal cylinders. Various customized applicators have been designed to give a high dose to vaginal lesions without giving excessive dose to the urinary bladder or rectum. The applicators are of different lengths, diameters, and shielding designs. In other words, individual application of treatment is optimized. Several designs, like the Delclos uterine-vaginal afterloading system, are designed for simultaneous treatment of the uterine cavity, cervix, and vaginal walls (Fig. 3-14).[1] Vaginal cylinders can be used in conjunction with interstitial implants. The cylinder can not only place sources in

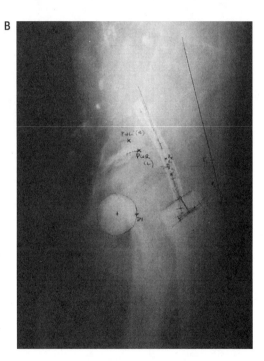

Fig. 3-10 Orthogonal radiographs of tandem and ovoid location. Note the packing that serves to stabilize the placement of the applicator as well as "push" the urinary bladder and rectum out of the way. **A**, Anterior. **B**, Lateral. (From Cox JD: *Moss' radiation oncology*, ed 7. St Louis, 1994, Mosby.)

proximity to diseased anatomy, it can also assist in the shielding of anatomy from radiation by both shielding material in the applicator and the application of the inverse square law. Fig. 3-15 shows an interstitial implant and vaginal cylinder used in the treatment of a posterior vaginal wall.

A specialized type of intracavitary brachytherapy places sources within body tubes such as the esophagus, trachea, and biliary tract. Obstructive lesions can be addressed by placing radioactive sources onto or adjacent to the lesions.

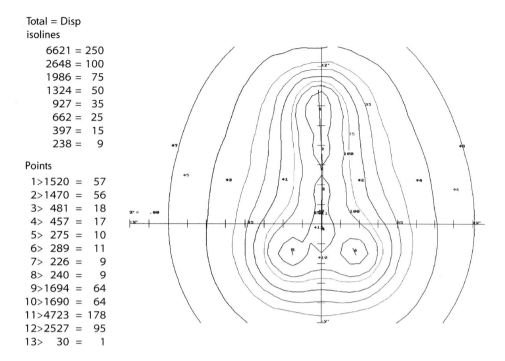

```
Total = Disp
isolines
    6621 = 250
    2648 = 100
    1986 =  75
    1324 =  50
     927 =  35
     662 =  25
     397 =  15
     238 =   9

Points
  1>1520 =  57
  2>1470 =  56
  3> 481 =  18
  4> 457 =  17
  5> 275 =  10
  6> 289 =  11
  7> 226 =   9
  8> 240 =   9
  9>1694 =  64
 10>1690 =  64
 11>4723 = 178
 12>2527 =  95
 13>  30 =   1
```

Fig. 3-11 Pear-shaped dose distribution. This was obtained with the use of a tandem and ovoid applicator. The fuller, inferior portion of the isodose distribution corresponds to the location of the ovoids.

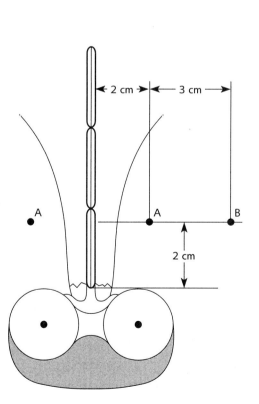

Fig. 3-12 Diagram of points A and B.

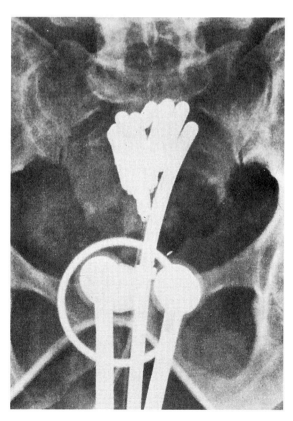

Fig. 3-13 Heyman capsules in the endometrium. (From Fletcher GH: *Textbook of radiotherapy*, Baltimore, 1980, Williams and Wilkins.)

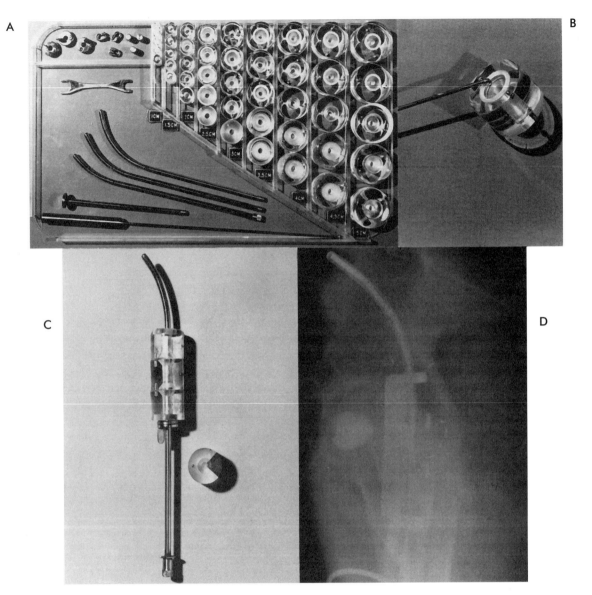

Fig. 3-14 **A**, Delclos cylindrical colpostat (diameter 1 cm to 5 cm). **B**, Detail of a selected cylinder. **C**, Cylinders mounted on intrauterine tandem and sample of leased cylinder. **D**, Leaded cylinders mounted on intrauterine tandem (*radiograph*). (From Delclos L, Fletcher GH, et al: Minicolpostats, dome cylinders, other additions and improvements of the Fletcher-Suit Afterloadable System: indications and limitations of their use, *Int J Rad Oncol Biol Phys*, 6:1195-1206.)

Pulsed high dose rate applications for these types of treatments using cesium 137 and iridium 192 have been done successfully. (For more information, review the high dose rate section of Chapter 15 in volume I of this series.)

BRACHYTHERAPY DOSIMETRY AND DOSE DISTRIBUTION

Dose distribution from radium 226 is the basis for all dose calculations in brachytherapy. As seen earlier, knowing the relationship of radium substitutes and radium allows the radiation therapy practitioner to deliver a dose to a patient accurately. A keen knowledge of anatomy and adherence to a few rules will provide the dosimetrist and radiation therapist

the ability to develop optimized treatment plans for patients. This section will provide basic rules and generalized discussion of dosimetry and dose distribution for interstitial implants. Three systems will be discussed: Paterson-Parker, Quimby, and Paris.

Paterson-Parker (Manchester) system

Using the gamma factor of radium, it is possible to perform radium dosimetry calculations, assuming the point source approximations stated previously. However, for patient dosimetry a number of sources are typically used, and the accurate calculation of the dose distributions from these implants is a complex procedure. Also, it requires that the

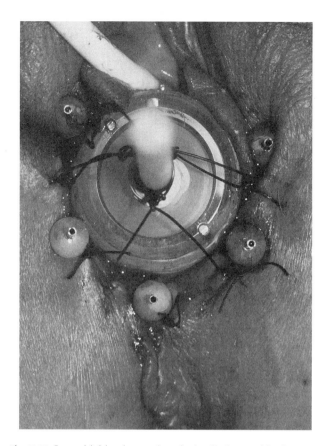

Fig. 3-15 Interstitial implant and vaginal cylinder used in the treatment of a posterior vaginal wall. (From Delclos L, Fletcher GH, et al: Minicolpostats, dome cylinders, other additions and improvements of the Fletcher-Suit Afterloadable System: indications and limitations of their use, *Int J Rad Oncol Biol Phys*, 6:1195-1206.)

radioactive sources be implanted in the patient before the calculations are done, so the physician, physicist, and dosimetrist have no idea how the patient is being treated until after the sources are already in place. In the 1930s Ralston Paterson and H.M. Parker at the Manchester Hospital in England developed a series of guidelines and dosimetry methods known as the Paterson-Parker or Manchester system of radium dosimetry to remove these difficulties.

The Paterson-Parker system establishes a set of guidelines that, if followed, will provide a dose of ±10% within the implanted area. Implantation philosophy strives to deliver a uniform dose to a plane or volume. This system uses a nonuniform distribution of radioactive material to produce a "uniform" distribution of dose. The system assumes the use of linear sources to be implanted in tissue in planes or other geometrical shapes and gives rules for placing the sources in each case. Then the system provides dose tables, which, if distribution rules have been followed, can be used to calculate the dose within the volume. Rules have been established for both planar and volume implants.[2,9]

Planar implants. Planar arrangements of sources are summarized in Table 3-6 for square and rectangular implants.

Table 3-6	Spacing sources in a Paterson-Parker planar implant
Area	**Activity in periphery/activity over area**
Area < 25 cm^2	$^2/_3$
25 cm^2 < area < 100 cm^2	$^1/_2$
Area > 100 cm^2	$^1/_3$

In multiple plane implants the planes should be 1 cm apart and parallel. If there is no crossing source at one or both ends, the area is reduced by 10% for each uncrossed end (Fig. 3-16). If the plane is not square, the mg-hrs are increased by the appropriate elongation factor for the ratio of long side to short side. Fig. 3-17 depicts a single plane implant.

For circular and near-circular areas the activity should first be placed on the periphery, preferably using more than five sources with spacing no greater than the treatment distance. Then more sources are arranged in an inner circle half the diameter of the original area. Remaining sources go in the center. The distribution of activity is governed by the ratio of the diameter to the treatment distance.[2] Parameters are outlined in Table 3-7.

Volume implants. If the shape of the implanted volume resembles a three-dimensional shape more than a plane, it is called a volume implant. Shapes defined by the Paterson-Parker system include cylinders, ellipsoids (football-shaped volumes), spheres, and cubes, among others. This type of calculation is usually done for seed implants of the prostate and other implants in which the activity is evenly spread out inside an organ or structure. Similar to the planar implants,

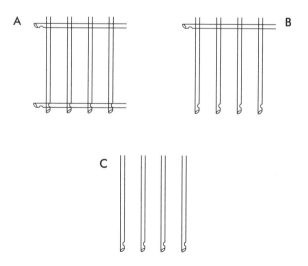

Fig. 3-16 Planar implants. **A**, Both ends crossed (reduce treatment area in calculation by 10%). **B**, One crossed end. **C**, No crossed ends (reduce treatment area in calculation by 20%).

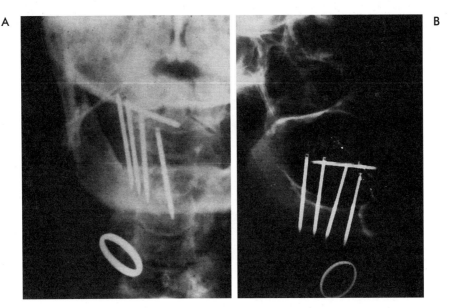

Fig. 3-17 Single plane implant. **A,** Diagram of a planar implant. **B,** Photograph of a single plane implant. (From Cox JD: *Moss' radiation oncology*, ed 7. St Louis, 1994, Mosby.)

Table 3-7	Circular source distribution in Paterson-Parker circular implants				
Diameter/distance (cm)	1-3	3-6	6	7.5	10
Outer circle (%)	100	95	80	75	70
Inner circle (%)	0	0	17	22	27
Center (%)	0	5	3	3	3

volume implants can have crossed ends. If there is no crossing source at one or both ends of the volume implant, the area used for calculations should be reduced by 7.5% for each uncrossed end. Fig. 3-18 shows a multiplane implant.

Quimby/Memorial dosimetry system

The Quimby system is similar in concept to the Paterson-Parker system. It provides a set of tables used to calculate dose given a number of implant parameters such as area, volume, or total activity. However, in the Quimby system the implant is assumed to be made up of a uniform distribution of activity within the implant, giving a nonuniform distribution of dose. The Quimby system is less frequently used than the Paterson-Parker system but has been adapted into a system called the Memorial system, whose tables are based on computer calculations that take into account filtration at all angles, modern units of activity, and dose.

Paris system

The Paris system was developed in the early 1920s and uses uniform distribution of the radiation sources, just as seen in the Quimby system.[1] The system is based on three principles:

1. The radioactive sources must be rectilinear and arranged so that their centers are in the same plane, which is perpendicular to the direction of the sources and is called the central plane. The dose is defined and calculated in this plane, but not restricted to the plane.
2. The linear activity must be uniform along each source and the same for all sources.
3. The radioactive sources must be spaced uniformly. This is the case even when more than one plane is used.[2]

This system is intended for use with removable long line implants, such as iridium 192 wires. The system uses wider spacing for longer sources or larger treatment volumes, typically implanted in parallel lines.[9]

Computer calculation methods

In the 1970s computers began to be used for calculating the dose distribution from a specific brachytherapy implant, using a method called the Sievert integral, which breaks a linear source into tiny components, calculates the dose at every point in the patient from every component, and adds these values to get the final result. Using computer methods, exact isodose distributions, like those from external beam treatments, can be obtained for brachytherapy, instead of relying on the somewhat general method of the Paterson-Parker tables. Today most implant procedures have a computerized dose distribution produced, and this has become an important tool in adjusting each implant to the individual patient's needs. As with all computer calculations, however, it must be cautioned that the doses obtained should be checked periodically by hand, using the Paterson-Parker tables or another method; reliance on a

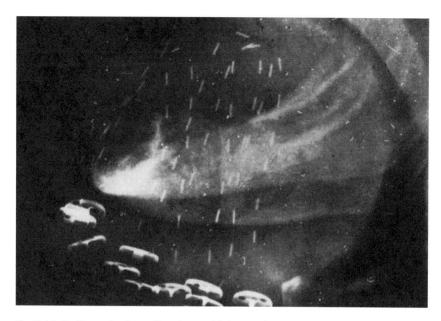

Fig. 3-18 Radiograph of a radioactive multiplane volume of the tongue and floor of the mouth. (From Cox JD: *Moss' radiation oncology*, ed 7. St Louis, 1994, Mosby.)

computer can have serious consequences if the results are not verified in some way.

RADIATION SAFETY AND QUALITY ASSURANCE

The safe handling of radioactivity has been a matter of concern in hospitals for many years.[1] Those small seemingly harmless ribbons and tubes can cause a great deal of hazard if not dealt with appropriately. While practical radiation safety of brachytherapy applications is covered in the chapter on radiation safety, the subject merits a few generalized thoughts concerning this important aspect of therapeutic administration.

A good place to start would be a complete description of all brachytherapy sources in use on file. The uniformity of the source materials distribution should be checked by autoradiograph. An **autoradiograph** is a signature exposure of a radioactive source obtained by placing the source on an unexposed x-ray film for a period of time long enough to darken the film. The film may be scanned to check for dose uniformity.[9] The storage of the sources should facilitate

source identification by type and strength. Appropriate documentation should be kept for source control from initial receipt through calibration, inventory, and disposal. Dose calculations should also be double-checked. A good quality assurance program can be the difference between safe administration of radiation and a massive radiation disaster.

SUMMARY

Brachytherapy is an art and a science that has evolved through the years into a specialized aspect of malignant disease management. The first brachytherapy procedure followed the discovery of radioactivity by only a few months. Today, brachytherapy is a standard technique in the treatment of a large number of malignancies through various means. Both naturally and artificially produced radioisotopes are used to deliver a high dose to the tumor while sparing normal tissues. Radiation therapy practitioners must be prepared to demonstrate a comprehensive knowledge of its uses, in that brachytherapy has resurged as an intricate part of cancer management.

Review Questions

Multiple Choice

1. When using both tandem and ovoids in a gynecological implant, the typical resultant dose distribution is of what shape?
   a. Oval
   b. Rectangular
   c. Butterfly
   d. Pear

2. Afterloading techniques were developed primarily to reduce:
   a. The possibilities of errors in loading
   b. The time required for the implant
   c. Exposure to personnel
   d. Exposure to nearby dose-limiting structures

3. Radium sources are leak tested as specified by state regulations to check for:
   a. Uranium 238
   b. Radon 222
   c. Radium 228
   d. Lead 208

4. The key relationship for radioactivity states:
   a. The change in the number of atoms per change in unit time is proportional to the number of atoms present.
   b. The change in unit time per change in the number of atoms is proportional to the number of atoms present.
   c. The change in the number of atoms per change in unit time is equal to the number of disintegrations per second.
   d. The change in unit time per change in the number of atoms is proportional to the number of disintegrations per second.

5. The decay constant describes:
   a. The half-life of a particular radionuclide
   b. The number of ionizations produced in tissue per unit time
   c. The fraction of the number of atoms that decay per unit time
   d. None of the above are true

6. When looking at the relationship between decay constant and activity, as the decay constant decreases, activity:
   a. Increases
   b. Decreases
   c. Remains the same
   d. Not enough information given

7. The time required for either the activity or the number of radioactive atoms to decay to half the initial value is the definition for:
   a. Activity
   b. Decay constant
   c. Half-life
   d. Exponential decay

8. A new batch of iridium 192 has arrived, and its calibration must be checked. The supplier states that the activity of the material was 0.351 mCi/seed 10 days earlier. What is the expected activity of the iridium 192 today (half-life = 74.2 days)?
   a. 0.002 mCi
   b. 9.97 mCi
   c. 0.320 mCi
   d. 0.007 mCi

9. The average lifetime for the decay of radioactive atoms is the definition of:
   a. Half-life
   b. Decay constant
   c. Specific activity
   d. Mean life

10. Packing in gynecological implants serves which of the following purposes?
    I.   Provides stability of applicator placement
    II. Aids in pushing dose-sensitive structures farther from sources
    III. Aids in spacing sources to even out dose distributions
    a. I and II
    b. I and III
    c. II and III
    d. I, II, and III

11. In which interstitial brachytherapy system is a uniform dose distribution to a plane or volume accomplished using a nonuniform distribution of sources?
    a. Quimby
    b. Paris
    c. Paterson-Parker
    d. All of the above employ the same system

12. For every uncrossed end in a Paterson-Parker planar implant the treated volume area is reduced by what percent?
    a. 5
    b. 7.5
    c. 10
    d. 12.5

13. The distance between the ends of radioactive material in a radium tube is known as:
    a. Permanent activity
    b. Active length
    c. Physical length
    d. Filtration factor

14. Which of the following is true of a radium needle autoradiograph?
    I. Assists in the determination of uniformity of activity distribution
    II. Allows visualization of the physical and active source dimensions
    III. Obtained by placing the source on an unexposed x-ray film for a period of time
    a. I and II
    b. I and III
    c. II and III
    d. I, II, and III

15. Isotopes used in permanent implants are most frequently:
    a. Iodine 125 and gold 198
    b. Gold 198 and cesium 137
    c. Cesium 137 and radium 226
    d. Radium 226 and iodine 125

Questions to Ponder

1. Compare and contrast the dose distribution rules of the Paterson-Parker and Quimby systems.
2. Compare and contrast the use of radium and cesium as brachytherapy sources for treatment.
3. Describe the necessary criteria for a radioisotope to be used as a permanent implant.
4. How does the mean life differ from the half-life of an isotope?
5. Describe the role of the inverse square law in the use of brachytherapy source applicators.

REFERENCES

1. Bentel GC: *Radiation therapy planning*, ed 2. New York, 1996, Macmillan.
2. Chapman J: Personal interview, 1994.
3. Clarke DH, Martinez A: An overview of brachytherapy in cancer management. *Oncology* 4(9):39-46, 1990.
4. Glickeman AS, Leith JT: Radiobiological considerations of brachytherapy. *Oncology* 2(1):25-32, 1988.
5. Hall EJ: Radiation dose rate: a factor of importance in radiobiology and radiotherapy. *Br J Radiol* 45:81-97, 1972.
6. Hilaris BS et al: *Atlas of brachytherapy*. New York, 1992, Macmillan.
7. Jordan LN, Mantravadi RV: Nursing care of the patient receiving high dose rate brachytherapy. *Oncol Nurs Forum* 18(7):1167-1171, 1991.
8. Joslin CA: *High dose rate brachytherapy—has it a future?* Royal College of Radiologists Annual Scientific Meeting and Exhibition, September 22-25, 1992, Southampton, UK.
9. Khan FM: *The physics of radiation therapy*, ed 2. Baltimore, 1994, Williams & Wilkins.
10. Mast DE, Mood DW: Preparing patients with breast cancer for brachytherapy. *Oncol Nurs Forum* 17(2):267-270, 1990.
11. Steel GG, et al: Dose rate effects and the repair of radiation damage. *Radiotherapy Oncol* 5:321-331, 1986.
12. Williams JR, Thwaites DI: *Radiotherapy physics in practice*. 1993, Oxford Medical.

BIBLIOGRAPHY

Ash D: Overviews of interstitial therapy. *Br J Radiol Suppl* 22:79-82, 1988.
Hall EF, Brenner DJ: The 1991 George Edelstyn Memorial Lecture: needles, wire and chips—advances in brachytherapy. *Clin Oncol* 4(4):249-256, 1992.
Hoefnagel CA: Radionuclide therapy revisited. *European Journal of Nuclear Medicine* 18(6):408-431, 1991.
Shiu MH, Hilaris BS: Brachytherapy and function-saving resection of soft tissue sarcoma arising in the limb, *Int J Radiation Oncol Biol Physics* 21(6):1485-1492, 1991.
Trott NG: Radionuclides in brachytherapy: radium and after. *Br J Radiol Suppl* 21:1-54, 1987.

C H A P T E R

4

Radiation Safety and Protection

Joseph S. Blinick
Elizabeth G. Quate

Outline

Key terms

Absorbed dose
Activity
Advisory
ALARA
Alpha particle
Beta particle
Dose equivalent
Effective dose equivalent
Exposure
Film badge
Gamma ray
Genetically significant dose

Ionizing radiation
LET
Natural background radiation
Occupancy factor
Photons
Pocket ionization chambers
Regulatory
Thermoluminescent dosimeters
Use factor
Workload
X-ray

The levels of radiation exposure in a radiation therapy department *can* be quite high. Thus it is important to consider the principles of radiation protection to avoid unnecessary exposure to patients, operators, and the general public.

In this chapter we will discuss types of radiation and their sources as well as the detection and measurement of levels of radiation in the environment of a therapy department. We will also discuss the risks of exposure to **ionizing radiation** (radiation with sufficient energy to separate an electron from its atom), the regulatory requirements for limits of exposure to radiation for various groups, and practical methods for individual radiation protection.

DETECTION AND MEASUREMENT
Types of radiation

Within a radiation therapy department, there are two major groups of radiation sources. The first comprises external beam therapy machines, such as cobalt teletherapy units or linear accelerators. These use gamma rays, x-rays, and sometimes electrons. The second group comprises brachytherapy sources, which use gamma rays and x-rays from sources such as ^{137}Cs, ^{192}Ir, and ^{125}I. Sources in this group may also emit alpha and beta particles. Table 4-1 summarizes types of ionizing radiation and some of their characteristics.

Alpha particles. Alpha particles consist of two protons and two neutrons and are therefore simply helium nuclei.

Table 4-1	Types of ionizing radiation		
Type of radiation	**Charge**	**Atomic mass number**	**Origin**
Alpha particles (α)	+2	4	Nucleus
Beta particles			
Negatron (ß⁻)	-1	0	Nucleus
Positron (ß⁺)	+1	0	Nucleus
Neutrinos (ν)	0	0	Nucleus
X-rays	0	0	Electron shells
Gamma rays (γ)	0	0	Nucleus

They are emitted from unstable heavy nuclei such as radium or radon during the decay process. Because of their charge and relatively heavy mass, alpha particles can only travel short distances (most can be stopped by a sheet of paper), but they produce intense ionization and are therefore high LET radiation. Thus they are extremely hazardous if ingested or inhaled but are less dangerous if the exposure is external. Alpha particles emitted by radium and radon are easily stopped by the material used to encapsulate the sources. If the integrity of the capsule is compromised, however, exposure to alpha particles is possible.

Beta particles. Beta particles are electrons emitted by the nucleus. They may be either negatively charged (negatron or ß⁻) or positively charged (positron or ß⁺). Positrons are not stable and may exist for only very short periods of time. Whenever beta particles are emitted, they are accompanied by a small, massless, chargeless particle known as the neutrino (see Chapter 2). Both types of beta particles have the same rest mass as an electron, and are usually emitted from the nucleus with high velocities. Beta particles and energetic electrons are more penetrating than alpha particles and may pose both an external and an internal threat. High energy (1 MeV) beta particles may have a range as long as 2 cm in soft tissue. Metals may be used for shielding, but bremsstrahlung radiation may result. The probability of bremsstrahlung x-ray production is directly proportional to the square of the atomic number of the absorber and inversely proportional to the square of the mass of the incident particle.[1] Thus bremsstrahlung radiation is much more likely to occur with beta particles than with alpha particles. It is often more suitable to shield beta particles with low atomic number materials, such as plastics or glass, than with metals, such as lead or steel.

X-rays and gamma rays. X-rays and **gamma rays** are both forms of electromagnetic radiation (**photons**). Photons have no mass and no charge. Gamma rays are photons emitted from a nucleus. X-rays are extranuclear and result from rearrangements within the electron shells or from bremsstrahlung radiation. Except for their origin, there is no difference between x-rays and gamma rays. X-rays and

gamma rays may be more penetrating than either alpha or beta particles, and substantial shielding may be required, depending on the energy of the photon.

Sources of radiation

People have been exposed to naturally occurring ionizing radiation since the beginning of time. However, it was not until the beginning of the 20th century that the general public had any exposure to manmade sources of radiation. In fact, even today, it is estimated that 82% of the exposure of the US population to radiation comes from natural background sources[5] (Fig. 4-1).

Natural background radiation. Natural background radiation comes from three sources: cosmic rays that bombard the earth, terrestrial radiation that emanates from radioactive materials naturally occurring in the earth, and internal deposits of radionuclides in our bodies.

1. *Cosmic rays.* Cosmic rays originate from nuclear reactions in space or from our own sun. Although the earth's atmosphere acts as a protective shield against much of the initial bombardment, the primary cosmic rays interact with molecules in the atmosphere to create other reactive agents, known as secondary particles. These include neutrons, protons, and pions (short-lived subnuclear particles), which go on to produce energetic electrons, muons (another subnuclear particle), and photons. The average annual effective dose equivalent at sea level in the United States from cosmic rays is about 0.26 millisieverts (mSv) (26 millirems [mrem]). The exposure from cosmic rays varies with solar sunspot cycles, latitude, and altitude. The magnetic nature of the earth accounts for the variation in dose resulting from latitude. The charged particles incident on the earth are drawn along the magnetic field lines, which are directed toward the poles. Thus exposure is higher at the polar regions than at the equator. Latitude, solar cycles, and other factors may account for a variation of 10% in exposure. The intensity varies even more with increasing elevation. The dose approximately doubles with each 2000-meter increase in altitude in the lower atmosphere, since there is less atmosphere to absorb the incident rays. People in Denver (elevation 1600 meters) receive about 0.5 mSv (50 mrem) from cosmic rays.[5]

2. *Terrestrial radiation.* The earth is made up of hundreds of materials, many of which are naturally radioactive because of the presence of small amounts of long-lived isotopes of uranium, thorium, and radium, among others. This is the source of terrestrial radiation. The distribution of these materials varies with geographical location and the composition of the soil in the area. In the United States the average annual effective dose equivalent is 0.16 mSv (16 mrem) along the Eastern Seaboard, but may be as high as 0.63 mSv (63 mrem) in the Rocky Mountains.[5] Additional exposure to the public occurs because many materials used in construction contain these radioactive elements. The largest exposure to terrestrial radiation involves radon. Radon may be particularly harmful because it is an easily inhaled gas and

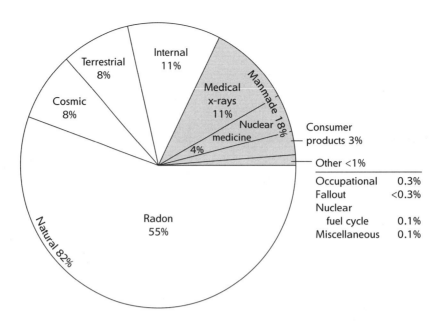

Fig. 4-1 The total average effective dose equivalent for the US population results from many sources of both natural and manmade radiation. This diagram illustrates the percentage that each of these sources contributes to the effective dose equivalent. (From National Council on Radiation Protection and Measurements: Report #93, *Ionizing radiation exposure of the population of the United States.* Bethesda, MD, 1987, NCRP Publications.)

it and its many progeny emit alpha and beta particles as well as gamma rays. Lung tissue can be damaged as deposited products decay. Radon concentration in houses varies greatly with the make-up of the soil, the design of the building, and the degree to which it is airtight. The average radon concentration in the United States is 37 millibecquerel/liter (1 pCi/liter), which yields about 2 mSv (200 mrem) to the bronchial epithelium per year.[2] The Environmental Protection Agency (EPA) estimates that radon exposure is the second leading cause of lung cancer in the United States (following smoking).[7]

3. *Internal exposure.* Internal exposure results from the radioactive materials that are normally present in our bodies. These include carbon-14, hydrogen-3, strontium-90, potassium-40, and very small amounts of uranium and thorium. Potassium-40 delivers the highest dose to the body (0.2 mSv/year or 30 mrem/year). Again, concentrations of these radioactive materials in the body depend on geographic location.

The average annual effective dose equivalent in the United States resulting from natural background radiation is estimated to be about 1.0 mSv (100 mrem) from all sources except radon. When radon is taken into consideration, the average increases to about 3.0 mSv (300 mrem).[5] These values can vary greatly. In the Kerala region of India, for example, the annual dose may be as great as 13 mSv (1300 mrem).[2]

Manmade sources. Manmade sources also contribute to the annual dose to individuals. These sources include medical x-rays; nuclear medicine procedures; consumer products such as televisions and tobacco products; nuclear reactors and the fuel cycle and fallout from above-ground nuclear weapons testing. These sources emit a broad spectrum of alpha and beta particles, electrons, x-rays, and gamma rays. The average annual effective dose equivalent from these sources to an exposed individual is about 0.60 mSv (60 mrem). Medical procedures contribute about 0.50 mSv (50 mrem) of that total, and consumer products contribute another 0.11 mSv (11 mrem).[5] The other sources together contribute less than 1% of the dose from manmade sources. However, the potential for much higher radiation exposure from these nuclear sources is evident in light of the atomic bomb explosions at Hiroshima and Nagasaki in 1945 and the Chernobyl power plant incident in the Soviet Union in 1986. The other significant dose from manmade sources is from tobacco products. Smokers inhale radioactive materials that are present naturally in tobacco (primarily polonium 210) and may receive an additional annual effective dose equivalent of 13 mSv (1300 mrem).[5]

The majority of the radiation to which the general population is exposed comes from natural background radiation, smokers excluded. It is not possible to effectively protect the entire population from these sources. That is why it is important to do all we can to minimize the radiation exposures from manmade sources, and why we strive to develop and implement valid radiation protection practices.

Units

Exposure is defined as the amount of ionization produced by photons in air per unit mass of air. The traditional unit for exposure is the roentgen. One roentgen (R) of exposure creates 2.58×10^{-4} coulomb (C) of charge per kilogram (kg) of air. The SI unit for exposure is C/kg of air (see Table 4-2 for conversions between conventional units and SI units). Exposure is only defined for ionization produced by photons interacting with air. For practical reasons, exposure is limited to photons whose energy is less than 3 MeV.

Absorbed dose is defined as the energy absorbed per unit mass of any material. The traditional unit for absorbed dose is the rad, defined as 100 ergs of energy absorbed per gram of absorbing material. The comparable SI unit is the Gray (Gy), which is defined as 1 joule of energy absorbed per kilogram of absorbing material (1 Gy = 100 cGy).

Dose equivalent takes into account the fact that different types of radiation produce different amounts of biological damage. Alpha particles and neutrons, for example, are high LET radiation and therefore have a greater biological effect than x-rays. Thus a 0.2 Gy (20 cGy) absorbed dose of alpha particles would be more damaging to a given mass of human tissue than a 0.2 Gy (20 cGy) absorbed dose of x-rays. To account for these differences in biological response, each type of radiation is assigned a quality factor (QF). The traditional unit, rem, is defined as the product of the absorbed dose in rads times the QF. The SI unit is the sievert (Sv), and it is defined as the absorbed dose in Gray times the QF.

Activity is the rate at which a radioactive isotope undergoes nuclear decay. The traditional unit of activity is the curie (Ci), which is defined as 3.7×10^{10} disintegrations per second. The SI unit is the becquerel (Bq), which is one disintegration per second.

Measurement devices

Many instruments and devices can be used to detect radiation, and several find use within the radiation oncology department. An instrument designed to calibrate the radiation output of a therapy machine will not necessarily be suitable for measuring low levels of radioactive contamination. It is important to understand the characteristics of each measuring device and the applications for which each is used.

Gas-filled detectors. One type of device is the gas-filled detector. This instrument has a chamber filled with a gas that is ionized in part or whole when radiation is present. Either the total quantity of electrical charge is measured or the rate at which charge is produced is measured. Two kinds of gas-filled detectors may be found in a radiation therapy department. These are the ionization chamber and the Geiger-Müller (G-M) detector.

The simplest of these, the ionization chamber, consists of two electrodes within a gas-filled chamber, an applied voltage across the electrodes, and electronics and a meter to amplify and measure the electrical signal (Fig. 4-2). The sensitivity of the chamber (smallest amount of radiation detectable) depends on the mass of gas within the chamber (chamber volume). The response of the chamber also depends on the applied voltage (Fig. 4-3). If there is no voltage, the positive and negative ions produced in the gas by the radiation will recombine instead of migrating to either of the electrodes. As the voltage across the electrodes is increased, more and more of the ions produced in the chamber will be collected on the electrodes; positive ions migrate to the cathode and negative ions to the anode. Ideally, ionization chambers should be operated at a voltage at which all of the ion pairs are collected and none recombine. Such a voltage (typically 100 to 300 volts) is said to produce saturation. When a positive ion reaches the cathode, it combines with one of the negative charges to form a neutral atom. This leaves a negative charge vacancy on the cathode, which is filled by a negative charge (electron) from the battery. The electrometer detects either the total charge that flows or the rate of charge

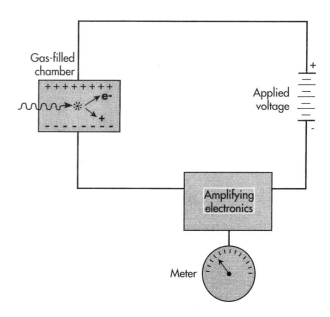

Fig. 4-2 An ionization chamber that consists of two electrodes within a gas-filled chamber. A voltage is applied across the electrodes. Electronics and a meter are used to amplify and measure the electrical signal.

Table 4-2	Traditional and SI unit equivalents		
Exposure	1 roentgen	=	2.59×10^{-4} C/kg
Absorbed dose	1 rad	=	0.01 Gy
Dose equivalent	1 rem	=	0.01 Sv
Activity	1 Ci	=	3.7×10^{10} Bq

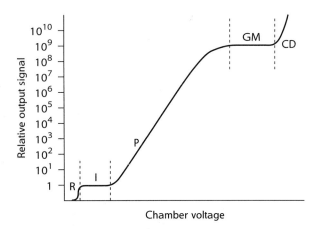

Fig. 4-3 The signal output from a gas-filled chamber depends on applied voltage. The stages of the chamber response are *R*, recombination region; *I*, ionization region; *P*, proportional region; *GM*, Geiger-Müller region; *CD*, region of continuous discharge. (From Bushong SC: *Radiologic science for technologists—physics, biology and protection*, ed 5. St Louis, 1993, Mosby)

flow and displays the value on the meter. The calibration can be set to read mR or mR/hour.

When properly calibrated, the accuracy of ionization chambers approaches 2%, which makes them suitable for measurement of the radiation output of therapy equipment. Ionization chambers with large air volumes are also suitable for environmental surveys around therapy rooms.

A form of ionization chamber, the pocket dosimeter, is used for personnel monitoring (Fig. 4-4). In this chamber the electrodes are arranged concentrically that is, one electrode is in the form of a thin rod and the other is a cylinder around it. When fully charged, a thin filament within the unit is displaced by static electricity to one end of a scale that can be viewed by holding the dosimeter up to a light. As radiation ionizes the air within the chamber, the ions deplete the charges on the electrodes and the filament is not displaced as far. The instrument is calibrated so that the position of the filament indicates the amount of exposure received by the chamber.

Because ionization chambers are not very sensitive, they are not suitable for the detection of very low levels of radiation or radiation contamination.

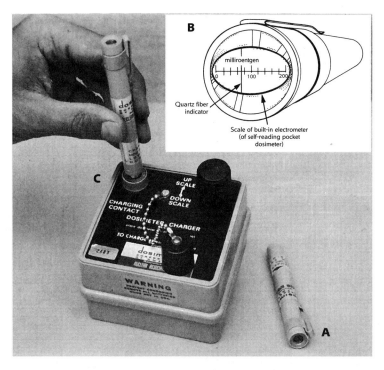

Fig. 4-4 Pocket ionization chamber. **A,** The pocket ionization chamber, or pocket dosimeter, resembles a fountain pen. **B,** The quartz fiber indicator of the built-in electrometer of the self-reading pocket dosimeter generally used in radiology indicates exposures of 0 to 5.2 x 10^{-5} C/kg (0 to 200 milliroentgens). **C,** Before use the pocket dosimeter must be charged to a predetermined voltage by a special charging unit so that the charges of the positive and negative electrodes will be balanced and the quartz fiber indicator reads zero. (Courtesy Dosimeter Corporation of America, Cincinnati, OH.)

If the chamber voltage is increased beyond that of the saturation region, the primary ions are energetic enough to produce additional ionizations, or secondary ions, in the gas. The Geiger-Müller region is reached as the voltage of the chamber is increased even further. An avalanche of secondary ions is produced for each primary ionization that occurs, so that individual events can be detected. This makes the G-M counter a very sensitive instrument and appropriate for detecting low levels of radiation or radioactive contamination (Fig. 4-5). G-M detectors tend to be strongly energy dependent, which means they respond differently to different photon energies. In addition, if a G-M detector is placed in a high level radiation field, it may produce a reading of zero because of overloading of the gas-filled detector. Increasing the voltage beyond the G-M range causes the gas insulation to break down. Electrical arcing occurs, and a continuous electrical discharge is produced. There is no useful reason for a detector to operate in this range, and damage to the chamber may result.

Thermoluminescent dosimeters (TLDs). Because of their small size, **thermoluminescent dosimeters (TLDs)** are widely used to measure radiation in a number of applications (Fig. 4-6). As the name implies, thermoluminescent materials give off light when heated. Whenever a crystalline material is irradiated, electrons are released from bound states in the valence band and become free to migrate in the conduction band. An energy gap separates these two regions, and it is this energy gap that must be overcome by the energy of the incoming radiation. In most materials, electrons immediately drop back from the conduction band to the valence band with the emission of characteristic photons. However, in some materials such as lithium fluoride (LiF) with some impurities deliberately introduced into the crystal structure, traps appear in the energy gap, and some of the electrons that would otherwise drop back to the valence band get caught in the traps. At a later time, if the crystal is heated to 100° to 200° C, the electrons will receive enough thermal energy to move back into the conduction band. Most of them immediately fall back to the valence band with the release of the characteristic photons. In the case of LiF (and other thermoluminescent materials), these characteristic photons are within the visible light range. In general, the more radiation absorbed by the crystal, the more electrons will be in traps, and the more characteristic photons will be released when the crystal is heated later. Thus the amount of light is a measure of the dose received by the crystal.

The atomic number of LiF is close to that of tissue (Li has an atomic number of 3, and F has an atomic number of 9), so LiF mimics tissue closely and is therefore useful as a patient or phantom dosimeter. If proper care is taken, doses can be measured with an accuracy of approximately 5%. TLDs are also used for mailed intercomparison of therapy unit calibration; in ring badges used for personnel monitoring; and for measurements of environmental levels of radiation. In these applications, TLDs have the advantage that the dose information can be stored for hours, days, or even weeks, until the dosimeter is heated. However, the readings may diminish with time because some of the electrons spontaneously leak

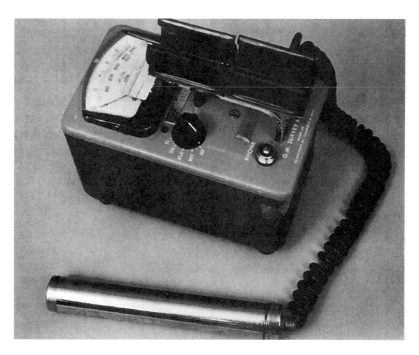

Fig. 4-5 Geiger-Müller detector. (Courtesy Baird Corporation, Nuclear Instruments Division, Bedford, MA.)

A

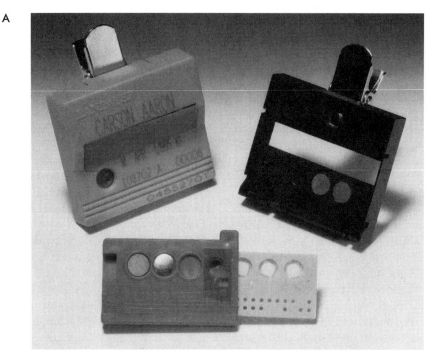

B

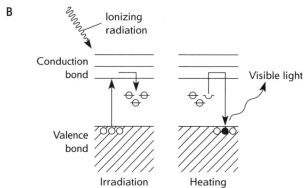

Conduction bond

Valence bond

Ionizing radiation

Visible light

Irradiation   Heating

Fig. 4-6 Thermoluminescent dosimeters. May be used in a number of applications in a radiation therapy department. **A,** A badge containing chips may be used for personnel monitoring. **B,** Electron transitions occurring when thermoluminescent LiF is irradiated and heated. (**A** Courtesy Landauer, Inc, Glenwood, IL; **B** From Bushong SC: *Radiologic science for technologists—physics, biology and protection,* ed 5. St Louis, 1993, Mosby.)

out of the traps. In addition, if the dosimeter is heated in transit, all the information may be lost. Despite this potential disadvantage, thermoluminescent dosimetry is a well-established technique for the measurement of radiation.

Film. After development, x-ray film exposed to radiation turns black. The amount of blackness is called the optical density, and the optical density is related to the amount of radiation received by the film. The actual relationship is not linear and depends on the type of film, the type and energy of the radiation, and the details of processing the film.

However, once calibrated, film is a convenient and inexpensive way to provide information about the doses received by individuals working in or visiting areas where radiation may be present.

A typical film badge has a slot in which the film (in its protective paper cover) may be placed and several thin metal filters that surround portions of the film (Fig. 4-7). The filters allow discrimination between different types and energies of radiation. Low energy radiation will not penetrate any of the filters but can reach the film in the area where no filters are present. Medium energy radiation will penetrate the no-filter and tin filter areas, but will not get through the lead filter. High energy radiation penetrates all areas. This discrimination is necessary because of the strong energy dependence of

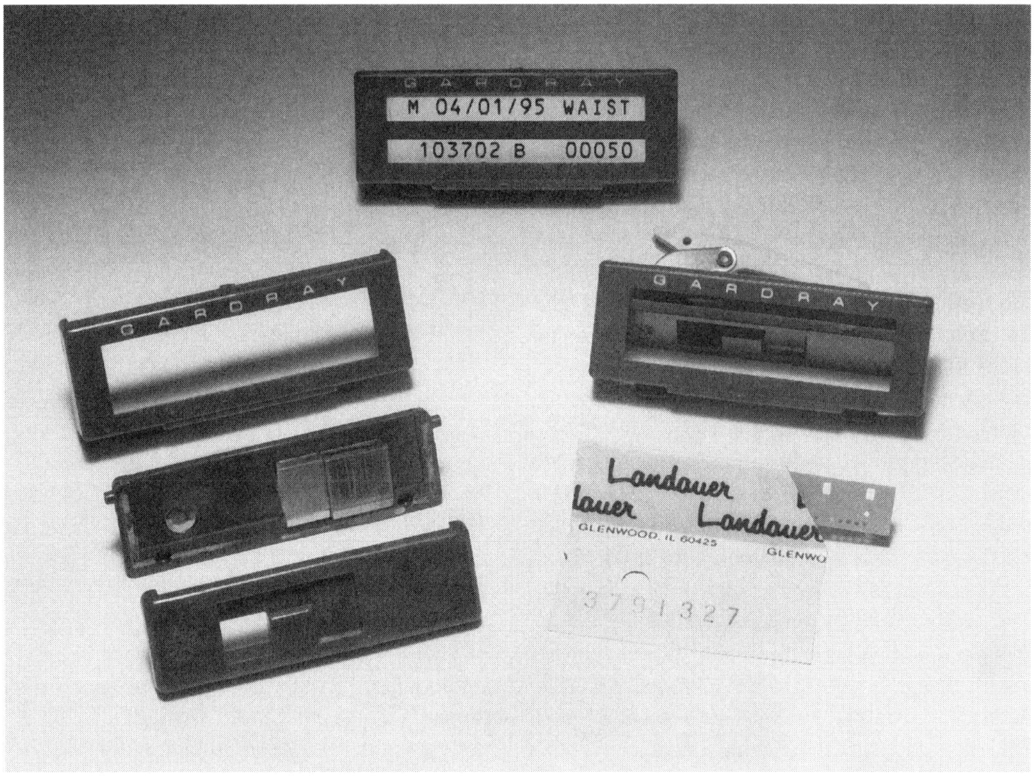

Fig. 4-7 Film badge. It consists of sensitive film, several thin metal filters, and a plastic holder. (Courtesy Landauer, Inc, Glenwood, IL.)

film. The response at high energies (1 MeV) may be up to 20 times less than the response at low energies (30 keV).

REGULATIONS AND REGULATORY AGENCIES
Advisory and regulatory agencies

The primary task of **advisory agencies** is to analyze the existing data related to radiation exposure and to assess the radiobiological risks associated with those exposures. These agencies can then develop recommendations for dose limits. Some of these agencies include the National Council on Radiation Protection and Measurement (NCRP), the International Commission on Radiation Protection (ICRP), the United Nations Scientific Committee on the Effects of Atomic Radiation (UNSCEAR), and the National Academy of Sciences Advisory Committee on the Biological Effects of Ionizing Radiation (NAS-BEIR). The recommendations may be acted on by Congress or state governments and made into law.

It is the role of the **regulatory agencies** to license users of radioactive materials and radiation-producing equipment, inspect such users, and enforce the appropriate laws. One of the leading federal regulatory agencies in the United States is the Nuclear Regulatory Commission (NRC), which oversees the use of isotopes produced in nuclear reactors. These isotopes are commonly used in nuclear medicine departments,

laboratories, and as sources for teletherapy (external beam radiation) and brachytherapy (internal implants). Many states have entered into agreements concerning licensing, inspection, and enforcement with the NRC and have become "agreement" states. As part of the agreement, states must maintain a certain level of compatibility with NRC regulations.

Transportation of radioactive materials is primarily the concern of the Department of Transportation (DOT) and the NRC. The use of machines that produce ionizing radiation, such as x-ray units and linear accelerators, falls under the jurisdiction of the Food and Drug Administration (FDA) and state agencies. The EPA and the Occupational Safety and Health Administration (OSHA) also have regulations that relate to the use of radiation.

Risk estimates

Estimating the risks of exposure to ionizing radiation is an extremely complex and difficult process. Although we probably know more about the effects of radiation on humans than is known about any other chemical or biological hazard, our knowledge is far from complete. Information about the risks of radiation has come from many sources, including victims of the bombs at Hiroshima and Nagasaki, Japan, at the end of World War II; people who received radiation for ankylosing spondylitis; women who received multiple fluoroscopic examinations for tuberculosis; and children treated with radiation for nonmalignant thymus and thyroid diseases.

In all of these cases, individual doses are not known precisely. In addition, individual variations are known to occur for any given radiation dose. Since there are no special effects attributable to ionizing radiation, the many effects that occur at low levels may be indistinguishable from those resulting from normal background levels.

We have a far greater knowledge of the effects of high doses of radiation than those of low doses. In sufficiently high quantities, radiation can be lethal. The lethal dose of whole body radiation, delivered acutely, to 50% of an exposed human population within 30 days is approximately 4.5 Gy (450 rads). This is known as the $LD_{50/30}$.

Even at levels below the lethal dose there are significant, long-term effects related to exposure to radiation. These fall into two general classifications: nonstochastic and stochastic. Nonstochastic effects are those for which a threshold exists and for which the *severity* of the effect increases with dose. Examples of such effects are erythema (skin reddening), epilation (loss of hair), cataract formation, and infertility. The threshold doses for these effects are relatively high, which is reflected in the higher permitted doses to the specific organs involved. Stochastic effects are those which have no threshold and for which the *probability* of occurrence is a function of dose. In this case, the severity of the effect is not a function of the dose. Either the effect occurs or it does not. Examples of stochastic effects are cancer induction, genetic effects, and embryological and teratogenic effects. Because of the lack of a threshold dose, these effects are of more concern at low levels of radiation exposure. The mechanisms by which these effects occur are discussed in Volume 1, Chapter 9, Radiobiology. Risk estimates for stochastic effects have been compiled by the NCRP in Report No. 115, "Risk Estimates for Radiation Protection" (1993). This publication assesses reports prepared by the UNSCEAR (1988), the Committee on the Biological Effects of Ionizing Radiations (BEIR V) (NAS/NRC, 1990), and Publication 60 of the ICRP. These reports discuss in length the methods by which risks associated with radiation exposure are estimated and what those risks are.

Cancer risks. The survivors of the atomic bomb explosions at both Hiroshima and Nagasaki are the primary source for estimating the cancer risks associated with ionizing radiation in NCRP No. 115, although data from other studies were considered. A linear-quadratic response for leukemias and a linear response for solid cancers were used in the estimation process (Fig. 4-8). No distinction was made between high dose rate and low dose rate exposures. The estimate for lifetime cancer risks for acute whole body exposure to low LET radiation is approximately 8 in 100 per Sv 8 in 10,000 per rem.[6]

Genetic risks. There are large uncertainties in assessing genetic risks. In part the uncertainties occur because the effects mutations have on life-threatening illnesses such as

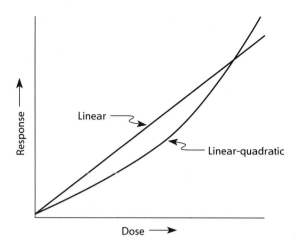

Fig. 4-8 Linear and linear-quadratic dose response curves. These are used for estimation of risks from exposure to ionizing radiation. (From Bushong SC: *Radiologic science for technologists—physics, biology and protection,* ed 5. St. Louis, 1993, Mosby.)

cancer and heart disease are unknown. As a model for radiation protection guidelines, a risk of 1 in 10 Sv^{-1} (1 in 10,000 per rem) has been assigned for the occurrence of severe hereditary effects for the general population by the reporting agencies, based only on animal data.[6]

Embryological and teratogenic effects. The effects of exposure to ionizing radiation on the embryo and fetus are discussed in Volume 1, Chapter 9, Radiobiology. NCRP No. 115 primarily addresses the probability of radiation effects on the fetal brain and the possible induction of childhood cancer. The NCRP assigned an overall risk estimate of 0.4 per Gy (4 in 1000 per cGy). Both linear and linear-quadratic responses were considered in forming this estimate. In addition, there may be threshold doses below which these effects will not be observed. The thresholds are related to gestational age and are estimated to be 0.12 to 0.23 Gy (12 to 23 cGy) for 8 to 16 weeks after conception and 0.23 Gy (230 cGy) for 16 to 25 weeks after conception.[6]

The NCRP further estimates that the total detriment from all causes resulting from exposure to low LET radiation is approximately 7 in 10^{-2} per Sv (7 in 10,000 per rem) for the general population and about 6 in 10^{-2} Sv (6 in 10,000 per rem) for the working population. This overall risk estimate includes fatal and nonfatal cancers, severe hereditary effects, and nonspecific life shortening.[6] These risks are higher than the previous estimates discussed in NCRP Report 91, "Recommendations on Limits for Exposure to Ionizing Radiation" (1987), which assigned a nominal lifetime somatic risk of 1 in 10^{-2} per Sv (1 in 10,000 per rem) for adults.[4] It is likely that these estimates will change again as more data become available.

There are many uncertainties in assigning risk estimates for the effect of ionizing radiation on humans. These include difficulties in assigning individual doses; choice of appropriate control groups; choice of an appropriate extrapolation model; determination of differences between effects at low dose rates compared to effects at high dose rates; and difficulties with the transfer of risk estimates from one population to another. However, these projections are necessary to develop recommendations for radiation protection standards.

Regulatory concepts

ALARA. Regardless of which models are used to estimate the risks of radiation exposure, it is universally agreed that the less radiation received, the lower the risk. For this reason, it is considered prudent to attempt to maintain exposures **as l**ow **as r**easonably **a**chievable (**ALARA**), in keeping with economic and social factors. In practice, this means that measures should be taken, whenever possible, to reduce individual exposures well below regulatory limits.

Comparable risk. The NCRP believes that a radiation worker should be at no higher risk of death from his or her employment than a worker in other "safe" industries. A "safe" industry is defined as one in which the annual accidental fatality rate is about 10^{-4} (or 1/10,000 per year). The NCRP has made an attempt to compare injuries, illnesses, and accidental death rates in various work places to the risks of ionizing radiation, specifically, cancer induction and severe hereditary effects. This is a difficult task, in part because of the latent nature of these effects. The effective dose equivalent limits specified by the NCRP reflect the average annual doses received by radiation workers and the risks associated with those doses that we have already discussed.

Genetically significant dose. The **genetically significant dose (GSD)** is a measure of the genetic risk to a population as a whole from exposure to ionizing radiation of some or all members of that population. It is the **effective dose equivalent** to the gonads weighted for age and sex distribution. The GSD is the gonadal dose that, if received by every member of the population, would be expected to result in the same total genetic effect on the population as the sum of the individual doses actually received. Everyone does not contribute equally to the GSD. For example, the dose received by a 60-year-old postmenopausal woman would have no impact on the genetic future of a given population. The weighting factor for that person would be zero. The dose received by a teenager would have a much higher impact, since there is a long reproductive life ahead for that person. The weighting factor assigned to the dose for the teenager would reflect the number of children he or she would likely produce. All sources of natural and manmade ionizing radiation contribute some dosage to the GSD. NCRP Report 93 ("Ionizing Radiation Exposure of the Population of the United States") reports the GSD for the United States circa 1980-1982 was 1.3 mSv (130 mrem), of which 1.0 mSv (100 mrem) results from natural sources.

Dose limits

The recommended effective dose equivalent limits for radiation workers and the general public are contained in NCRP

Report 91 and have been adopted by the NRC and most states. These limits are summarized in Table 4-3.* There are two important points to note about these values: (1) the limits are exclusive of medical exposures for both radiation workers and the general public and (2) the limits are a summation of both internal and external exposures.

Radiation workers. It can be seen from Table 4-3 that the effective dose equivalent (whole body) limit for radiation workers is more than that for the general public. There are relatively few radiation workers, and it is felt that a slightly increased risk to this group is worth the benefits of radiation to society at large. The same situation occurs in other occupations, such as nursing, driving a truck, or doing construction work, where the amount of risk is similar or even higher.

The effective dose equivalent, which is the limit for stochastic effects, is 50 mSv (5 rem) per year. Nonstochastic limits are set at 150 mSv (15 rem) for the lens of the eye and 500 mSv (50 rem) for all other tissues and organs, including extremities. There are special guidelines for planned special exposures and emergency situations. In general, if the limit for the whole body dose is met by adherence to radiation safety standards at a medical facility, then the nonstochastic limits will also be met.

General public. The NCRP recommends that the annual effective dose equivalent limit for this population be 1 mSv (0.1 rem) for persons who are exposed continuously or frequently and 5 mSv (0.5 rem) for persons who are infrequently exposed. These limits do not include doses from natural background radiation or medical procedures, which in most cases cannot be controlled.

Embryo/fetus. The total dose equivalent for an embryo or fetus is 5 mSv (0.5 rem) during the gestational period. It is recommended that the exposure be distributed uniformly with respect to time and should not exceed 0.5 mSv (0.05 rem) in any month.

Personnel monitoring

Monitoring of the radiation dose received by individual radiation workers serves several purposes: (1) It allows the worker to know how much radiation he or she is receiving (at least in the area where the monitor is kept or worn); (2) it allows the facility safety officer and administration to determine if certain areas or workers are receiving more radiation than expected; and (3) it provides a permanent record of radiation received if questions arise at a later time. The NRC and most state regulatory agencies require individuals to be monitored if it is expected that 10% of the effective dose equivalent limit will be exceeded.

*The NCRP has published a more recent report (NCRP #116, Limitation of exposure to Ionizing Radiation, 1993) Which has some minor changes in the methodology and recommendations compared to NCRP #91. However, the recommendations on NCRP #116 have not yet been adopted by most regulatory bodies.

Table 4-3	Summary of NCRP recommendations*		
A. Occupational exposures (annual)[†]			
1. Effective dose equivalent limit (stochastic effects)		50 mSv	(5 rem)
2. Dose equivalent limits for tissues and organs (nonstochastic effects)			
a. Lens of eye		150 mSv	(15 rem)
b. All others (e.g., red bone marrow, breast, lung, gonads, skin, and extremities)		500 mSv	(50 rem)
3. Guidance: cumulative exposure		10 mSv × age in years	(1 rem × age in years)
B. Planned special occupational exposure, effective dose equivalent limit[†]			
C. Guidance for emergency occupational exposure[†]			
D. Public exposures (annual)			
1. Effective dose equivalent limit, continuous or frequent exposure[†]		1 mSv	(0.1 rem)
2. Effective dose equivalent limit, infrequent exposure[†]		5 mSv	(0.5 rem)
3. Remedial action recommended when:			
a. Effective dose equivalent[‡]		>5 mSv	(>0.5 rem)
b. Exposure to radon and its decay products[§]		>0.007 Jhm^{-3}	(>2 WLM)
4. Dose equivalent limits for lens of eye, skin, and extremities[†]		50 mSv	(5 rem)
E. Education and training exposures (annual)[†]			
1. Effective dose equivalent limit		1 mSv	(0.1 rem)
2. Dose equivalent limit for lens of eye, skin, and extremities		50 mSv	(5 rem)
F. Embryo-fetus exposures[†]			
1. Total dose equivalent limit		5 mSv	(0.5 rem)
2. Dose equivalent in a month		0.5 mSv	(0.05 rem)
G. Negligible individual risk level (annual)[†]			
Effective dose equivalent per source or practice		0.01 mSv	(0.001 rem)

From National Council on Radiation Protection and Measurements: Report #116. *Limitations of exposure to ionizing radiation*, 1993, Bethesda, MD.
*Excluding medical exposures.
[†]Sum of external and internal exposures.
[‡]Including background but excluding internal exposures.
[§]WLM stands for working level month and refers to a cumulative exposure for a working month (170 hr). As applied to radon and its daughter products, 1 WLM represents the cumulative exposure experienced in a 170-hour period caused by a radon concentration of 100 pCi/L. The occupational limit for miners is 4 WLM/yr, which results in an absorbed dose equivalent of approximately 0.15 Sv (15 rem) per year.

To be effective, devices used for personnel monitoring must be reasonably accurate, inexpensive, and easy to use. Three examples of such devices are the film badge dosimeter, the TLD, and the pocket ionization chamber (pocket dosimeter). The methods by which these devices work were described earlier in this chapter.

A **film badge** is the most commonly used personnel monitoring device in medical facilities, especially if only one monitor is to be used. It is relatively inexpensive and is certainly easy to use. The filters within the film holder allow energy discrimination to be made, which in turn allows estimates to be made of the doses received at different tissue depths. In particular, film badge readings may be used to estimate the deep dose equivalent (the dose received at a depth of 1 cm), the eye dose equivalent (that received at the depth of the lens of the eye, taken to be 0.3 cm), and the shallow dose equivalent (that received at a depth of 0.007 cm). The overall accuracy of the film badge is about ± 20%, and erroneous readings can result if the badge is not read for a long period of time or if the film is exposed to heat and/or humidity. In addition, for most facilities the film badges cannot be read immediately, so there is always a lag between the time of exposure and the receipt of the readings.

Thermoluminescent dosimeters respond to radiation more like tissue than film does, which results in readings that are potentially more accurate. However, it is not possible to estimate the energy (or energy components) of the radiation beam. The TLD is less susceptible to the effects of temperature and humidity compared to film, but the individual dosimeters are more expensive than film. TLDs are primarily used in ring and wrist badges because of their small size. Like film, TLDs are usually sent out to be read, with a waiting period for receipt of the results.

Pocket ionization chambers (pocket dosimeters) can be read immediately, which is a significant benefit, but they are subject to erroneous readings if exposed to humidity or mechanical shock. Their initial cost is high, but once obtained, the operating cost is low, so use of pocket dosimeters over a long period can be cost-effective when compared to the use of film badges.

PRACTICAL RADIATION PROTECTION— EXTERNAL BEAM

The radiation beams produced by radiation therapy equipment, such as linear accelerators, betatrons, and even cobalt 60 units, are much more intense than those produced by conventional x-ray units. In addition, the energy of the beams is much higher, and thus the radiation is more penetrating. For these reasons, extra care must be taken by facility designers and operators to be sure that the radiation exposure to patients, personnel in the department, and the general public is kept ALARA. The time-honored methods of radiation protection are *time, distance,* and *shielding*. In addition, there are several safety devices that contribute to the safe operation of radiation therapy facilities.

Time

As expected, the less time one is exposed to radiation, the less dose is acquired. From a practical point of view, there is little opportunity to use this method in a radiation therapy department, since all personnel are outside the therapy room when the equipment is operated. However, cobalt 60 units continuously emit small amounts of radiation even when the source is in the off position (by regulation the *maximum* level cannot exceed 10 mR/hr at any point 1 meter from the source, and the *average* level cannot exceed 2 mR/hr at 1 meter from the source). Therefore it is prudent to spend as little time near the head of a cobalt 60 unit as practicable, consistent with the need to properly position the patient and any accessories. Brachytherapy patients also emit radiation after the sources have been implanted, so that the time spent near such patients should be minimized.

Distance

Increasing the distance from a source of radiation can drastically reduce the radiation exposure. If the source is small, the inverse square law applies, and doubling the distance from the source reduces the exposure to one quarter its original level (Fig. 4-9). If the distance is tripled, the reduction factor is nine. Even if the source is relatively large, the radiation level will fall off with distance. Again, the major applications of this method of protection are around cobalt 60 units and brachytherapy patients, since for all other therapy units the operator will be outside the treatment room during operation of the unit.

Shielding

Shielding is the most important method for protection of operators and members of the general public in a radiation therapy department. The shielding requirements for superficial x-ray therapy units are similar to those for conventional x-ray units, since the energies are similar. However, all other external beam therapy units produce radiation beams of higher energy, and the shielding requirements are consequentially greater. The choice of shielding material depends on the energy of the beam. Lead is the preferred material for

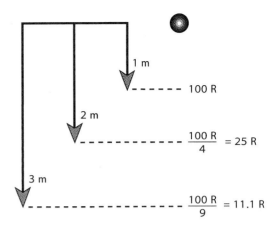

Fig. 4-9 Radiation exposure. Radiation exposure from a small source is dependent on the inverse square of the distance from the source. For example, if the distance is doubled, the exposure is reduced to one-fourth its original value.

superficial units because it is more effective than concrete or steel at stopping photons at these low energies, where photoelectric collisions dominate. At higher energies, where Compton interactions dominate (which includes cobalt 60 units, linear accelerators, and betatrons), all materials attenuate radiation equally gram for gram, and the choice of material is usually based on economic and space factors. Stated another way, a given wall may be shielded by equal *masses* of concrete, steel, or lead. Because of the different densities of these materials, the *thickness* required will be different for each material. Half-value layers for several materials at different energies are listed in Table 4-4. For cobalt 60 radiation, a 1-meter (3.28-feet) thick wall of concrete may be replaced by 0.30 meter (1.0 foot) of iron or 0.21 meter (8.2

| Table 4-4 | Half-value layers: approximate values obtained at high attenuation for the indicated peak voltage values under broad beam conditions* | | |

| Peak voltage (kV) | Attenuation material HVL | | |
	Lead (mm)	Concrete (cm)	Iron (cm)
50	0.06	0.43	
100	0.27	1.6	
300	1.47	3.1	
500	3.6	3.6	
1000	7.9	4.4	
6000	16.9	10.4	3.0
10,000	16.6	11.9	3.2
Cesium 137	6.5	4.8	1.6
Cobalt 60	12.0	6.2	2.1
Radium	16.6	6.9	2.2

Data obtained from National Council on Radiation Protection and Measurements: Report #49, *Structural shielding design and evaluation for medical use of x-rays and gamma rays of energies up to 10 MeV,* Bethesda, MD, 1976, NCRP Publications.
*Note: With low attenuation these values will be significantly less.

inches) of lead (Fig. 4-10). If space is at a premium (for example, when an existing room is being upgraded), lead or steel may be preferred, even though they are usually much more expensive than concrete. On the other hand, for new construction, concrete is usually the material of choice because of its relatively low cost.

In calculating the shielding requirements for any radiation-producing machine, several factors must be taken into account. These include the **workload** (W) of the machine (how many patients will be treated per week and how much radiation will be given to each one); the primary beam **use factor** (U) for each wall (the fraction of time of use the beam will be aimed at the wall); the **occupancy factor** (T) for each area adjacent to the therapy room (the fraction of time the area will be occupied); the distance (d) from the source of radiation to the occupied area; and the effective dose equivalent limit (P) for the occupied area (radiation worker or general public). Table 4-5 summarizes the parameters that must be considered in shielding design. Consideration must be given to scatter radiation from the patient and leakage radiation from the head as well as to the primary beam. If the primary beam is intercepted by a beamstopper, the transmission through the beamstopper must be taken into account.

Workload. Workloads for superficial and orthovoltage x-ray units are usually specified in mA-min/week and may be determined from an estimate of the beam on time for each patient, the mA used, and the number of treatments per week. For cobalt 60 units and other high energy units, the workload

Table 4-5	Summary of shielding parameters
Workload (W)	Number of patients per week × Amount of radiation for each
Primary beam use factor for each wall (U)	Fraction of time the beam is aimed at a particular wall
Occupancy factor (T)	Fraction of time area will be occupied
Distance (d)	Distance from the source of radiation to occupied area
Effective dose equivalent limit	Limit for occupied area; radiation worker or general public

is usually specified in cGy per week at the isocenter. This number can be determined from the number of treatments given per week and the dose delivered to the isocenter for each one. For a typical linear accelerator, 200 patients may be treated per week (40 per day) and the isocenter dose may be 300 cGy, which yields a workload figure of 60,000 cGy per week at isocenter.

Use factor. In conventional x-ray rooms the equipment is pointed down most of the time, and, except in chest rooms, the primary beam is rarely aimed at the walls and almost never at the ceiling. Even in fluoroscopy rooms when the beam is aimed up, it must be intercepted by a barrier so no radiation reaches the ceiling. In radiation therapy rooms, on the other hand, the situation is very different. During anteroposterior or posteroanterior (AP/PA) treatments, for example, the primary beam is alternately aimed down and up. Furthermore, many treatments are given with lateral, oblique, and even rotational beams, so radiation may be aimed at the floor, ceiling, and at least two of the four walls within the room. For these reasons the **use factors** for therapy differ from those used with conventional x-rays. Ideally the use factors (which can range from 0 to 1) should be determined from knowledge about how the equipment is actually used. However, if these values are not known, the use factors recommended by the NCRP in Report No. 49, "Structural Shielding Design and Evaluation for Medical Use of X Rays and Gamma Rays of Energies Up to 10 MeV" (1976), may be used. These are 1 (100%) for the floor, ¼ for each wall that may be struck by the primary beam, and ¼ for the ceiling, if the beam can be pointed at the ceiling.[3] It can be seen that these figures add up to more than 100%. This overestimate of use is one of many conservative assumptions used in shielding design. It should also be noted that the use factors just discussed apply to the *primary* beam. Both scatter and leakage radiation impact all surfaces of the room, so the use factor for these sources of radiation is always 1.

Occupancy factor. If the area on the other side of a treatment room wall were totally unoccupied (for example, if it were below grade and the earth extended for a distance of many meters), no shielding would be required. Similarly, an

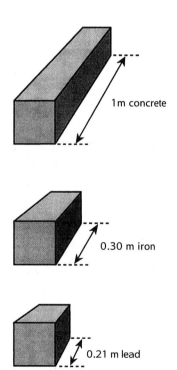

Fig. 4-10 Thicknesses of various materials. These thicknesses provide equal attenuation for a cobalt 60 source.

area that will be occupied all the time the machine is in operation would require considerable shielding. The **occupancy factor** is the fraction of time an area adjacent to the therapy room is occupied. Values can range from 0 to 1. Again, the best occupancy factors are those derived from knowledge about the occupancy of surrounding areas (including allowance for changes in the future). In the absence of such knowledge the recommendations of NCRP Report 49 may be used. These are 1 for offices, laboratories, nurses' stations, etc.; ¼ for corridors, rest rooms, unattended parking lots, etc; and 1/16 for waiting rooms, toilets, stairways, outside pedestrian areas, etc.[3]

Distance. As already mentioned, the greater the distance a person is from a source of radiation, the less radiation is received. Thus adjacent areas that are far from the sources of radiation in a treatment room will receive less radiation than those which are closer, and less shielding will be required. The primary beam distance is measured from the source to the appropriate surface when the machine is pointed toward that surface. For scatter radiation, both the distance from the source to the patient and the distance from the patient to the appropriate surface must be considered. In addition, the fraction of the radiation incident on the patient that is scattered must also be considered. This fraction depends on the incident beam energy and the scatter angle. Values are tabulated in NCRP Report 49. For leakage radiation, the most appropriate distance is the distance from the source to the appropriate wall, when the head of the machine is *closest* to that surface.

Effective dose equivalent limits. As discussed earlier, radiation workers have different effective dose equivalent limits than members of the general public. In general, the shielding requirements for areas that will only be frequented by radiation workers or areas under positive control by a radiation worker (restricted areas) will not require as much shielding as areas accessible to the general public (unrestricted areas). However, in many cases the shielding design for restricted areas is based on the limits for unrestricted areas in the name of ALARA.

The application of the values obtained for each of the factors already discussed to determine actual thicknesses of shielding materials is a complex process for which training, experience, and judgment are required. In the case of shielding designs for cobalt 60 units, the person performing the design must be approved by the NRC or an agreement state. Similarly, shielding designs for linear accelerators must be performed, in most cases, by persons approved by the state.

Partly as a result of the recent reductions in the effective dose equivalent limit for the general public, several groups have reexamined the conservative assumptions that have been made in obtaining values for workloads, use factors, and occupancy factors, and changes in the methodology for performing shielding calculations may be published in the near future.

Safety equipment

Because of the high levels of radiation that exist within the treatment room, no one but the patient is allowed to be in the room during the treatment. The NRC and virtually all states have additional regulations designed to protect both the operator of the equipment and the patient.

Warning signs. Entrance doors to therapy rooms must be posted with signs to warn anyone about to enter the room that radiation might be present. Because the levels in the room can exceed 1 mSv (100 mrem) in 1 hour, the room must have a sign posted that says "Caution, High Radiation Area." In some cases the radiation levels may be in excess of 5 Gy (500 cGy) in 1 hour, in which case the sign is supposed to read, "Grave Danger, Very High Radiation Area." This wording seems singularly inappropriate for a medical facility.

Warning lights. Beam on light indicators are required on the control panel, at the entrance door, and on the treatment unit itself. These lights should be illuminated whenever the therapy unit is energized to alert personnel that the beam is on. In the case of cobalt 60 units a mechanical indication that the source is in the on position is also required on the head of the unit.

Door interlocks. Entrance doors to therapy rooms must be equipped with an interlock that will shut off the machine (or in the case of a cobalt 60 unit, return the source to the off position) if the door is opened during treatment. The circuit design must be such that the unit will not produce radiation when the door is closed unless the operator deliberately turns it on. In addition, it is common to have interlocks on access doors to the machine stands so that if someone is working on the unit it cannot be accidentally energized.

Visual and aural communication. It is necessary for the operator to be able to see the patient throughout the treatment. If the patient moves or shows signs of distress, the operator can turn the unit off and enter the room. For superficial and orthovoltage units, visual monitoring may be by means of a leaded glass window. However, for high energy machines the thickness of glass required usually makes this method impractical. In these cases, monitoring is usually done by means of closed circuit television systems. Care must be taken to position the camera so that the patient is in view no matter what the position of the gantry. Frequently, two separate television systems are used. In fact, regulations require that visual communication be available at all times, so that if only one system is used and it fails, the treatment room cannot be used until the television system is repaired. Regulations also require the availability of aural communication between operator and patient. Again, this is primarily a safety measure for the patient, as it allows the patient to notify the operator if he or she is in distress.

"Beam on" monitors. High energy therapy units are required to have an independent beam on monitor in the room to alert the operator if he or she enters the room when the beam is on. This monitor must not be connected to the therapy machine in any way and must have provision for battery operation in the event of an electrical failure.

Emergency off controls. In the unlikely event that a high energy therapy machine may be energized when an operator is in the room, emergency push buttons are located at several points within the room and on the machine itself that will remove all power to the unit when pressed. The circuits are designed so that the machine will not be energized when the buttons are released unless the operator proceeds through the normal start procedure at the control panel. In the case of cobalt 60 units, means and instructions are also provided to operators so they can mechanically return the source to the off position should it become stuck. This is also an unlikely event. In all cases the operator must be concerned first with the care of the patient and next with his or her own welfare. The dose received by an operator standing 1 meter to the side of a patient being treated at 300 cGy/min will be approximately 0.5 cGy/min. While all unnecessary radiation is to be avoided, the few seconds required to move the table to remove the patient from the beam if it cannot be shut off will be unlikely to deliver a dose to the operator in excess of the effective dose equivalent limit.

Quality assurance. No safety device is effective if it is not working, so frequent testing of the devices on a regular basis is necessary. Such tests are required either by regulation or by recognized protocols. The television and aural communication systems are easy to test daily. Testing of emergency off buttons may cause harm to the treatment unit, so manufacturer's recommendations should be followed carefully. Testing of beam on monitors can be done either by turning the television camera to visualize the monitor or by using a mirror so that an image of the monitor can be seen by the television camera.

PRACTICAL RADIATION PROTECTION— BRACHYTHERAPY

The sources used for implants require special consideration, since, like cobalt 60, they are always "on." A license from either the NRC or an agreement state is required to receive, possess, and use such sources. Sources may be obtained only from facilities or firms licensed to distribute them. Sources must be stored in heavily shielded "safes" in an area secure from theft or loss.

Written directives and inventory

Before an implant is prepared, a written directive must be completed by the requesting physician, and certification must be made that the implant was assembled in accordance with the directive. A careful inventory must be maintained of all sources, and any time sources are removed or returned, a log entry must be made and a complete inventory performed. Inventories are also required at least weekly, even if no sources have been removed from or returned to the safe.

Transportation

If sources must be transported within the hospital, shielded carriers must be used. In most cases the required shielding makes the carriers too heavy to carry by hand, and wheeled carriers are necessary. Whenever sources are moved within the hospital—either in carriers or already implanted within a patient who is being moved—the route should be chosen to minimize exposure to other hospital personnel or members of the general public.

Patient rooms

The room used by a patient with a radioactive implant also requires special consideration. A private room with a bath (if the patient will be allowed to use the bath) should be provided. Placement of the patient's bed should be such that a patient in an adjoining room will not receive a dose in excess of the effective dose equivalent limit for the general public. This usually implies that the bed be placed by a wall adjacent to a stairway or other little occupied area. In some cases shielding may be required on the wall. Radiation exposure to the areas above and below the patient's room should also be considered.

Training of personnel

All personnel who may care for the patient must be thoroughly instructed in radiation safety procedures and the actions to take if the implant is dislodged or other emergencies occur. Nurses should use personnel monitors. Ancillary personnel such as dietary aides, maintenance personnel, and housekeeping personnel also need to receive instruction about radiation safety at a level commensurate with their risk. Personnel monitors are usually not required for such personnel.

Warning signs and surveys

The entrance door to the patient's room must be posted with a caution sign, and visiting periods should be limited (typically to 20 minutes per visitor/day), with the visitor remaining behind a line established by the radiation safety officer. Radiation warning signs are also placed on the patient's wrist, bed, and chart to ensure that no one will be inadvertently exposed because he or she was not aware that the patient contained radioactive materials. After the patient returns to his or her room and/or after placement of the radioactive material in the patient, a survey must be performed of the environs of the patient's room. After removal of the implant, a survey must again be performed to ensure that no sources have been inadvertently left behind. Nothing should be removed from the patient's room, nor should the patient be discharged until this survey is done.

Leak tests

Because it is possible for the material encapsulating the radioactive material in implant sources to sustain damage and leak, brachytherapy sources must be leak tested at intervals not to exceed 6 months. The method used must be sensitive enough to detect removable contamination at a level of 0.005 μCi (11,100 disintegrations per minute [dpm]). Leak tests must also be performed on cobalt 60 units every 6 months. In this case, however, the limit for removable contamination is 0.05 µCi.

High dose rate brachytherapy

Conventional low dose rate brachytherapy procedures require the patient to be hospitalized for 24 to 72 hours. Recently, high dose rate units have become available that allow the treatment time to be shortened. The sources in these units have considerably greater activity than those used in low dose implants (10 Ci iridium 192 vs 65 mCi cesium 137) and therefore cannot be handled manually. This implies less exposure for those who would normally prepare and insert low dose rate implants. But it also implies the need for computer control of the position and dwell time of the sources and the possibility of error or the loss of control of the source. For these reasons, special procedures are required to ensure the safe operation of such devices.

Review Questions

Matching

1. Match the following forms of ionizing radiation and quantities associated with radiation with the descriptions on the right.

___ Exposure	a. Produced by electron rearrangement
___ Activity	b. Produced during nuclear decay; has no charge or mass
___ Absorbed dose	c. Short range, relatively heavy mass, high LET particle
___ Dose equivalent	d. Rest mass is same as an electron, but has a positive charge
___ Gamma ray	e. Product of absorbed dose and QF
___ X-ray	f. Rate of nuclear decay
___ Positron	g. Ionization per unit mass of air by photons
___ Alpha particle	h. Energy absorbed per unit mass

Multiple Choice

2. The source of ionizing radiation that contributes the most to exposure of the general population in the United States is:
   a. Medical procedures
   b. Nuclear power plants
   c. Natural background radiation
   d. Above-ground nuclear testing
3. Which type of device is best suited for output measurements of radiation therapy equipment?
   a. TLDs
   b. Ionization chamber
   c. G-M detector
   d. X-ray film

4. Stochastic, or non-threshold, effects of radiation exposure do not include:
   a. Cancer induction
   b. Cataract formation
   c. Genetic effects
   d. Birth defects
5. Exposure of which of the following people would contribute the most to the genetically significant dose?
   a. 50-year-old woman
   b. 70-year-old man
   c. 20-year-old woman
   d. All contribute equally
6. The annual effective dose equivalent limit for radiation workers is:
   a. 0.5 mSv
   b. 5 mSv
   c. 50 mSv
   d. 500 mSv
7. A G-M detector is 2 meters from a small brachytherapy source and has an exposure rate of 10 milliroentgens/hour. What exposure rate would you expect to measure if the detector were moved to 4 meters from the source?
   a. 5 milliroentgens/hr
   b. 20 milliroentgens/hr
   c. 2.5 milliroentgens/hr
   d. 1 milliroentgens/hr

Questions to Ponder

1. What are some of the sources of natural background radiation? Is it possible or reasonable to attempt to shield or protect the general population from these sources?
2. What are the factors that must be considered in designing the shielding for a linear accelerator facility?

3. Why is it important that regulatory agencies such as the NRC or state agencies oversee the operation of radiation therapy facilities?
4. What are the primary reasons for implementing a radiation protection program? How does the concept of ALARA affect the development of such a program?

REFERENCES

1. Bushberg JT et al: *The essential physics of medical imaging*. Baltimore, MD, 1994, Williams & Wilkins.
2. Hall EJ: *Radiobiology for the radiologist*, ed. 3. Philadelphia, 1988, JB Lippincott.
3. National Council on Radiation Protection and Measurements (NCRP): Report #49, *Structural shielding design and evaluation for medical use of x-rays and gamma rays of energies up to 10 MeV*. Washington, DC, 1976, NCRP Publications.
4. National Council on Radiation Protection and Measurments (NCRP): Report #91, *Recommendations on limits for exposure to ionizing radiation*. Bethesda, MD, 1987, NCRP Publications.
5. National Council on Radiation Protection and Measurements (NCRP): Report #93, *Ionizing radiation exposure of the population of the United States*. Bethesda, MD, 1987, NCRP Publications.
6. National Council on Radiation Protection and Measurements (NCRP): Report #115, *Risk estimates for radiation protection*. Bethesda, MD, 1993, NCRP Publications.
7. Statkiewicz-Sherer MA, Viscounti PJ, Ritenour ER: *Radiation protection in medical radiography*, ed 2. St. Louis, 1993, Mosby.

Quality Improvement in Radiation Oncology

Judith M. Schneider
Beverly A. Buck

Outline

Key terms

Quality improvement (QI) in health care is "an approach to the continuous study and improvement of the processes of providing health care services to meet the needs of patients and others. Synonymous terms include continuous quality improvement (CQI), continuous improvement (CI), and total quality management (TQM)."[11] It is premised on Dr. W.E. Deming's 14 principles of management, which were first introduced in Japan's industry after World War II and into the United States' health care industry in the early 1980s. The Deming principles of management emphasize continuous quality improvement in a product (service) through proactive employee participation in a "customer-responsive" environment.[14,16-18] According to Deming, quality is not only achieved but maintained by the following[16,17]:

- Delineating the health care organization's mission and goals, so that there is a reason for improving
- Instead of setting thresholds, which are expected levels of compliance, always strive for improvement no matter how good the product (service)
- Improve the process rather than "inspect for errors"
- Plan for the future by analyzing "long-term costs" and "appropriateness of product (service)"

- Allow the employee to contribute to the improvement process
- Encourage and support employees through education
- Ensure qualified leaders for the improvement system
- Eliminate fear by encouraging employees to offer suggestions
- Eliminate staffing barriers by helping employees understand the needs of other departments or sections
- Require management to always keep employees informed of what is happening
- Emphasize quality first rather than quantity
- Promote and encourage teamwork versus individual performance
- Encourage and support an employee's educational and self-improvement program
- Support and train all employees in the "transformation process"

Today's **health care organizations** are facing the same dilemmas as industry did a few years ago involving quality control and cost containment. Appropriate utilization of continuous quality improvement assists the health care organization in responding to the problems of "increased competition," "escalating costs," "quality concerns," and "demands for increased accountability."[17] Participation in CQI has been demonstrated to decrease costs, increase customer satisfaction, and ensure quality throughout the health care organization.[14,16]

Traditionally, quality assurance activities were used by health care organizations to systematically analyze the quality of health care services rendered and to meet the criteria for accreditation by the **Joint Commission on the Accreditation of Healthcare Organizations** (JCAHO), an independent, not-for-profit organization dedicated to improving the quality of care in health care settings.[11,26] **Quality assurance** focuses on performance measurement, which is based on the comparison of processes with **outcomes** to **quality indicators**, the measurable dimension of quality that defines what is to be monitored.[5,14] It stresses control and assessment of performance, hence the terms **quality control**, providing standards of measurement, and **quality assessment**, involving the systematic collection and review of quality assurance data.

A continuous quality improvement plan integrates quality assurance, quality control, and assessment into a complex, system-wide improvement program revolving around the health care organization's mission and goals.[14] It eliminates duplication of quality assurance and quality improvement efforts, but still provides assurance that services are of high quality.[18]

Quality improvement in radiation oncology involves ongoing activities encompassing the three major areas of treatment—clinical, physical, and technical—as defined by the American College of Radiology (ACR) and the American Association of Physicists in Medicine (AAPM).[6,13,15] It includes a quality control program to measure the radiation

output and mechanical integrity of the treatment and simulation units and brachytherapy sources as well as quality assessment programs to measure all aspects of the treatment delivery and patient care process. Even the patient care givers are evaluated through a **peer review** program.

Only through continuous evaluation of all aspects of the radiation therapy process can the ultimate goal to deliver quality radiation and patient care be achieved. However, this is not accomplished without the cooperative efforts and commitment to quality of each member of the **radiation oncology team**.

EVOLUTION OF QUALITY IMPROVEMENT
Radiation measurement

Before the process of quality improvement can be implemented, standards must be developed by which one can compare, evaluate, and establish quality control.[20] From the time of the discovery of the x-ray, standards for its measurement have been proposed, starting with the original erythema dose as the unit of measurement and evolving into exact scientific standards for the measurement of the Gray as specified by national and international agencies. During the Second International Congress of Radiology held in Stockholm, Sweden in July, 1928, several recommendations were made, including that an "International Unit of X-radiation" be adopted and that the unit be called the "Roentgen" designated by a small "r." The complete recommendations were published in the report entitled *Recommendations of the International X-Ray Unit Committee,* published in 1929.[21] This earmarked the beginning of quality control in radiation measurements, although it was not defined as such. As technology advanced in radiation oncology, the number of governing regulations increased. There is no comparison between this simple two-page document and the volumes of regulations that currently exist. With the advent of the unit of measure came the standardization of equipment performance with an increased emphasis on quality control. Thus quality improvement in radiation oncology was initially focused on the physical aspect of treatment equipment performance.

Hospital oversight and accreditation

The oversight of patient care in hospitals began in 1917 when the American College of Surgeons (ACS) established the Hospital Standardization Program, and in 1919 "Minimum Standards" were developed (JCAHO, The Joint Commission: *Who We Are and What We Do, Historical Background*, 1987). From 1917 until 1951 the ACS worked to improve the hospital-based practice of medicine. In 1952 the Joint Commission on Accreditation of Hospitals (JCAH) was formed through the efforts of the ACS, the American Medical Association (AMA), the American Hospital Association (AHA), the American College of Physicians (ACP), and the Canadian Medical Association (CMA). With the passage of Medicare in 1965, JCAH accreditation of hospitals increased in importance when the United States

Congress determined that JCAH-accredited facilities would be recognized for purposes of Medicare reimbursement. In 1988 the name of the JCAH was changed to the Joint Commission on Accreditation of Healthcare Organizations (JCAHO) to broaden its scope to include ambulatory centers, group practices, health maintenance organizations, community health centers, emergency and urgent care centers, and hospital-based practices under its accreditation umbrella.

While the original mission of the JCAH was to ensure plant safety in hospitals, that mission has evolved and expanded to include quality improvement based on the measurement of patient outcomes. Initially, JCAHO standards for radiation oncology were included in those for the radiology departments, since the majority of radiation therapy departments came under the auspices of that department, but rarely were the radiation therapy facilities visited. In 1987, however, the JCAHO developed separate standards for radiation oncology, and a dedicated quality improvement plan is now required for each department. The original emphasis was on the quality control aspects of radiation oncology and concentrated on the treatment units themselves and the process used to deliver patient care. Now the emphasis is on "doing the right thing" and "doing the right thing well."[10] Doing the right thing refers to delivering effective and appropriate treatment, and doing the right thing well refers to providing patient care effectively, accurately, in a timely manner, and with respect and caring for the patient.

Definitions

Multiple definitions exist regarding the various components of quality improvement; the definitions used throughout the rest of this chapter are those developed by the International Standards Organization (ISO)[7] and accepted as the American National Standard.[2]

Quality, in reference to radiation oncology, is defined as "the totality of features and characteristics of a radiation therapy process that bear on its ability to satisfy stated or implied needs of the patient." To determine whether quality standards are met, each feature or characteristic of the radiation therapy process must be identified and measured and the results analyzed.

Quality assurance is defined as "all those planned or systematic actions necessary to provide adequate confidence that a product or service will satisfy given requirements for quality." The term is used to refer to the planned and systematic actions to ensure that a radiation therapy facility consistently delivers high quality care in the treatment of patients leading to the best outcomes with the least amount of side effects. All aspects of the radiation therapy process must be routinely and continuously measured, the results analyzed, and corrective action taken as required to ensure quality patient care. This type of review is referred to as a quality audit.

Quality control is defined as "the operational techniques and activities used to fulfill requirements of quality." The term is typically used to refer to those procedures and techniques used to monitor or test and maintain the components of the radiation therapy quality improvement program, such as the tests performed to measure the mechanical integrity of the treatment units.

Measurement of patient outcomes is now required by the JCAHO. This measurement includes not only areas such as morbidity, mortality, recurrence of disease, and survival rates, but also patient satisfaction and quality of life.

JCAHO has replaced the term *quality assurance* with terms such as *quality assessment* or *quality improvement*, since the emphasis is now on the ongoing evaluation of all aspects of care for the purpose of determining areas where improvement is needed. A key word is "ongoing;" hence this program is frequently referred to as **continuous quality improvement** (CQI) or **total quality management** (TQM).

COMPONENTS OF QUALITY IMPROVEMENT
Quality improvement team

The quality improvement team is composed of all personnel in the radiation oncology department who interact with the patient and family. Each individual makes a contribution to the quality of care and level of patient satisfaction.

The JCAHO requires that the departmental medical director be responsible for the establishment and continuation of a quality improvement program. The director may meet this responsibility by appointing a quality improvement committee to develop and monitor the program, collect and evaluate the data, determine areas for improvement, implement changes when areas for improvement have been identified, and evaluate the results of the actions taken. Table 5-1 delineates the responsibilities of the quality improvement committee.

It is also the responsibility of the director to ensure that all employees are qualified for their jobs. Job descriptions must clearly state the qualifications, the credentials or license required, continuing education requirements, and the scope of practice for each position. Institutional requirements regarding maintenance of qualifications in cardiopulmonary resuscitation (CPR) and attendance at infectious disease, fire, and safety seminars are to be strictly adhered to, as well as all radiation safety standards.

Staff physicians are required to actively participate in departmental quality improvement activities, and documentation of participation is reviewed as part of the medical staff recredentialing process. The radiation oncologists participate in these activities during chart review, morbidity and mortality conferences, review and development of departmental policies and procedures, portal film review, patient and family education, and the completion and review of incident reports.

Members of the physics division (physicists, dosimetrists, and engineers) develop and carry out the quality control program to meet the needs of the department and to be in compliance with nationally accepted or mandated standards. They also conduct weekly and final physics reviews of the treatment records.

	Responsibilities of members of the quality improvement (QI) committee		

Table 5-1

QI activity	Goals	Frequency	Reporting mechanism
Develop and monitor a CQI program	Oversee departmental peer review activities	Ongoing	QI committee meeting minutes
Collect and evaluate data	Develop and implement new policies and procedures as needed	Monthly meetings	Chart rounds reports
Determine areas for improvement	Oversee implementation of and adherence to departmental policies and procedures		Policies and procedures
Implement change as necessary			Incident reports
Evaluate results of actions taken			

The radiation therapists perform warm-up procedures on the treatment units, perform quality control tests on the simulation and treatment units, verify the presence of completed and signed prescription and consent forms, review the prescription and treatment plan on each patient before the initiation of treatment, deliver accurate treatment adhering to the prescription, accurately record treatment delivered, take initial and weekly portal films, evaluate the health status of the patient daily before treatment delivery to ensure there are no adverse reactions to treatment or other impending physical or psychological problems that require assistance, participate in patient and family education, and provide care and comfort to meet the needs of the patient.

The oncology nurses perform a nursing assessment on each new patient to determine overall physical and psychological status; evaluate the educational needs of each patient and family to determine any barriers to education; develop an educational program to meet the needs of the patient and family; evaluate the effectiveness of the entire educational program, including the education given to the patient by the radiation oncologist, nurses, and radiation therapists; monitor the patient's health status on a routine or as needed basis throughout the course of treatment; and order, evaluate, and record blood counts and weights according to departmental policy.

The departmental support staff gathers pertinent information and prepares the treatment chart before the patient's initial visit; contacts the patient and/or family to set up appointments and give instructions regarding information or diagnostic studies to be brought with the patient; greets and assists the patient and family daily; informs the radiation oncologists, nurses, and/or radiation therapists of the patient's arrival; answers the patient's questions and gives assistance whenever possible or refers the patient to an individual who can help; completes and files treatment records; and sets the tone for the entire radiation therapy treatment encounter.

Development of a quality improvement plan

A quality improvement plan or program lists the organizational structure, responsibilities, procedures, processes, and resources for implementing a comprehensive quality system. Included in the plan is an audit mechanism to document measurement and evaluation activities to verify that all aspects of the radiation oncology process meet institutional or departmental quality standards, as well as a mechanism to institute change when quality standards are not met.

The plan may be developed and overseen by a departmental Quality Improvement Committee. The objectives of the program are to:

- Establish a program that promotes an ongoing collection of information about important **aspects of care**.
- Utilize the information gathered to substantiate that high standards of care are being met or to identify opportunities to improve patient care.
- Implement action as necessary to modify and improve the quality of patient care.
- Assess the effectiveness of actions taken to improve the quality of patient care
- Report quality assessment activities to the Radiation Oncology staff, hospital Quality Improvement Department, and other departments or committees as requested.[8]

Refer to the box on p. 73 for a summary of the elements in a quality improvement plan.

The first step in the development of such a plan is to identify all aspects of departmental activities that affect the patient's care. Only by following the patient's progress, or flow, through the department can the activities to be evaluated be identified. This process might be facilitated by the use of a **flow chart** (see the box on p. 73). Quality indicators can then be developed for each important aspect of care. As stated previously, indicators are tools used to measure over time, a department's performance of functions, processes, and out-

Components of a Continuous Quality Improvement (CQI) Plan

Evaluation of both quality and appropriateness of care
Evaluation of patterns or trends
Assessment of individual clinical events
Action to be taken to resolve identified problems
Identification of important aspects of care for assessment
Identification of indicators to monitor and acceptable thresholds
Methods of data collection
Annual review of quality improvement plan for effectiveness

comes.[11] Well-defined and measurable indicators help focus attention on opportunities for improved patient care.

QUALITY IMPROVEMENT PROCESS

It is the responsibility of each individual radiation oncology center to formulate and implement quality improvement standards, based on its own "strengths and needs, in accordance with previously developed national, state, and professional guidelines."[13,15] Due to the variations in the "strengths and needs" of each individual radiation oncology center, this chapter will not address the step by step technical procedures for specific quality improvement processes, but instead will refer the reader to reports generated by various professional organizations such as the American College of Radiology (ACR), the American Association of Physicists in Medicine (AAPM), the American College of Medical Physics (ACMP), and the Nuclear Regulatory Commission (NRC).*

Clinical evaluation, therapeutic decision-making, and informed consent

The first phase of the process occurs when a patient is referred to the radiation oncologist for evaluation and consideration of treatment. The radiation oncologist makes a decision regarding whether or not the patient will benefit from radiation therapy based on the pathological diagnosis, clinical extent of disease, physical status of the patient, and the patient's and/or family's wishes. Treatment recommendations are made to the patient and/or family along with details regarding the type of treatment recommended, alternatives to the recommended treatment, the consequences of receiving no treatment, and potential side effects of radiation therapy. A patient can be asked to give informed consent only after a thorough explanation has been given and the patient's questions have been answered.

The validity of informed consent has been, and continues to be, questioned regarding whether it is possible to obtain fully informed consent, since most patients are not able to

*References 1-4, 13.

Patient Flow Chart with Quality Indicators

Consultation and informed consent quality indicators

History and physical report in treatment record
Pathology report in treatment record
Consent form signed by patient or legal guardian
Consent form signed by radiation oncologist

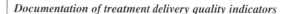

Treatment planning quality indicators

Quality control program for simulator, imaging processing equipment, immobilization devices, and accessory equipment
Quality control program for treatment planning computer systems
Adherence to departmental policies and procedures
Target volume indicated on planning films
Treatment parameters accurately recorded
Setup information, diagrams, and photographs in treatment record
Calculations and graphic plans double-checked

Treatment delivery quality indicators

Quality control program for treatment unit, imaging processing equipment, immobilization devices, accessory equipment, and safety equipment
Written and signed prescription
Approved treatment plan
Comparison of portal films with simulation films
Weekly review of portal films by radiation therapist
Initial and weekly portal films signed by radiation oncologist

Documentation of treatment delivery quality indicators

Adherence to the prescription
Documentation of weekly physics review
Adherence to professional and departmental standards
Completeness of treatment record
Incident/unusual occurrence reports

Patient outcomes and quality indicators

Completion notes/treatment summary filed in chart
Follow-up notes filed in chart
Documentation of treatment outcomes, including:
- Morbidity
- Mortality
- Recurrence
- Survival
- Patient satisfaction
- Quality of survival

understand all the information given them. While various types of forms are used in an attempt to relay information to the patient and/or family, risk managers support the use of forms listing the information necessary for an ordinary person to make a decision based on knowledge of the benefits and risks of the proposed treatment. An informed consent document specifies the area to be treated; states the anticipated side effects of treatment; obtains the patient's permission to perform routine blood tests, to mark the skin with tattoos, to take photographs, and to review the record as part of future studies; and asks female patients to declare whether or not they are or might be pregnant. In addition, there is a statement that no guarantees have been given regarding treatment outcome. The patient or legal guardian signs the form along with the radiation oncologist presenting the information. The possible side effects of radiation therapy to this specific area are listed according to whether they are immediate or long-term reactions.

After the consultation a detailed report is generated that includes a patient history, the results of the physical examination, and the treatment recommendations made to the patient and/or family. The report is signed by the radiation oncologist and filed in the treatment record.

In this aspect of patient care, the quality indicators to be evaluated are as follows:

- History and physical report in treatment record
- Pathology report in treatment record
- Staging form in treatment record
- Consent form signed by patient or legal guardian
- Consent form signed by radiation oncologist

Treatment planning and target volume localization

Once consent for treatment has been given, the patient goes through the treatment planning process. Quality control procedures are routinely performed, documented, and evaluated on the simulator, image processing equipment, immobilization devices and accessory equipment, and treatment planning computer systems to ensure that all is in proper working order according to manufacturer, departmental, or national specifications. Table 5-2 offers a listing of commonly performed quality control procedures and their tolerances for the simulator.

Using information available from diagnostic studies and surgical reports, the target volume is localized. Decisions are made regarding the recommended treatment technique according to departmental policies or protocols, and the treatment fields are simulated. Once the simulation films have been approved and signed by the radiation oncologist, the prescription is written, signed, and filed in the treatment record.

All treatment parameters are recorded, diagrams drawn, immobilization and positioning devices described, and photographs taken to enable reproducibility of the setup on the treatment unit. All physics information is recorded and contours are taken to enable dose calculations and/or the generation of isodose distributions. A system of double checks is

Table 5-2	Commonly performed quality control procedures and recommended tolerances for the simulator (as established by the AAPM)[2,13]	
Procedures		**Tolerance (+/-)**
I. Daily		
Lasers		2 mm
Distance indicator (ODI)		2 mm
II. Monthly		
Field size indicator		2 mm
Gantry/collimator angle indicators		1 degree
Cross-hair centering		2 mm diameter
Focal spot-axis indicator		2 mm
Fluoroscopic image quality		Baseline
Emergency/collision avoidance		Functional
Light/radiation field coincidence		2 mm or 1%
Film processor sensitometry		Baseline
III. Annually		
A. Mechanical checks		
Collimator, gantry, couch rotation isocenter		2 mm diameter
Coincidence of collimator, gantry, couch axes, and isocenter		2 mm diameter
Table top sag		2 mm
Vertical travel of couch		2 mm
B. Radiographic checks		
Exposure rate		Baseline
Table top exposure with fluoroscopy		Baseline
Kilovolt peak and milliamperage calibration		Baseline
High and low contrast resolution		Baseline

From AAPM: Comprehensive QA for radiation oncology: Report of AAPM Radiation Therapy Committee Task Group 40, *Med Phys* 21(4):518-616, 1994 and Khan FM: *The physics of radiation therapy*, ed 2, Baltimore, 1994, Williams & Wilkins.

in place to ensure that all calculations are accurate before filling in the information on the treatment record. The isodose distribution is signed by the radiation oncologist before the initiation of treatment.

Beam-modifying devices, such as shielding blocks or compensating filters, are constructed as prescribed.

In this aspect of patient care the quality indicators to be evaluated are as follows:

- Results of quality control tests performed on simulator, imaging processing equipment, immobilization devices, and accessory equipment
- Results of quality control program for treatment planning computer systems
- Adherence to departmental policies and procedures
- Target volume indicated on treatment planning films
- Treatment parameters accurately recorded
- Setup information, diagrams, and photographs filed in treatment record

- Calculations and graphic plans double-checked
- Beam-modifying devices matched to prescription

Treatment delivery

Quality control procedures are routinely performed, documented, and evaluated on the treatment unit, image processing equipment, immobilization devices, and accessory equipment, as well as on all safety equipment such as emergency switches, door interlocks, and communication devices to ensure that all is in proper working order according to manufacturer, departmental, or national specifications. Tables 5-3 and 5-4 list commonly performed quality control procedures on the cobalt and medical accelerator.

Before the patient is escorted into the treatment room for the initial treatment, the radiation therapist reviews the written and signed prescription, beam-modifying devices, and all physics data to ensure a thorough understanding of the treatment plan. In addition, the therapist performs a final check on all treatment parameters and transcription of numbers. The importance of having a written and signed prescription before the initiation of treatment cannot be overemphasized.

Using the setup parameters and information provided during simulation, the patient is positioned for the initial treatment. Portal films are taken and compared with the simulation films to ensure reproducibility of setup and accuracy of shielding block shape, size, and position. The radiation oncologist reviews and signs the portal films. Portal films of every field are repeated once per week, or whenever there is a change in field position or arrangement, to document continued reproducibility and accuracy of field position. The radiation therapist and the radiation oncologist review the films, making setup changes as necessary.

In this aspect of patient care, the quality indicators to be evaluated are as follows:

- Results of quality control tests performed on treatment unit, image processing equipment, immobilization devices, accessory equipment, and safety equipment
- Written and signed prescription
- Approved and signed treatment plan
- Initial portal films compared with simulation films
- Weekly portal films taken and compared with simulation films
- Initial and weekly portal films signed by radiation oncologist

Documentation of treatment delivery

Each treatment is accurately and legibly recorded in the treatment record, along with documentation of the use of prescribed beam-modifying devices such as compensators, wedges, and bolus. In addition, the taking of portal films is documented along with any change in field size, patient position, or dose to the tumor.

The increasing use of electronic record and verification systems (R&V) has changed the way treatments are recorded

Table 5-3	Commonly performed quality control procedures and recommended tolerances for the cobalt 60 unit (as established by the AAMP and NRC)[2,13]

Procedures	Tolerance (+/-)
I. Daily	
A. Safety devices	
Audiovisual monitor (camera, television, intercom)	Functional
Door interlock	Functional
Radiation room monitor	Functional
B. Mechanical devices	
Lasers*	2 mm
Distance indicator (ODI)*	2 mm
II. Weekly	
Source positioning check	3 mm
III. Monthly	
A. Dosimetry	
Output constancy	2%
B. Mechanical checks	
Light/radiation field coincidence	3 mm
Field size indicator (collimator setting)	2 mm
Gantry and collimator angle indicator	1 degree
Cross-hair centering	1 mm
Latching of wedges, trays	Functional
C. Safety checks	
Emergency off buttons	Functional
Wedge interlocks	Functional
Beam orientation restriction interlocks	Functional
Beam condition indicator interlocks	Functional
IV. Annual	
A. Dosimetry checks	
Output constancy	2%
Field size dependence and output constancy	2%
Central axis dosimetry parameter constancy	2%
Timer linearity and error*	1%
B. Safety interlocks	
Follow test procedures of manufacturer	Functional
Distance indicator (ODI)*	2 mm
C. Mechanical checks	
Collimator, gantry, and couch rotation isocenter	2 mm diameter
Coincidence of collimator, gantry, and couch axes with isocenter	2 mm diameter
Table top sag	2 mm
Vertical travel of table	2 mm
Field light intensity	Functional

From AAPM: Comprehensive QA for radiation oncology: Report of AAPM Radiation Therapy Committee Task Group 40, *Med Phys* 21(4):518-616, 1994 and Khan FM: *The physics of radiation therapy*, ed 2, Baltimore, 1994, Williams & Wilkins.
*NRC recommends a monthly check.

Table 5-4	Commonly performed quality control procedures and recommended tolerances for the medical accelerator (as established by the AAMP)[2,13]

Procedures	Tolerance (+/-)	Procedures	Tolerance (+/-)
I. Daily		**III. Annual**	
A. *Dosimetry checks*		**A. *Dosimetry checks***	
X-ray output constancy	3%	X-ray/electron output calibration constancy	2%
Electron output	3%	Field size dependence of x-ray output constancy	2%
B. *Mechanical checks*		Output factor constancy for electron applicators	2%
Lasers	2 mm	Central axis parameter constancy	2%
Distance indicator	2 mm	Off-axis factor constancy	2%
C. *Safety checks*		Transmission factor constancy for all treatment accessories	2%
Door interlock	Functional	Wedge transmission factor constancy	2%
Audiovisual monitor (television, cameras, intercom, etc.)	Functional	Monitor chamber linearity	1%
		X-ray output constancy vs. gantry angle	2%
II. Monthly		Electron output constancy vs. gantry angle	2%
A. *Dosimetry checks*		Off-axis factor constancy vs. gantry angle	2%
X-ray and electron output constancy	2%	Arc mode	Manufacturer's specifications
Backup monitor constancy	2%	**B. *Safety interlocks***	
X-ray beam flatness constancy	2%	Follow manufacturer's test procedures	Functional
Electron beam flatness constancy	3%	**C. *Mechanical checks***	
B. *Safety interlocks*		Collimator, gantry, couch rotation isocenter	2 mm diameter
Emergency off buttons	Functional	Coincidence of collimator, gantry, and couch axes with isocenter	2 mm diameter
Wedge, electron cone interlocks	Functional	Coincidence of radiation and mechanical isocenter	2 mm diameter
C. *Mechanical checks*		Table top sag	2 mm
Gantry/collimator angle indicators	1 degree	Vertical travel of table	2 mm
Light/radiation field coincidence	2 mm or 1% on side		
Wedge position	2 mm		
Tray position	2 mm		
Applicator position	2 mm		
Field size indicators	2 mm		
Cross-hair centering	2 mm diameter		
Treatment couch position indicators	2 mm/1 degree		
Latching of wedges, blocking tray	Functional		
Jaw symmetry	2 mm		
Field light intensity	Functional		

From AAMP: Comprehensive QA for radiation oncology: Report of AAMP Radiation Therapy Committee Task Group 40, *Med Phys* 21(4):518-616, 1994 and Khan FM: *The physics of radiation therapy*, ed 2, Baltimore, 1994, Williams & Wilkins.

in many departments. The verification portion of the system ensures that the daily treatment setup parameters match pre-entered parameters before allowing the radiation beam to be turned on. The recording portion documents all treatment parameters actually used and the total dose delivered. Since all treatment data are retained in the computer, it is possible to eliminate the paper chart treatment record. As with a paper chart, however, there must be a checking system in place to ensure accurate entry of the prescription and treatment information. It is also necessary to have a computer backup system to ensure that data are not lost should the computer fail.

Any and all variations from a prescribed course of treatment are to be reported immediately to the radiation oncologist. Treatment misadministrations can generally be easily corrected, since a fraction of the total dose is delivered daily,

and adjustments can be made in subsequent treatments to make up for any over- or under-dosage. A departmental policy should be available that describes the circumstances under which a dose misadministration should be formally reported to the quality improvement committee for evaluation and recommendations to prevent similar incidents from occurring in the future.

A physics review of the treatment charts is conducted weekly and at the completion of the course of treatment to check for mathematical accuracy and adherence to the prescription. In addition, charts and portal films are reviewed weekly as part of the peer review process to check for adherence to professional standards and departmental policies and procedures, as well as to check for correlation between simulation and portal films. During this chart review the charts are also audited for inclusion of all required documentation. A check list may be used to ensure that all required documentation is included in the treatment record, as well as to document all chart reviews performed on the treatment records.

In this aspect of patient care, the quality indicators to be evaluated are as follows:

- Adherence to prescription
- Documentation of weekly physics review
- Documentation of physics review at completion of treatment
- Adherence to professional and departmental standards
- Completeness of treatment record
- Incident/unusual occurrence reports

Patient evaluation during treatment and outcomes

The radiation therapist assesses the medical condition of each patient daily before treatment. Any untoward reactions are evaluated and reported immediately to determine whether these conditions warrant delay of treatment until the patient has been seen by the radiation oncologist.

Throughout the course of treatment the patient undergoes a weekly status check with the radiation oncologist to evaluate the tumor response and tolerance to radiation. In response to the patient's reaction to treatment, the patient may be placed on a treatment break to allow normal tissue reactions to subside, the daily dose fraction may be lowered, or the treatment fields may be rearranged to spare normal tissues.

On completion of a course of treatment, a summary note stating the details of the treatment delivered is dictated and filed in the patient's chart, and the patient's return appointment for follow-up evaluation is documented. During the follow-up visit the patient is evaluated for tumor response, as well as acute and chronic reactions to treatment. A follow-up note is dictated and filed in the chart with a copy sent to the referring physician.

Quality of life assessment is a valuable tool in radiation oncology, since survival among this patient population is frequently not a valid measure. How the patient and family evaluate the quality of the patient's life before, during, and after treatment is a more important quality indicator. Areas that may be assessed include relief of symptoms, ability to return to a normal lifestyle, intensity of treatment reactions that interfere with normal lifestyle, or the impact of hair loss on the patient's self-image.

Patient satisfaction surveys are a tool commonly used to determine whether the care received in the radiation oncology department meets the patient's and/or family's expectations and needs. Questions may be asked about various aspects of the treatment experience, including, for example, whether the education provided prepared the patient and/or family for the radiation treatment experience, how much time was spent waiting for treatment or for the radiation oncologist, or the availability of parking. Responses can provide information about the wants and needs of the patient along with information regarding areas that need to be addressed to improve the level of satisfaction and quality of care.

In this aspect of patient care, the quality indicators to be evaluated are as follows:

- Completion note/treatment summary field in chart
- Follow-up notes filed in chart
- Documentation of outcomes of treatment:
  Morbidity
  Mortality
  Recurrence
  Survival
  Patient satisfaction
  Quality of survival

ASSESSMENT OF THE DATA

An integral part of implementing the quality improvement process in radiation oncology is a continual statistical assessment of the data collected. Each of the aspects of care delineated under the quality improvement process discretely collects data through the use of check sheets, data sheets, and check lists. These data should then be statistically analyzed against "internal and external customer satisfaction and placed in a meaningful format such as charts, graphs and histograms and distributed to all employees.[14,16,17] The selection of the appropriate solution or response should be substantiated by the data analysis. This task may be appropriately delegated to the quality improvement committee. However, in a large health care facility/organization, this might necessitate the procurement of the assistance from other "organization-wide systems such as strategic planning, performance management, measurement, budgetary, and management information." By doing that, the health care organization becomes a true "quality organization which continues to improve."[14]

SUMMARY

The transition from quality assurance to continuous quality improvement in radiation oncology is a slow process. The literature indicates that it may take as long as 5 years before any benefits are gained or recognized.[16,18] With the integration of quality assurance into the continuous quality improvement plan, focus must be diverted specifically from the level of performance to the process. This process requires total commitment and involvement from all staff members at all times. Linked to cost containment, increased quality, and the JCAHO accreditation criteria, continuous quality improvement is an unlikely trend. It will not dissipate with the resolution of the factors that led to its creation. It is therefore the responsibility of the radiation therapist and every other radiation oncology team member to become educated about and involved in continuous quality improvement as it evolves because the ultimate benefit goes to our customers, especially our patients.

Review Questions

Essay

1. Indicate who is responsible for overseeing the departmental quality improvement plan.

2. Why are quality improvement programs important in a radiation oncology facility?

3. Discuss the role of the radiation therapist in a quality improvement program.

4. Explain the differences between quality assurance and quality improvement.

5. Describe what should be done with the data collected in a quality improvement plan.

Questions to Ponder

1. Explain why the phrase "If it ain't broke, don't fix it" cannot be applied in a quality improvement program.
2. An initial step in improving a process is defining those activities used in completing the process. Develop a flow chart outlining the steps necessary to complete a specific process in the radiation therapy oncology department (for example, simulation, delivering a radiation treatment, taking a portal film, developing a portal film).
3. Referring to Deming's principles of management, what suggestions would you give a coworker who consistently complains about a specific problem relating to the treatment delivery process in radiation oncology?

REFERENCES

1. AAPM: *Report No. 13: physical aspects of quality assurance in radiation therapy. AAPM Radiation Therapy Committee Task Group 24.* 1984, The American Association of Physicists in Medicine.
2. AAPM: Comprehensive QA for radiation oncology: report of AAPM Radiation Therapy Committee Task Group 40. *Med Phys* 21(4):518-616, 1994.
3. ACMP: *Radiation control and quality assurance in radiation oncology: a suggested protocol. Report No. 2.* Reston, VA, 1986, American College of Medical Physics.
4. ACR: *Physical aspects of quality assurance.* Reston, VA, 1990, American College of Radiology.
5. Earp KA, Gates L: A model QA program in radiation oncology. *Radiol Tech* 61(4):297-304, 1990.
6. ISCRO Subcommittee: Radiation oncology in integrated cancer management. *Blue Book,* Dec 1991.
7. ISO: *International Standards Organization Report ISO-8402-1986.* 1986.
8. JCAHO: *1990 Accreditation Manual for Hospitals.*
9. JCAHO: *Quality assurance standards.* 1992, Joint Commission on the Accreditation of Healthcare Organizations, Radiation Oncology Services.
10. JCAHO: *1994 Accreditation Manual for Hospitals.*
11. JCAHO: *1995 Accreditation Manual for Hospitals.*
12. The Joint Commission: *Who we are and what we do, historical background,* 1987, JCAHO.
13. Khan FM: *The physics of radiation therapy,* ed 2. Baltimore, 1994, Williams & Wilkins.
14. Kirk R: The big picture: total quality management and continuous quality improvement. *J Nurs Admin* 24(3):37-41, 1994.
15. Levitte SH, Khan F: Quality assurance in radiation oncology. *Cancer* 74(Suppl 9):2642-2646, 1994.
16. Lapresti J, Whetstone WR: Total quality management: doing things right. *Nurs Management* 24(1):34-36, 1993.
17. Nelson MT: Continuous quality improvement (CQI) in radiology: an overview. *Applied Radiol* 23(7):11-16, 1994.
18. Sherman J, Malkmus MA: Integrating quality assurance and total quality management/quality improvement. *J Nurs Admin* 24(3):37-41, 1994.
19. Thwaites D, Scolliet P, Leer, JW: Quality assurance in radiotherapy. *Radiotherapy Oncol* 35:61-73, 1995.
20. Van der Schueren E, Hariot JC, Leunens G: Quality assurance in cancer treatment. *Europ J Cancer* 29A(2):172-181, 1993.
21. Wambersie A: The role of the ICRU in quality assurance in radiation therapy. *Int J Radiation Oncol Biol Phys* 10(Suppl 1):81-86, 1984.
22. Wizenberg MJ, editor: *Quality assurance in radiation therapy: a manual for technologists.* Chicago, 1982, American College of Radiology.

Simulation

6

Simulator Design and Operation

Dennis T. Leaver
Patton Griggs
Jeremy Myles

Outline

Key terms

Beam restricting diaphragms
Central axis
Collimation
Collimator assembly
Fiducial plate
Field defining wires
Gantry
Grid
Image intensifier
Isocenter
Optical distance indicator (ODI)
Patient support assembly (PSA)

Pendant
Positioning lasers
Protractor
Simulation
Simulator
Table top
Tensile strength
Treatment verification
Tumor localization
Virtual simulation
X-ray generator

The clinical application of radiation therapy is a complex process requiring the use and involvement of many professionals and high technology equipment.[6] The effective use of the treatment **simulator** is important in achieving the goal of delivering a lethal dose of radiation to the cancer tissue and at the same time reducing the dose to the normal surrounding tissue. In most cases this requires a high degree of precision and accuracy. It is the right combination of high technology equipment, like the simulator, and the involvement of dedicated professionals that can sometimes make the difference between a geographical miss and curing the patient of cancer.

The primary purpose of the simulator is to assist the physician and other members of the radiation therapy team in the treatment planning process. It can be assumed that patients treated for cure may have 30 to 40 separate treatments, and those who are treated for palliation may have between 10 and 20 treatments.[32] Therefore reproducibility of treatment is a critical factor for all patients. A modern simulator, which can support up to two or three treatment units in the radiation oncology department, helps to achieve this goal.[6] Ideally, the simulator should imitate all of the mechanical and geometrical features of the treatment unit. It must do so accurately and reliably. To do this, a radiation therapy simulator uses a diagnostic x-ray tube to duplicate the geometrical, mechanical, and optical properties of the treatment unit.* All the information gathered during a simulation procedure, such as treatment distances, field size, and gantry angles, must be reproduced on the therapy machine.

Although there are various simulators manufactured, the basic elements of each unit are similar. A mechanical C-

*References 2, 14, 15, 24, and 27.

shaped device called a gantry allows the duplication of treatment unit motions. It supports the x-ray tube and collimator device at one end and an image system at the other. The **patient support assembly** (treatment couch) allows the positioning of a patient within the open part of the C-shaped gantry (Fig. 6-1). Essentially, these two pieces of equipment along with an x-ray generator are the major components of the simulator. Additional optical devices, such as positioning lasers and a field defining light, assist in the duplication and reproducibility of the patient's setup on the treatment unit.

HISTORICAL PERSPECTIVE

Historically, radiation oncology began as a subsection of diagnostic radiology. The simulation process also has its roots in diagnostic radiology (remember, the simulator uses an x-ray tube as one of its primary components). Before the widespread commercial availability of the simulator, most patients' treatment planning occurred on the cobalt unit, betatron, or linear accelerator. Competition for space and capital budget requests within the radiology department may have contributed to this initial approach (in the early days) of setting up new patients on the treatment unit.

In the past a "simulation time" was scheduled on the treatment unit or a conventional diagnostic x-ray unit to "set up" new patients.* There were several problems associated with this type of procedure. First, it took time away from treating patients. "Room simulations" (treatment room) required a fair amount of time to adequately estimate the target volume and provide some parameters to ensure repro-

*References 3-5, 13, 17, 20, and 21.

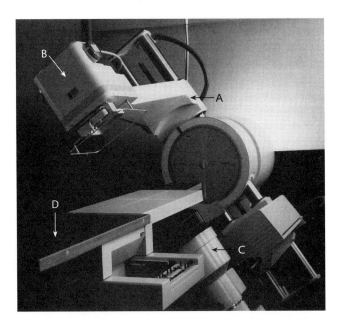

Fig. 6-1 Components and motions of a radiation therapy simulator. These include: the gantry (*A*) (including the collimator head [*B*] and image intensifier [*C*]) and patient support assembly (*D*) (treatment couch). (Courtesy Oldelft Corporation, Fairfax, VA.)

ducibility on subsequent days of treatment. Second, the quality of the planning radiographs (which were a type of port film) were very poor. High energy x-rays and gamma rays do not produce good quality images. In addition, the initial estimates of the target volume (without the aid of fluoroscopy) depended to a large degree on the radiation team's understanding and application of topographical anatomy. Fig. 6-2 illustrates the difference between a simulation radiograph and a port film. The simulation radiograph (*A*), which is exposed using x-rays in the diagnostic range (70 to 120 kVp), demonstrates overall improved contrast and visibility of detail as compared to the corresponding portal localization radiograph (*B*), which was produced using a 6 MV x-ray beam.

The development of the modern radiation therapy simulator was prompted by the introduction of linear accelerators and other high energy treatment units.[14] It was thought that if a machine could be built that duplicated the mechanical and geometrical features of a treatment unit, then the treatment unit could be used for its original purpose—to deliver a prescribed dose of radiation to the patient. Initially, it was thought, the cobalt unit, betatron, and linear accelerator deserved most of the credit for curing or effectively palliating a patient's cancer. It was not long before the benefits of the treatment simulator were also established.

Simulator justification

In the early days of radiation therapy it may have been difficult for a radiation oncologist or radiologist to justify to the radiology administrator the cost-effectiveness of a simulator. Many more patients were treated for relief of symptoms such as obstruction, bleeding, and pain than were cured. In the 1960s, only about one in three patients was cured of their cancer. Today, it may be well over 50%.[7] When radiation therapy began, it was considered a small ancillary part of most radiology departments.

It could be argued that the addition of a simulator would increase the number of patients treated on the therapy machine. Additionally, the cost to society of serious side effects from less than optimal and sometimes ineffective simulation was also a factor.

The cost-effectiveness, increased efficiency, and accuracy of a radiation therapy simulator have been documented.[12,14,15,23] One group of researchers reviewed the records of 97 patients (1970 to 1975) with lung cancer who had survived at least 18 months. All patients were treated with irradiation at one of two Boston hospitals. Three spinal cord injuries were observed in nonsimulated patients, and none were observed in those patients whose treatment planning involved the use of a treatment simulator. This is a small group of patients, but it obviously documents the benefits of a simulator. Spinal cord injuries not only decrease the quality

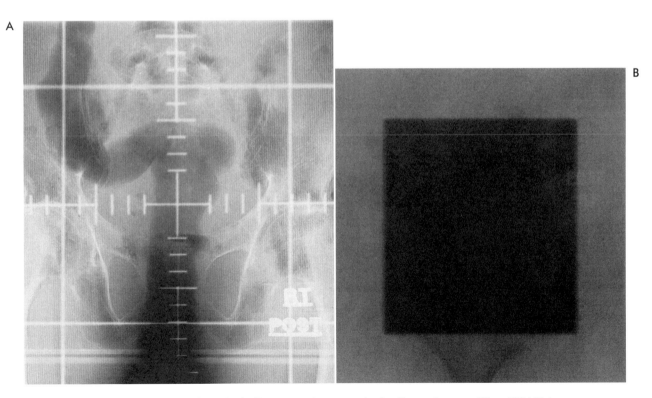

Fig. 6-2 Simulation radiograph. **A,** Exposure using x-rays in the diagnostic range (70 to 120 kVp) demonstrates overall improved contrast and visibility of detail as compared to the corresponding portal localization radiograph (**B**), which was produced using a 6 MeV x-ray beam.

of life for the patient, but also add a considerable financial burden to society.[14]

Increased simulator usage

If a department had a simulator in the 1950s and 1960s, it was most likely homemade or custom built. Fig. 6-3 illustrates a custom built simulator first introduced in Newcastle, England in 1955.[16] This unit had a C-shaped gantry incorporating the x-ray tube and imaging system. A patient support assembly pivoted around a magnetic clutch embedded in the floor.[13] This was probably one of the first simulators used; even in the early days of radiation therapy, some understood the simulators' usefulness and importance.

Since the late 1960s, there has been a gradual increase in the application and use of the treatment simulator. Today all radiation therapy facilities should have access to at least one simulator, whatever the total number of new patients treated.[32] Fig. 6-4 documents the increased usage of simulation equipment through several studies in radiation facilities throughout the United States from 1978 to 1995.[22,31]

SIMULATION PROCESS

The general responsibility for the patient's clinical progress and proper treatment belongs to the radiation oncologist. The technical aspects of treatment such as simulation, dose delivery, and computerized treatment planning are the responsibility of the radiation therapist, clinical physicist, and dosimetrist. The simulation process, which is an initial step in the treatment planning process and involves several members of the team, is an indispensable element that contributes to the effective and accurate practice of radiation oncology.

As a first step in treatment planning, the *simulation process* can be simple or complex, depending on the type of cancer, the extent of the tumor, and its proximity to normal surrounding tissue. However, before any planning begins, the diagnosis of a patient's cancer must be established. This is a crucial step. It may involve a complete clinical workup, including histology, staging, grading, and various studies such as x-rays and laboratory work. Fig. 6-5 illustrates the steps, from diagnosis to patient follow-up, involved in the radiation therapy process. Only after a diagnosis has been established does the radiation oncologist discuss with the patient and family (during a consultation) the treatment options, along with the risks and benefits of such treatment. Simulation and treatment planning may follow, if a decision to use radiation therapy alone or in combination with surgery and/or chemotherapy has been made.

Treatment planning consists of tumor localization (simulation), computation of dose distribution, and fabrication of treatment aids. Karzmark outlines two setup functions of **simulation**: (1) **tumor localization**, which may involve determining the extent of the tumor and location of critical structures, and (2) **treatment verification** using diagnostic quality radiographs of each treatment field from the initial simulation procedure.[8,22] These radiographs, taken during

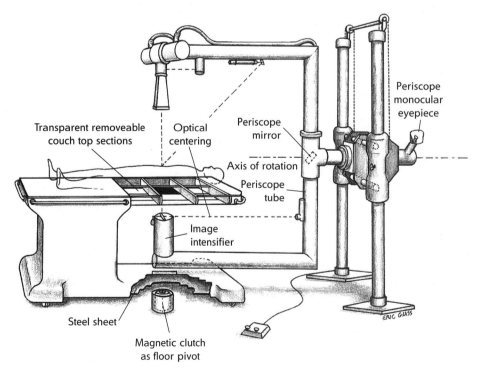

Fig. 6-3 Custom built simulator. This device, used in Newcastle, England, in 1955, shows isocentric capabilities and a periscope system for imaging purposes. (Redrawn with permission from Farmer ET, Fowler JF, Haggith JW: *Brit J Rad* 36:426-435, 1963.)

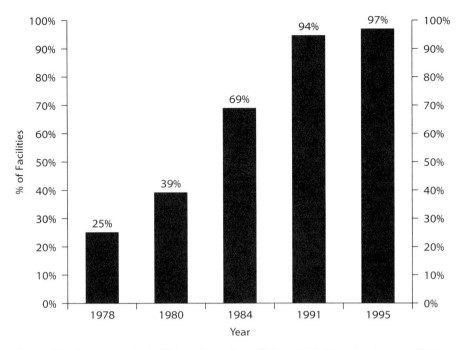

Fig. 6-4 Simulator usage in the United States from 1978 to 1995. (Data for the years 1978 to 1984 from Karzmark CJ, Nunan CS, Tanabe E: *Medical electron accelerators.* Princeton, NJ, 1993, McGraw-Hill, Inc. Data for 1991 obtained from Owen J, Coia L, Hanks G: *Recent patterns of growth in radiation therapy facilities,* poster presentation at the meeting of the American Society of Therapeutic Radiologists and Oncologists, Washington, DC, Nov 1991. Data for 1995 were obtained from Owen J at the American College of Radiology, as an estimate from 1995 data on recent patterns of growth in radiation therapy facilities.)

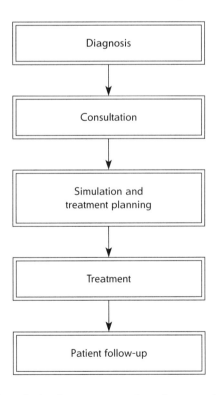

Fig. 6-5 The radiation therapy process. Several steps are involved in treating a typical patient with radiation therapy. The process begins with diagnosis and includes consultation, simulation and treatment planning, treatment, and patient follow-up.

simulation, become the "masters" to compare subsequent port films, which are taken on the treatment unit.

As we will see, the treatment simulator is an important tool in optimizing the radiation therapy process. The following discussion includes the design of a radiation therapy simulator, its theory, and its operation.

SIMULATOR DESIGN

Conventional simulators are designed to simulate the mechanical, geometrical, and optical conditions of a variety of treatment units.[2,14,15,24] This is their basic purpose. It is critical that the mechanical parameters and geometrical characteristics of the simulator match those of the treatment unit. If they do not, a simulator may as well not be used in the treatment planning process.

Simulators have evolved to allow the practice of more aggressive and curative radiation therapy. Design improvements have played a major role in this evolution. Improvements in x-ray characteristics and mechanical performance have contributed greatly to more effective tumor localization and simulation procedures. To ensure that the critical mechanical parameters of the simulator match the geometry of the treatment unit, each department needs a comprehensive quality assurance program. The purpose of a *quality assurance program* is to objectively and systematically monitor the quality and appropriateness of the simulation process as it relates to patient care.[35] The British Standards Institution, which represents the United Kingdom's view on standards in Europe and at the international level, has published a guide to functional performance values for the radiation therapy simulator.[9] The guide, which is based on International Electrotechnical Commission (IEC) standards for the safety of medical electrical equipment,* may be useful in establishing specific elements for a quality assurance program.

The guidelines provided are recommendations both to manufacturers and to users. They provide guidance to manufacturers on the needs of radiation oncologists and radiation therapists in respect to the performance of radiation therapy simulators. They also provide guidelines to users wishing to check the manufacturer's declared performance characteristics. In addition, users can establish and carry out acceptance tests and quality assurance tests to check periodically the performance throughout the life of the equipment.[9]

To create some uniformity in the design of a simulator, certain criteria and specifications should be followed by the manufacturer. Specific design features and performance specifications of the simulator are also outlined in the *British Journal of Radiology* Supplement 23 and an assessment by McCullough and Earle.[6,26] Table 6-1 summarizes the simulator performance specifications in the *BJR* Supplement 23. The box on pp. 87-89 provides British Standard Institution guidelines for the functional performance values of radiation therapy simulators.[9]

*IEC 601-1: 1988, from BSI Medical electrical equipment–Part1: General requirements for safety, and Amendment 1, 1991. In addition, IEC 601-1 is supplemented by IEC 1168: 1993, Radiotherapy simulators—Functional performance characteristics.

Table 6-1	A summary of the simulator specifications	
	Specification	**Description**
Gantry		
Height of isocenter above the floor	≤115 cm	
Angle of rotation at ≤100 cm SAD	>360°	0.03-1.0 rpm
Angle of rotation at >100 cm SAD	±90°	
Isocenter accuracy, diameter	2 mm	
Clearance between gantry and isocenter	≥110 cm	
X-ray head and collimator		
Source-to-axis distance	80-100 cm*	0.5-5 cm s[-1]
Beam limiting diaphragms at 100 cm	50 cm × 50 cm max	
Diaphragm rotation	>220°	0.01 rpm
Beam delineating wires at 100 cm	50 cm × 50 cm max	
Source-to-skin distance indicator	60-150 cm	
X-ray tube and generator		
Focal spot size	0.3 mm × 0.3 mm	
Target angle	≥20°	
Continuous rating of target	500 HU s[-1]	
Generator	3 phase	
Radiographic output (minimum)	500 mA, 90 kV	
Fluoroscopic output (minimum)	6 mA, 125 kV	
Imaging device		
Film cassette and grid	≥35 cm[2]	Manual rotation
Image intensifier	12 inch	
Scanning movements of the image intensifier	±20 cm	3 cm s[-1]
Radial movements of the image intensifier	−10 to −60 cm	3 cm s[-1]
Couch		
Couch top	220 cm × 45 cm	
Rotation about couch support	360°	Manual rotation
Rotation about isocenter	±100°	0.003-0.05 rpm
Vertical movement	+2 to −50 cm	0.1-3.0 cm s[-1]
Minimum couch movement	<50 cm	
Longitudinal movement	−30 to +100 cm	Manual, 2 cm s[-1]
Lateral movement	±20 cm	Manual, 2 cm s[-1]

Used by permission from Bomford CK et al: *BJR* supplement 23: *Treatment simulators*. London, 1989, British Institute of Radiology.
*Extending to 175 cm source-to-couch distance when the beam is vertical.

Functional Performance Values of the Radiation Therapy Simulator

X-ray tube (4.3)*

Focal spot size
    Large   _____ mm
    Small   _____ mm
Target angle   _____ degrees
Anode speed
    With high speed starter   _____ rpm
    Without high speed starter   _____ rpm
Nominal x-ray tube voltage   _____ kVp
Continuous mode
    Without fan   _____ joules
    With fan   _____ joules
Inherent filtration   _____ mm Al

Indication of delineated radiation fields (5)*

Delineated radiation field size at 100 cm
    Maximum   _____ cm × cm
    Minimum   _____ cm × cm

Numerical field indicator (5.1)*

Maximum difference between the numerical delineated radiation field indication and the dimensions of the delineated radiation field

			Values			
		Declared				**Suggested**
	SAD : min	80 cm	100 cm	max		
3 cm × 3 cm to 20 cm × 20 cm	: _____ mm	_____ mm	_____ mm	_____ mm		[2]†
From 20 cm × 20 cm to max, squared	: _____ %	_____ %	_____ %	_____ %		[1]

Light field indicator (5.2)*

Maximum distance between any edge of the delineated light field and the corresponding edge of the delineated radiation field at 100 cm SAD:

Focal spot size	Large	Small	
3 cm × 3 cm to 20 cm × 20 cm	: _____ mm	_____ mm	[1]
From 20 cm × 20 cm to max, squared	: _____ mm	_____ mm	[0.5]

Maximum distance along the major axes between the delineated light field edge and the delineated radiation field edge at 1.5 times the above SAD

Focal spot size	Large	Small	
3 cm × 3 cm to 20 cm × 20 cm	: _____ mm	_____ mm	[2]
From 20 cm × 20 cm to max, squared	: _____ mm	_____ mm	[1]

Maximum distance between the center of the delineated light field and the delineated radiation beam axis for each focal spot size

Focal spot size	Large	Small	
At 100 cm SAD (or nearest)	: _____ mm	_____ mm	[1]
At 1.5 times this SAD	: _____ mm	_____ mm	[2]

Reproducibility (5.3)*

Differences between the measured delineated radiation field sizes at 100 cm SAD for repeated settings of the same numerical field indication of 20 cm × 20 cm   _____ mm   [1]

Geometry of the delineator (5.4)*

Maximum deviation from parallelism of opposing edges   _____ degrees   [0.5]
Maximum deviation from orthogonality of adjacent edges   _____ degrees   [0.5]

Illuminance of the delineated light field (5.5)*

Average illuminance at 100 cm SAD   _____ lux   [50]
Edge contrast ratio at points 3 mm apart   _____ %   [400]

Modified from British Standard Institution, Medical electrical equipment; part 3. Particular requirements for performance, section 3.129, Methods of declaring functional performance characteristics of radiotherapy simulators, Supplement 1. Guide to functional performance values. London, 1994, 1-14.
*Clause or subclause of the International Electrotechnical Commission (IEC); IEC 1168:1993.
†Value in bracket is the suggested value from British Standard Institution; section 3.129:1994

Functional Performance Values of the Radiation Therapy Simulator—*cont'd*

Maximum deviation of the delineated radiation beam axis from the measured delineated radiation beam axis (6.1-3)[*]

	Values		
	Declared		Suggested
Over 100 cm (or nearest) ± 25 cm SAD (or working range if smaller) at entrance surface		_____ mm	[1]
Over 100 cm SAD to 130 cm SAD (or working range if smaller) at exit surface		_____ mm	[2]
Over the maximum range of source axis distance at the isocenter		_____ mm	[2]

Maximum displacement of the delineated radiation beam from the isocenter (7.1)[*]

	Shadow blocks		
At min SAD	0 kg _____ mm		[1]
At 100 cm SAD	0 kg _____ mm		[1]
At max SAD	0 kg _____ mm		[1]
At min SAD	max kg _____ mm		[2]
At 100 cm SAD	max kg _____ mm		[2]
At max SAD	max kg _____ mm		[2]

Maximum displacement from the isocenter of any device for indicating the position of the isocenter (7.2)[*]

Device A		
At min SAD	_____ mm	[1]
At 100 cm SAD	_____ mm	[1]
At max SAD	_____ mm	[2]
Device B		
At min SAD	_____ mm	[1]
At 100 cm SAD	_____ mm	[1]
At max SAD	_____ mm	[2]
Device A		
At min SAD	_____ mm	[1]
At 100 cm SAD	_____ mm	[1]
At max SAD	_____ mm	[2]

Displacement of the delineated radiation beam with changes in focal spot (7.3)[*]

Maximum shift of the center of the delineated radiation field at the isocenter at 100 cm SAD (or nearest) when changing from one focal spot to another _____ mm [0.5]

Device for indicating distance from isocenter (8.1)[*]

Maximum difference between the indicated and the actual distance over the working range of the indicating device (For isocentric equipment, the reference point shall be the isocenter.)

At min SAD	_____ mm	[1]
At 100 cm SAD	_____ mm	[1]
At max SAD	_____ mm	[1]

Device for indicating distance from the radiation source (8.2)[*]

Maximum difference between the indicated and the actual distance over the working range of the indicating device

At min SAD	_____ mm	[2]
At 100 cm SAD	_____ mm	[2]
At max SAD	_____ mm	[2]

Indication of image receptor plane to isocenter distance (8.3)[*]

Maximum difference between the numerical distance indication and the actual distance

At min distance	_____ mm	[2]
At min distance	_____ mm	[2]

[*]Clause or subclause of the International Electrotechnical Commission (IEC); IEC 1168:1993.
[†]Value in bracket is the suggested value from British Standard Institution; section 3.129:1994

Functional Performance Values of the Radiation Therapy Simulator—*cont'd*

*Numerical indication of the radiation source to isocenter distance (8.4)**

	Values		
	Declared		**Suggested**
Maximum difference between the numerical distance indication and the actual distance			
At 75 cm or min SAD	_____ mm		[2]
At 100 cm SAD	_____ mm		[2]
At 125 cm or max SAD	_____ mm		[2]

*Movements of patient support (11.1-4)**

Maximum horizontal displacement of the table top for a change in height of 20 cm when loaded with 30 kg distributed over 1 m and when loaded with 135 kg distributed over 2 m, both weights acting through the isocenter

30 kg load	_____ mm		[2]
135 kg load	_____ mm		[2]

Maximum displacement of the axis of isocentric rotation of the patient support from the isocenter

30 kg load	_____ mm		[1]
135 kg load	_____ mm		[1]

Maximum angle between the axis of isocentric rotation of the patient support and the axis of rotation of the table top

	_____ mm		[0.5]

Maximum difference in the table top height near isocenter between 30 kg load at retracted condition and 135 kg load at extended condition

	_____ mm		[5]

Maximum angle of lateral tilt from horizontal of the plane of the table top as it is laterally displaced

	_____ mm		[0.5]

Maximum deviation of the height of the table top as it is laterally displaced

	_____ mm		[5]

*Clause or subclause of the International Electrotechnical Commission (IEC); IEC 1168:1993.
†Value in bracket is the suggested value from British Standard Institution; section 3.129:1994

Mechanical components

The mechanical components of the simulator include the gantry, patient support assembly (treatment couch), and controls. A number of simulators are on the market today and the choice depends on the need and budget of the radiation oncology department. Some are highly sophisticated computer-assisted models, and others have more basic functions, including some without fluoroscopy. An introduction to the essential components of the radiation therapy simulator will reveal many similarities, especially in their mechanical functions. This may include the gantry, treatment couch, controls, and other ancillary devices such as the blocking tray and safety features. Each of these components will be discussed separately in this section.

Gantry. The *gantry arm* is the rigid C-shaped structural support of the **gantry**. It provides support for both the x-ray tube, located within the *head of the gantry* at one end of the open part of the C, and the image-intensifying/film holder

system, located at the opposite end. These components of the gantry should be constructed in such a way that their alignment with the central axis of the beam can be maintained over the life of the simulator.[6] Fig. 6-1 illustrates the three gantry components, including the gantry arm, gantry head, and image intensifier/film holder. Through 360° rotation the gantry can potentially direct the beam toward the patient from any angle. Its speed of rotation is variable and may be from less than 10°/min up to 720°/min.[28] On more basic models, it may be adjusted manually. In addition, the head of the gantry moves in a radial direction, or up and down, much like the periscope on a submarine.

Before looking at each of the components of the gantry in more detail, an explanation and description of the motions of the simulator, as illustrated in Figs. 6-6 and 6-7, may be helpful to understanding this complex piece of equipment. Table 6-2 describes each of the motions of the simulator illustrated in Fig. 6-6.

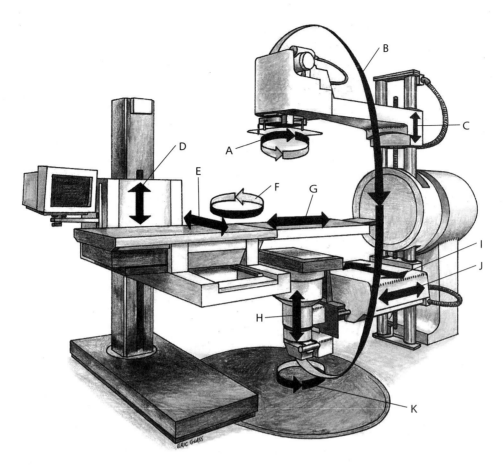

Fig. 6-6 Motions of the simulator. Each letter corresponds to one of the 11 motions described in Table 6-3.

Isocenter. The gantry rotates around a fixed point in space, called the **isocenter**. The isocentric method, proposed by Howard-Flanders and Newbery in 1950, is still used today in radiation oncology.[13] This is an abstract concept. The isocenter should be considered as a reference point in space, a fixed distance (80 to 100 cm) from the focal spot on the anode. If the isocenter is placed either on the surface of the patient (fixed source-to-skin distance [SSD] treatment) or at some location within the patient (isocentric source-to-axis distance [SAD] treatment) in the simulator room, then it can also be reproduced on or within the patient in the treatment room.

In searching for this invisible point in the simulator or treatment room, it would take some understanding to locate it. It could be measured. The isocenter is generally located 80 to 100 cm from the focal spot and between 100 and 130 cm above the floor, depending on the manufacturer's specifications. The distance from the isocenter to the source of x-ray production (focal spot) will be the same from any gantry angle.

The treatment couch, sometimes mounted on a turntable, allows rotation about a fixed axis that passes through the isocenter. Thus there are three axes of rotation—the central

axis of the beam, the axis of rotation of the gantry, and the treatment couch axis—that all meet at a point known as the isocenter.[13] The **central axis** is the central portion of the beam emanating from the target. It is the only part of the beam that is not divergent. In a treatment plan with multiple fields, the central axes of each beam are directed toward the isocenter.

Each part of the gantry revolves around the isocenter. It is like the axle of a bicycle wheel. All the spokes of the wheel have a relationship with the axle. The head of the gantry is always, like the spokes of the wheel, the same distance from the isocenter regardless of its position in space.

The **protractor** (gantry angle scale), located at the central point of rotation of the gantry arm, is an instrument in the shape of a graduated circular device. It is used to measure the gantry angle, which may range from 0° to 360°. Because of a lack of agreement among manufacturers of simulators and treatment equipment on the angular specifications of the protractor, some simulators and treatment units do not correspond in this area. One unit may indicate a 0° reading when the gantry is in the vertical position, and another may read 360°. The International Electrotechnical Commission (IEC) has developed recommendations for linear and angular scale placement

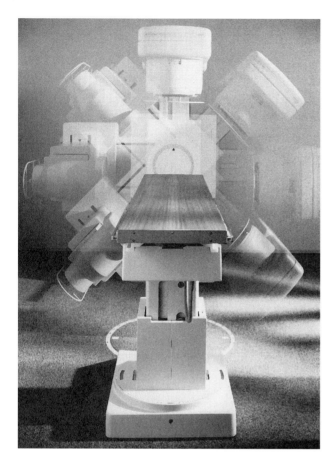

Fig. 6-7 Radiation therapy simulator movements. (Used by permission. Philips Medical Systems, Shelton, CT.)

field defining wires, beam limiting diaphragm (also called shutters or blades), and accessory holder. Fig. 6-8 illustrates the components of the gantry head. Each of these features will be discussed in this section.

Design features of the **collimator assembly** allow it to provide support for the x-ray tube aperture, field defining wires, light field indicator, beam limiting diaphragms, and an accessory holder. Essentially the collimator assembly comprises most of the gantry head, except for an optical beam directing device mounted at the head of the gantry. The **optical distance indicator** (ODI), sometimes called a rangefinder, projects a scale onto the patient's skin, which corresponds to the SSD (Fig. 6-9). This is generally mounted near the collimator. The motorized collimator assembly should rotate around the central axis of the x-ray beam through at least a 220° collimator rotation angle.[6] For example, this allows a 10 × 10 cm square shaped field, projected on the patient's skin, to become a 10 × 10 cm diamond shaped field, if the collimator is rotated 45°. The collimator assembly also directs the path of the x-ray beam toward the patient, after it emerges from the x-ray tube.

Mounting the simulator's x-ray tube onto the diaphragm system is recommended. When or if the x-ray tube needs to be replaced, the alignment of the geometric axis of the diaphragm system is made easier if it is mounted onto the gantry and not the x-ray tube.[6] The x-ray tube used for simulation must have a large and small focal spot; preferably, the small focal spot is no greater than 0.6 mm. To obtain a sharp image of the 0.5 mm diameter field defining wires that are located in the collimator assembly, a small focal spot is necessary. For this reason and others, careful selection of the x-ray tube and generator is significant

Field defining wires are located in the collimator assembly. It is recommended that the remote and locally controlled field defining wires (also called delineators) simulate a maximum field size up to 40 × 40 cm at 100 cm SSD on any treatment unit available. The wires represent the edge of the treatment

and 0° location on the protractor for treatment units as well as simulators.[19] A conversion chart, located near the simulator work area, may be helpful in matching gantry angle readouts.

Gantry head. The gantry also provides stability for the collimator assembly, optical distance indicator, x-ray tube,

Table 6-2	The mechanical motions of the simulator*		
Location	**Motion**	**Major component**	**Description**
A	Collimator rotation	Gantry head	
B	Gantry rotation	Gantry arm	Variable speed
C	SAD adjustment	Gantry arm	
D	Vertical movement	Patient support assembly	
E	Lateral movement	Patient support assembly	
F	Pedestal rotation	Patient support assembly	Not found on all simulators
G	Longitudinal movement	Patient support assembly	
H	Radial movement	Image intensifier	
I	Lateral movement	Image intensifier	Scanning ability
J	Longitudinal movement	Image intensifier	Scanning ability
K	Rotation about isocenter	Patient support assembly	

*Each letter (A to J) corresponds to the components illustrated in Fig. 6-6.

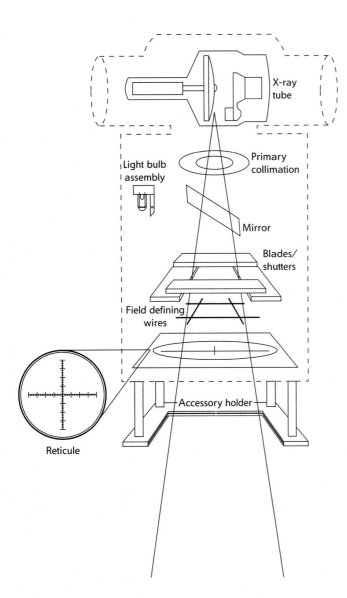

Fig. 6-8 Components of the gantry head. These include the port of the x-ray tube housing, the field light mirror, collimator blades (shutters), field defining wires, central axis crosshairs, and the accessory holder.

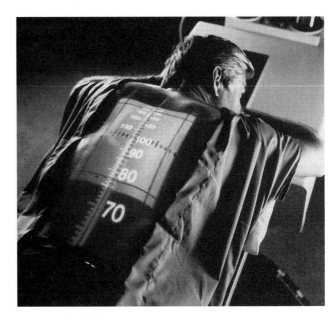

Fig. 6-9 Use of the optical distance indicator (ODI). It projects a graduated light beam, in centimeters, on the patient's skin, which allows for accurate measurements of source-to-skin distance (SSD). (Courtesy of Oldelft Corp, Fairfax, VA.)

field within the larger image that is defined by the beam limiting diaphragms (Fig. 6-2, *A*). To simulate a variety of field sizes from zero to 40 × 40 cm (or larger) at 100 cm, the four extremely narrow wires, each representing a field border, must move symmetrically within tolerance. The scale indicating the range of field sizes at this distance should be displayed accurately within ±2 mm inside the simulator room and remotely at the control panel.[6] Some simulators provide independent motorized movement of each of the field defining wires and beam limiting diaphragms. This allows for the simulation of half field blocks and asymmetric beams. One can understand

the strict tolerance and routine quality assurance that are necessary if you are to depend on this definition of the beam edge.

Also located within the collimator assembly are the **beam restricting diaphragms**, which are made of 2 to 3 mm of lead.[29] They are one of the most important parts of the simulator because the diaphragms define both the size and the axis of the x-ray beam.[6] Beam restricting diaphragms (also called x-ray shutters, blades, or collimators) operate much the same way as the field defining wires. These thin blades of lead define the simulator's x-ray beam during fluoroscopy or during a radiograph by limiting the area exposed. To minimize the amount of unwanted scatter reaching the film or image intensifier, the irradiated field must be kept as small as possible. The diaphragms serve this purpose. Every radiograph should show evidence of **collimation** (restricting the beam with the diaphragms) by displaying a 1 to 2 cm clear border of unexposed film (Fig. 6-2, *A*). Primarily, the beam restricting diaphragms restrict the coverage of the x-ray field.

A secondary purpose of the beam restricting diaphragms is to optically indicate the coverage of the x-ray field. The field light represents the radiation field, so one can see on the patient's skin where the x-ray field will be directed. It does this much the same way it restricts the x-ray field on a radiograph. In addition to restricting the radiation on a radiograph, it restricts a light field on the patient's skin. A special light bulb (usually a quartz-iodine projector lamp), located within the collimator assembly, is used for this purpose.[13] An angled mirror, located above the field defining wires and beam restricting diaphragms, projects an image from the filament of the light bulb through the diaphragms and onto the patient, as demonstrated in Figs. 6-9 and 6-10. Critical care should be taken when replacing this bulb. In fact, each time a field light bulb is replaced (both on the simulator and on the treatment unit), a special test is performed called a light field/radiation field coincidence test. This type of quality assurance test evaluates the maximum distance between the light field edge and the x-ray field edge. At the normal treatment distance for field sizes 5 × 5 cm to 20 × 20 cm the coincidence should be 1 mm or 0.5% for field sizes greater than 20 × 20 cm.[6] It is only through careful evaluation that one can be certain that the light field actually represents the x-ray field.

Fiducial plate. Plexiglas or plastic trays imbedded with lead markers at regular intervals are called **fiducial plates** or beaded trays.[34] These trays, sometimes referred to as a reticule, are positioned in the head of the gantry between the field defining wires and the accessory holder. Because the lead markers, which may be shaped like BBs or small lines, are spaced to represent the geometry of the field at the treatment distance, a separate tray is necessary on most simulators to represent 80 and 100 SSD treatments (Fig. 6-11). Other trays are also available from some manufacturers. Tray selection should be checked before each simulation procedure to ensure accurate geometric representation of the treatment unit (if the simulator supports multiple treatment units with different treatment distances). Magnification can be determined using this type of tray system, since the hash marks or lead beads represent 1 or 2 cm at the isocenter. On some simulators the fiducial tray serves a second purpose. The tray not only helps to document the field size on the simulation radiograph, but it also protects the delicate tungsten wire crosshairs (Fig. 6-10), which are located within the collimator assembly and mark the center of the field radiographically.[29]

Accessory holder. On most simulators an adjustable accessory holder is mounted on the collimator or gantry head. It appears to hang down (when the gantry is positioned vertically) from the head of the gantry (Fig. 6-12). The accessory holder may serve two purposes: a block tray holder and an electron cone adapter.

As a block tray holder, a specific block tray distance must be set on the simulator for each treatment unit to provide geometric duplication of shielding blocks. This distance generally ranges from 40 to 60 cm. It is adjustable to accommodate a number of different treatment units within a single department. There are two purposes to the blocking tray. One is to simulate shielded areas during the simulation process. Thin lead foil blocks or small solder wires can be placed on a Plexiglas tray, which cast a shadow onto the patient's skin. In this way, coverage of any critical external structures such

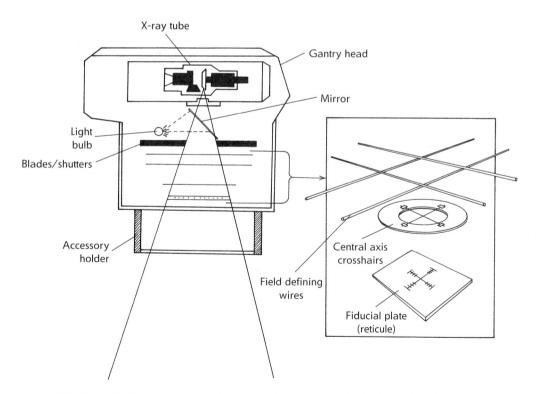

Fig. 6-10 X-ray field coverage. An angled mirror, located above the field defining wires and beam restricting diaphragms, projects an image from the filament of the light bulb through the diaphragms, field defining wires, and central axis crosshairs and onto the patient.

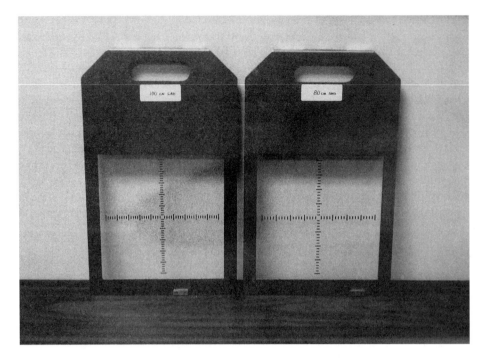

Fig. 6-11 Fiducial plates. Sometimes called beaded trays or reticules, these plates are inserted into the head of the gantry to represent various geometries ranging from 80 to 100 SAD. Notice the lead marks are embedded in the plastic trays and spaced at regular intervals. They are spaced closer together on the 100 SAD tray as compared to the 80 SAD tray and project 1 cm divisions at either distance.

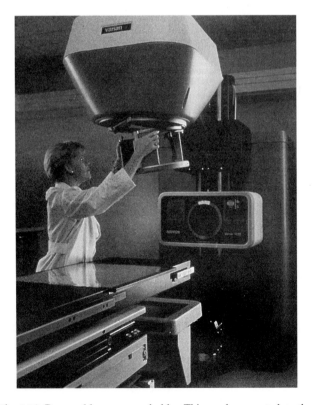

Fig. 6-12 Removable accessory holder. This can be mounted on the collimator head of the gantry to accommodate custom blocks or an electron cone. (Courtesy of Varian TEM, Ltd., UK.)

as the lens of the eye or an involved surgical scar is evaluated (otherwise the blocked area can be determined from a computed tomography [CT] scan or drawn directly on the film). A second purpose is to verify the geometry of individualized custom shielding blocks on the simulator before they are used during an actual treatment. Some individual shielding blocks, which are constructed after the initial simulation procedure, can weigh up to 35 to 45 pounds. The average weight of a set of custom blocks realistically averages around 10 to 15 pounds. If actual block verification is performed on the simulator, the blocking tray should rotate with the collimator head and support this amount of weight.

An accessory holder should also support the weight of various electron cones because it may be necessary to simulate electron setups for the treatment unit. This can easily be accomplished on the simulator if the accessory holder can support the weight of an electron cone and reproduce the geometry of the desired treatment field.

Image intensifier system. Another valuable component, located at the opposite end of the gantry arm, is the image intensifier. This complex device receives and processes the created image, which is a result of radiation interacting with the patient, field defining wires, beam restricting diaphragms, crosshairs, and accessory holder.

A typical image intensifier system contains four major components: the film holder, the image intensifier, television camera, and video monitor. As illustrated in Fig. 6-13, the image intensifier system can scan in several directions. Besides its scanning design during fluoroscopy, the image intensifier also provides mechanical support as a film holder in the radiography mode.

The image intensifier has a frame mounted onto it, which can accommodate a 35 × 43 cm radiographic cassette. The cassette slides into a groove in the film holder, which supports it at right angles to the central axis of the x-ray beam, regardless of the gantry position. This is an important feature that reduces distortion (elongation and foreshortening) in the production of radiographs. Some film holders provide 180° rotation of the 35 × 43 cm (14 × 17 inch) cassette. This is a feature found on some simulators in the United States, so the cassette may be positioned crosswise instead of lengthwise, if necessary, during a radiographic exposure. In most European countries, 35 × 35 cm cassettes are used.

Some film holders also provide a slot for positioning an optional **grid** in front of the cassette to help control scatter radiation. As a rule of thumb, any time the thickness of the body part exceeds 10 to 12 cm, a grid should be employed. All tissues of the foot, hand, lower leg, forearm, and elbow can be adequately demonstrated without the use of a grid. In many cases the knee and upper arm may also be examined using only screen-type radiographic techniques. Beyond this, a grid should be employed both to absorb the scattered radiation emitted from the thicker body parts and to allow the use of beam energies needed to maximize differential absorption between similar tissues.

The image intensifier also reduces object-film distance (OFD). It should be remembered that the image intensifier

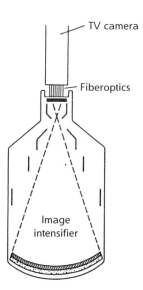

Fig. 6-13 Image intensifier. This device is made up of a glass envelope containing an input screen, photocathode, electrostatic lenses, anode, and output screen. (From Bushong S: *Radiologic science for technologists: physics, biology and protection*, ed 5. St. Louis, 1993, Mosby.)

can move radially (closer to and away from the gantry head). In doing so, OFD is reduced to a minimum during fluoroscopy or for a radiographic exposure. Fig. 6-14 illustrates two radiographs, taken at 100 SSD and the same radiographic exposure technique. However, the source-film-distance (SFD), thus the OFD, has been increased for radiograph B. Note two things as a result. The image in radiograph B is considerably larger because of magnification from the increased OFD. Also, note the overall density of radiograph B is decreased because of the inverse square law (the same amount of radiation has been spread out over a larger area).

The **image intensifier** is a useful tool during fluoroscopy because it converts an x-ray image into a light image. There are several design components that enable it to accomplish this task. Structurally, it is made up of a glass envelope containing an input screen, photocathode, electrostatic lenses, anode, and output screen, as shown in Fig. 6-13. It amplifies the brightness of an image, usually between 500 and 8000 times.[11] The ultimate purpose of an image intensifier is to convert the x-ray image into a video image, which is then viewed on a television monitor. Let us examine that process in more detail.

The primary x-ray beam exiting the patient passes through the table top and strikes the *input screen* of the image intensifier. A fluorescent screen, which is built into the image intensifier as the input screen, absorbs x-ray photons. It can range in size from 12.5 to 35 cm in diameter.[35] The larger the diameter, the less scanning is required during fluoroscopy. During fluoroscopy, light photons, emitted by the input screen (much like the photons emitted from an intensifying screen in a radiographic cassette) are then absorbed by the photocathode. Electrostatic lenses, positioned inside the perimeter of the unit, focus and accelerate the converted electrons. As the electrons are focused, they gain more speed as they near the end of their journey through this vacuum tube containing the cathode and anode. The focusing lens helps direct the electrons toward the anode at the opposite end of the image intensifier tube. As the electrons accelerate and focus toward the anode, they increase in their energy and their ability to emit light at the *output screen*. The output is significantly greater than the input. For example, one 50 keV photon striking the input screen may produce 200,000 light photons at the output screen.[11] Light photons produced at the output screen are then processed electronically through a video system. Located in a small shielded area of the simulator room, the video image appears on a television monitor. The image intensification process simply changes the quantity of photons and electrons, representing the image, at each stage of the process.

During fluoroscopy the x-ray tube current is usually less than 10 mA. This is in contrast to the 100 to 500 mA used for producing radiographs. The kilovoltage (or kVp) used during fluoroscopy depends on the body section examined. Most image intensifiers have an automatic brightness system

A

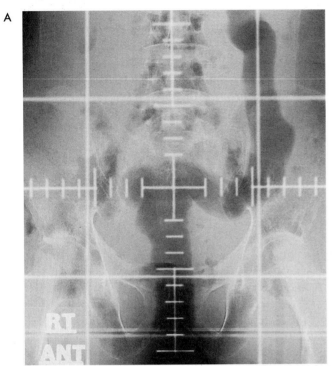

B

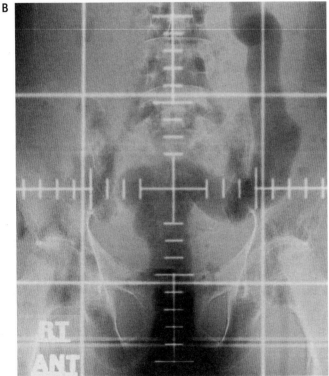

Fig. 6-14 Effect of increasing OFD. These two radiographs **A and B** were taken at 100 SSD and with the same radiographic exposure technique. The source-film-distance (SFD), thus the OFD, has been increased for radiograph **B** from 140 to 155 cm SSD. Note two things as a result. The image in radiograph **B** is considerably larger because of magnification from the increased OFD. Also note the overall density of radiograph **B** is decreased as a result of the inverse square law (the same amount of radiation has been spread out over a larger area).

maintained by varying the kilovoltage (kVp) or milliamperes (mA) automatically during fluoroscopy. Such features may be referred to by different names, such as automatic brightness control (ABC), automatic brightness stabilization (ABS), automatic exposure control (AEC), or automatic gain control (AGC).[10]

Storage of a "still" fluoroscopic image is possible with some systems. This allows the members of the treatment planning team to study and evaluate an image without continuous exposure to the patient. Some systems also allow the electronic image, available for video display, to be digitized through computer enhancement and stored for later use. Digitized images may then be available for treatment planning purposes involving dosimetric calculation. They may also be available at the treatment unit for verification and comparison to portal images created on the therapy machine. The storage and retrieval of electronic images may open the door to even more efficient and accurate treatment of the patient in the future.

The image intensifying system must have a collision avoidance system. This may take the form of a mechanical touchbar/microswitch system, which will prevent the image intensifier from colliding with the patient or treatment couch.[23] A combination of electronic position sensors and some type of computer logic may accomplish the same objective. A computer, integrated with the simulator, can prevent the collision of gantry or image intensifier with the floor or treatment couch by plotting and constantly evaluating the position of each component. Some simulators also come equipped with audio alarms as part of their collision avoidance system.

Patient table top. The device in which a patient is positioned during treatment or simulation may be called a *treatment couch* or *patient table top* (Fig. 6-1). It is essential that the patient table top on the simulator provide support identical to that of the patient table top on the treatment unit in order to maintain reproducibility. Many table tops will support up to 140 kg (300 lb) and range in width from 45 to 50 cm. If the couch width in the simulator is not similar to that of the treatment unit, then reproducibility may become a problem, especially with larger patients.

It is desirable for the table top to be a hard flat surface that minimally attenuates the x-ray beam. Part of the table should enable the therapist to view the patient through the table top when the beam is directed up vertically through the table. This is important in recording posterior and posterior oblique SSDs. Some simulators provide a table top with a segment that can be removed and a section of more supportive transparent material substituted in its place. This may be a square or rectangular section of plastic, or a frame with strings, similar to a tennis or racquetball racquet woven tightly together (Fig. 6-15). After extended use this "tennis racquet" section should be restrung to provide more patient support and reduce the amount of "sag" during simulation. The "tennis racquet" insert, if used on the simulator, may more accu-

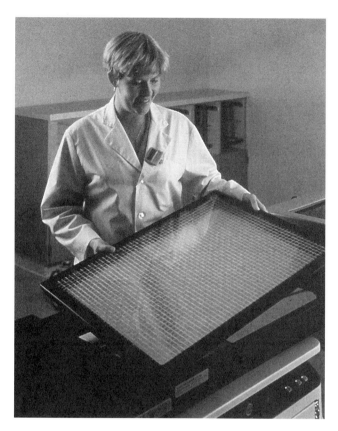

Fig. 6-15 Couch top accessory. This may include a square or rectangular frame with strings, similar to a tennis or racquetball racquet, woven tightly together. After extended use, the "tennis racquet" section should be restrung to provide more patient support and reduce the amount of "sag" during simulation. (Courtesy of Varian TEM, Ltd., UK.)

rately represent the potential for "sag" during actual treatment conditions, where a similar insert can be used. This process may reduce the number of discrepancies between simulation and treatment. Table top manufacturers have developed some models that are hard, flat, and radiolucent and come without metal supports. These table tops are mostly constructed out of a carbon fiber material.

What is carbon fiber material? The material used for radiological purposes, such as table tops and cassettes, is made by binding a fabric of pure carbon fiber with a resin. The result is a material that is extremely supportive with a low density and x-ray absorption. It also has a high **tensile strength** (resistance in lengthwise stress, measured in weight per unit area). Carbon fiber is used in table tops as the outside support around a plastic foam center.[18]

There are several unique features of the **patient support assembly** (PSA), which allows the table top its mobility. A standard feature allows the table top to mechanically move in a horizontal and lengthwise direction. It must do this smoothly and accurately with a patient in the treatment position. This permits the precise and exact positioning of the

isocenter during simulation. Some table tops, mounted on the PSA, may provide the opportunity through rotation of the PSA for patient positioning in two additional directions. One direction allows the table top to be rotated horizontally (laterally) 90° in either direction. For example, if the table top were the big hand of a watch at the 6 o'clock position, it could be rotated to either the 3 or the 9 o'clock position, while maintaining the same isocenter. This type of positioning limits gantry rotation to about 30° from vertical because of the possible collision of the image intensifier with the PSA. The amount of gantry rotation depends on the thickness of the patient and the level of the isocenter. A second motion on some models also allows the PSA to extract the patient from the C-shaped opening in the gantry by rotating the patient on another axis. This other axis is located several meters from the isocenter within the PSA. Experimenting with the various motions of the PSA will demonstrate its versatility and range of motion.

Additionally, a set of local controls may be located on the PSA. These can mimic those of the treatment units as a **pendant** (hand-held control) suspended from the ceiling or attached to the treatment couch through a telephone-like cord. In some models the control panel can also be located on one side of the PSA. In either case, these controls should allow access to the mechanical movements and optical features of the simulator.

Simulator controls. Control of simulator movements should be possible through local control within the simulator room and through remote control, usually located behind a separately shielded area. Local and remote control of the mechanical simulator functions should provide for all motor-driven motions, specifically, the field defining wires, beam restricting diaphragms, collimator rotation, radial movement of the gantry head, as well as linear and rotation movements of the PSA. Scanning and radial movements of the image intensifier should also be located within the simulator room. Activation of the optical features of the simulator, such as the field light, optical distance indicator, positional lasers, and room lights, should be available along with several emergency off switches, positioned strategically throughout the simulator room.

Remote controls, located in the shielded control room, should duplicate those within the simulator room. This includes all of the optical features and motor-driven movements of the simulator along with digital indicators for field size, SAD, SSD, gantry, and collimator angle. Familiarity with all of the simulator's features will allow for efficient and accurate treatment planning. This can become more critical, especially when simulating certain palliative cases in which the patient is experiencing severe pain.

Control area. Within the shielded control area, several components are strategically positioned (Fig. 6-16). This includes the x-ray generator (along with a circuit breaker for the incoming voltage), a television monitor, the remote control panel, and an observation window. It is important that this room be large enough to hold several members of the radiation therapy team, students, and other interested observers.

An observation window, installed along the wall facing the simulator, allows the operator and others involved in the simulation process to view the patient and the mechanical motions of the equipment. Whether the window is made of thick plate glass or lead glass depends on the distance it is located from the simulator and/or whether it is inclined to be irradiated by the primary beam. A 0.7 × 1.5 m (2.3 × 5 ft) size is recommended.[6] Usually, larger sizes can adapt to additional staff and students without overcrowding. The control panel should be located close enough to the observation window so the operator can observe the patient while the simulator is moving.

In addition, a video monitor positioned near the control panel provides ready access to the fluoroscopic image during the simulation process. A dimmer switch, which can control the lighting level in the simulator and control area, is also necessary. Monitoring a fluoroscopic video image without the distraction of overhead lighting is more efficient. It might be compared to watching television in a dark room (sometimes while watching television, the image may appear sharper and more detailed when the room lighting is kept low or turned off). X-ray view boxes mounted in the control room are helpful in comparing radiographs or scans during the simulation process.

The **x-ray generator** is another important component, which provides radiographic and fluoroscopic control of the simulator. Exposure reproducibility, which should be maintained within 5%, is an important consideration for guaranteeing radiographic image quality.[36] The *BJR* Supplement 23 recommends that the tube and generator ratings be 8 to 10 times greater than for general diagnostic radiography.[6] In part, this may be because of the increased distance used in radiation therapy simulation (70 cm in diagnostic imaging to between 130 and 200 cm on the simulator). A three-phase generator is recommended. It should be capable of radiographic outputs of up to 500 mA at 90 kVp, 300 mA at 150 kVp, and 6 mA at 125 kVp for fluoroscopy.[6] A single-phase generator may limit the higher exposure factors needed for some examinations, especially a large lateral pelvis—a most challenging body part to image effectively.

Kilovoltage and milliamperage exposure factors are controlled by the radiation therapist at the operating console. By adjusting the voltage and current of the x-ray generator, exposure factors can be selected. It may appear intimidating to the novice at first, with its many buttons and control knobs, although some systems are equipped with anatomically programmed radiography (APR). Bushong describes the process from a diagnostic radiography perspective: "Rather than have the radiologic technologist select a desired kVp and mAs, graphics on the control panel guide the technologist. To produce an image the technologist simply touches a picture or a written description of the anatomy to be imaged and another indication of body habitus. The microprocessor selects the appropriate kVp and mAs automatically. The whole process is phototimed, resulting in near-flawless radiographs...".[10]

In more conventional radiation therapy settings, the therapist must select the appropriate kilovoltage, milliamperage, and time manually. Most x-ray control panels provide a range of steps (buttons) for the selection of each of the radiographic controlling factors. Technique charts, with suggested exposure factors, are required by some state and local laws. Additional features located on the x-ray control panel include the exposure switch, a possible digital heat unit display, and fluoroscopic specifications. Fluoroscopic specifications may include zoom modes, automatic brightness control, and a mandatory 5-minute timer. The timer is a carryover from diagnostic radiology. It is set at the start of each fluoroscopic procedure and attempts to limit patient exposure (when an audible alarm sounds at the end of 5 minutes) during lengthy fluoroscopy procedures.

It is easy to see why the control room should be large enough to accommodate several members of the radiation therapy team along with students and other interested observers. Field size, gantry angle, exposure technique, and several other important parameters can be manipulated from within the shielded walls of the control room. If the components within the control room are well positioned and accessible, the entire simulation process is more efficient. Detail to room design is a wise investment that will provide many dividends, especially during peak times of the simulator's use.

ROOM DESIGN

The design of a simulator room is a process that must involve the expertise of numerous professionals, including an architect, an engineer, and a radiological physicist. Input should also be encouraged from the therapists and the radiation oncologists in the department. Before designing the room, the site must be chosen. The ideal location is close to the treatment machines. This facilitates communication among all parties involved in the patient's treatment.

Space allocations

The simulator room should be of sufficient size to accommodate not only the machine and all of its components, but also its full range of motions. The equipment will have a longer life if enough space is provided to avoid collisions, such as bumping into walls with the table. It will also be a more pleasant work area if personnel have enough room to comfortably perform their duties. It is recommended that a minimum size be approximately 400 square feet.[6]

Space must also be allocated for a good-sized counter that should include a sink and a work space/writing area. The work space should be of sufficient size to allow for the manufacture of various immobilization devices used in radiation therapy. Cabinets and drawer space for the storage of simulation equipment, contour-taking devices, and spare simulator parts are necessary in any simulator room.

The control area is normally set in one corner of the room, usually near the entrance. This area is designed to protect the operators from radiation and to house the simulator's controls and x-ray generator. It must be large enough for several pieces of equipment, which might include a record and verify system, work area, and numerous personnel. It is important that the operator have full visual and aural contact with the patient at all times. A lead glass window may be installed for patient visualization. Fig. 6-16 illustrates a typical simulator room design.

If space allows, a film processing area should be included in the area. This could be in the form of an adjacent darkroom or a daylight film system. The daylight system eliminates the need for additional walls.

Other considerations

There are several other considerations worth mentioning concerning the simulator. Simulator manufacturers have very specific requirements for ventilation of the room. They reserve the right to negate the warranty if these requirements are not met. The lighting system is also important. The intensity must be adjustable, with independent control of the room and the control area. Visualization of the light field is easier in low light, as is the fluoroscopy image. On the other hand, certain simulation duties need maximum light, such as recording pertinent information, preparing contrast materials, or designing an immobilization device. Task lighting in certain areas, as under cabinets, is very beneficial.

Positioning lasers, which project a small red or green beam of light toward the patient during the simulation process, will need to be installed. There are several types

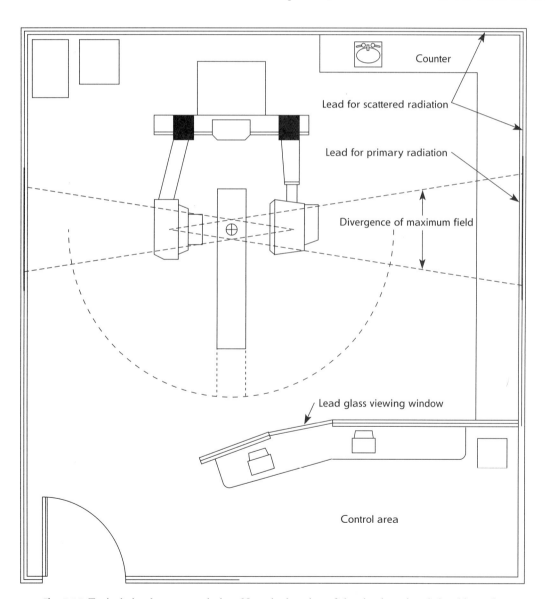

Fig. 6-16 Typical simulator room design. Note the location of the simulator in relationship to the primary barriers and control area with lead glass window.

available, and the department personnel will need to choose the style they feel best suits their needs. Side lasers are more stable if they are recessed in the wall to prevent inadvertent collisions. A third overhead laser is installed and represents the anterior central axis or midsagittal plane when the gantry is rotated from its vertical position. These lasers provide the therapist several external reference points in relationship to the position of the isocenter. Daily checks, which provide strict quality control of the positional lasers, are a must.

Shielding requirements

As with all radiation equipment, room shielding is an important consideration. Shielding radiation rooms is done most commonly with lead or concrete or a combination of the two. Lead is the denser of the two, and less is needed to stop an equal amount of radiation. Lead is also more expensive than concrete and very difficult to support structurally. This is the reason one finds many diagnostic and radiation therapy departments in the basements of hospitals. Shielding costs are reduced significantly by the surrounding earth, and precious space is gained when thick concrete walls need not be built.

All walls may not have the same amount of shielding. **Primary walls** are those that the radiation will aim at directly and therefore need more shielding than **secondary walls**, which have only scattered radiation impinging on them.

Several factors are taken into consideration in determining the required wall thickness. The time the machine is normally aimed at a wall or ceiling is called the **use factor** (U). A standard use factor for a simulator's primary walls and ceilings is $1/4$. Floors are usually 1 because more exposures are made with the simulator in the vertical position. An **occupancy factor** (T) takes into consideration how an area on the other side of an irradiated wall is going to be used. An office where someone could be sitting for 40 hours a week would require more shielding in the wall than a storage closet where workers would spend 10 minutes once or twice a week.

Another important factor is workload. **Workload** (W) for a simulator is defined as the current (mA) times the time (min) a department expects to run the machine in a normal week. These estimates are always on the high side to calculate the largest possible scenario. A value in units of mA-mins is used to describe workloads of diagnostic machines.

The **weekly permissible dose** (P) is 10 times higher (under normal conditions) for people who have chosen a career in the radiation field (radiation workers) compared to members of the general public. The most recent recommendations are 1 mSv/week for the occupationally exposed and 0.02 mSv/week for the general public.[30] Controlled areas are made off-limits to members of the general public for this reason. **Uncontrolled areas** (areas where access is not limited) will have a lower P value and therefore need more shielding.

The calculation of barrier thickness is much more complicated than is shown here, but the following formula is the basis of most shielding calculations:

$$B = \frac{P(d)^2}{WUT}$$

The distance (in meters) from the source to the opposite side of the barrier is symbolized by d. The transmission of radiation through the barrier required to meet the weekly permissible dose is shown as B. This value is then used as a reference (to a graph or chart) to determine the barrier thickness relative to the maximum photon energy and the type of shielding that will be used. See Fig. 6-17 for a sample graph using 125 kVp x-rays.

Many of the factors used in consideration of the simulator room design, such as space allocations, equipment motions, and shielding design, provide for more efficient use of this essential piece of equipment. Because the time invested during the simulation process can seriously affect the outcome of a patient's treatment plan, a thorough knowledge of the simulator, its use, and its limitations is necessary if the simulator's maximum potential is to be reached.

The effective use of the treatment simulator, which can greatly assist in the delivery of a tumoricidal dose of radiation, is important in achieving the goal of delivering a lethal dose to the cancer tissue and at the same time reducing the dose to the normal surrounding tissue. To help reach this goal, simulator design and its use in treatment planning have expanded in the last two decades. As radiation therapy continues to become a more effective tool in the treatment of cancer, there will be a growing need for even more precise and accurate tumor localization.

Simulators with CT mode

Simulators with a CT mode are based on cross-sectional anatomy. They can provide an external contour of the patient and additional information on the location, size, and thickness of some internal structures. These types of simulators incorporate the conventional benefits of a simulator with the benefits of cross-sectional information obtained during the simulation process. In contrast, conventional simulators provide information from orthogonal projections (two radiographs taken at right angles).

To produce a reconstructed image similar to a conventional CT image, the imaging device (x-ray tube and receptor) on the simulator must record information while the gantry rotates.[7] This recorded information consists of transmitted beam intensities that correspond to tissue densities (Fig. 6-18).

The cost, compared to purchasing a conventional CT scanner for this purpose, is an advantage with this type of simulator. Disadvantages include poor image quality compared to that of a conventional CT scanner, increased amount of time to simulate a patient, and the limitation that the x-ray tube can only tolerate a specific amount of heat

Transmission 125 kVp

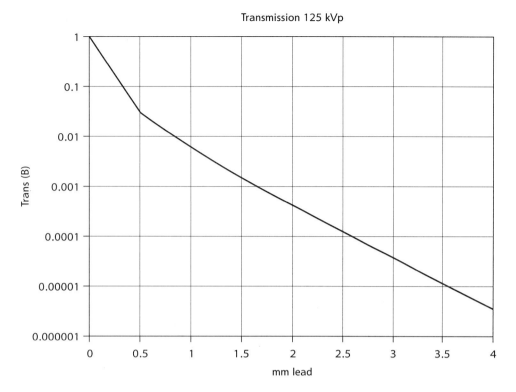

Fig. 6-17 Barrier thickness. This graph shows the thickness of lead (in mm) needed for 125 kVp x-rays using a transmission factor (*B*) in the workload formula.

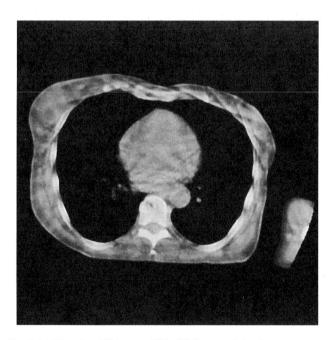

Fig. 6-18 Planning CT image. This CT image of the thorax, generated by a simulator, is used for treatment planning purposes. (Courtesy of Varian TEM, Ltd, UK.)

(each scan generates more heat units than a conventional x-ray, so delays may be encountered waiting for the tube to cool down). The differences in image quality between a conventional CT scanner and a CT simulator are very noticeable. However, the geometry produced with a simulator using a CT mode is not restricted by the conventional CT aperture opening (the opening where the patient passes through the scanner) and is more representative of the treatment unit geometry.

While this type of CT simulator is being perfected, others are working on a type of "virtual simulation" (see Applied Technology on p. 102). McCollough's description of such a CT simulator provides a glimpse into the future: "It can be argued the most desirable (non treatment) piece of equipment for radiation therapy planning is something that combines the convenience and perspective of the x-ray simulator (delineator of borders on high quality, divergent beam's eye view images), the exquisite cross-sectional delineation of soft tissues of the computed tomography (CT) scanner and the isodose generation/overlay capabilities of the modern treatment planning system. There are a number of groups working on such systems as well as several early commercial manifestations."[25]

Virtual Simulation

Virtual simulation, a type of CT simulation that operates along with a three-dimensional geometric planning computer, is a newer method of treatment planning. Still in its infancy, it is a tremendous leap forward compared to the small diagnostic C-arm used many years ago as a simulator in the radiation therapy department. The application of the treatment simulator has gained more importance in recent years. Today it is an essential piece of equipment for precise and accurate treatment planning.

Gradually it was accepted that the use of a diagnostic C-arm (a small piece of mobile radiography equipment with fluoroscopy capabilities) was a very inaccurate method of planning a highly accurate radiation therapy treatment. Commercial radiation therapy simulators were introduced in the early 1960s to overcome this problem of inaccuracy. It was also felt by many that a simulator was better able to reproduce the same setup as the treatment machine. Fluoroscopy was added to allow the operator to look around at the patient's anatomy and accurately set the required field before taking the radiograph. At this time, to obtain a contour (a representation of the external shape of the patient's body at a specific level), the patient outline was hand drawn using plaster or a solder wire bent around the body. It was then transposed to paper. The outline then had added to it the tumor volume and major organs transposed from the simulation radiograph before a plan (usually manual) was carried out.

In the mid-1980s the treatment simulator became computer controlled and also acquired the ability to exactly simulate all aspects of the treatment unit, including the beam shaping devices and treatment accessories. Now the information obtained from the simulator could be combined with that from a diagnostic CT scan to formulate a computerized geometric plan. However, the use of a diagnostic CT scanner created unique problems for radiation therapy departments. Very few radiation therapy departments had a dedicated CT unit, and the amount of time available on one in the diagnostic department was very limited. In addition, because of the size of the aperture, some patient treatment setups were impossible to obtain.

To overcome these problems, several manufacturers introduced Sim CT/Simulated CT. CT images created on the simulator were of poor quality and limited for radiation therapy treatment planning purposes. Four recent developments occurred in the early 1990s that affected radiation therapy treatment planning:

1. CT images on a standard treatment simulator were dramatically improved to the point where they could be used for planning purposes, in place of diagnostic CT images. These had the added advantage of a larger aperture size (up to 100 cm), allowing the scanning of patients in the treatment position.
2. Treatment planning computers were developed that could carry out true three-dimensional treatment planning.
3. Virtual simulation was introduced, which provided the ability to use a diagnostic-type CT scanner to take multiple images (Fig. 6-19). CT simulation/virtual simulation was enhanced with the advent of spiral CT acquisition, where 100 slices could be acquired in a matter of seconds.[33] The images were then sent to a special viewing station where they were reconstructed to form a three-dimensional image. Viewing of overlaid treatment beams could be provided by the computer. These beams could then be manipulated to cover the appropriate tumor volume. Parameter readouts from a graphic simulator could then be transferred to the treatment machine setup.
4. A true virtual simulator provides the ability to generate high resolution (minimum of 512^2) digitally reconstructed radiographs (DRR) (Fig. 6-19) to serve as high quality simulation radiographs.[33]

Many hospitals today are considering, or are about to consider, purchasing a treatment planning computer capable of carrying out three-dimensional planning. To make use of this type of equipment, the radiation therapy department needs access to a diagnostic CT scanner to acquire the 30 to 80 slices needed for this type of planning.

The virtual simulator links with a geometric planning computer to provide physicians with the means to define the target volume in three dimensions. This can be carried out on an off-line terminal where each slice is identified with the tumor volume, the patient outline (contour), and any bony structures or landmarks. Once the process has been accomplished, then the virtual simulator work station sends the information back to the CT scanner (where the patient is still waiting) to control the position of lasers that identify on the patient's skin the superior, inferior, and lateral field borders and/or the isocenter. The whole process can take anywhere from 30 to 60 minutes, utilizing the recently developed fast spiral CT acquisitions.[33] Still others report the entire process can sometimes take up to 2 hours, utilizing CT acquisition techniques.[29]

The virtual simulator is extremely useful for planning complicated treatments and, with the three-dimensional treatment planning computer, is already altering some types of conventional treatment. Anatomic treatment positions not possible on conventional simulator systems (vertex views) can be generated using virtual simulation.[33] It provides the option of delivering a more con-

Virtual Simulation—*cont'd*

centrated dose to the tumor volume while sparing normal surrounding tissue. However, there are some drawbacks that have yet to be overcome:

- The size of the aperture is still too small to accommodate all treatment positions. It's use may require change in the treatment planning process and position.
- The use of certain beam shaping devices and treatment accessories is limited. For example, custom shielding blocks cannot be checked for accuracy and reproducibility before their use on the treatment machine. In addition, irregular electron fields cannot be checked accurately.
- Simulation of mechanical clearance of the treatment machine is limited.
- Deflection characteristics of the table ("sag") and consequently the patient setup are different from those on the treatment machine. Although deflection characteristics of some systems have been matched to the accelerator couch "sag" within 2 mm, even with the heaviest patients.[33]
- The digitally reconstructed radiographs (DRR), which were used as "masters" to compare to the portal images, are of very poor quality compared to conventional simulation radiographs. However, today similar quality "masters" can be obtained using DRR. Two things are necessary. First, the CT platform must provide high spatial resolution and the data acquired must

utilize spiral acquisition techniques within thin slices. Secondly, the information gathered is viewed on a high performance 3D geometric planning computer system capable of generating images in full spatial and contrast resolution with a minimum matrix of 512×512.[33]
- Simple simulations, which account for about 60% of all patients, may take twice as long on the virtual simulator as on a conventional simulator.

A conventional simulator still has an essential place in any radiation therapy department. It is generally accepted that a conventional simulator is required to check any plan produced by the virtual simulator before the patient is treated.[29] However, with the increased utilization of virtual simulation, conformal therapy and isocentric 3D therapy delivery, many leading academic departments and general radiation therapy departments have eliminated the use of conventional simulation as a final "check" of virtual simulation. Their extensive tests have identified that CT based virtual simulation is as accurate as conventional simulation in many anatomical areas.[33] Some simulators today can digitize the fluoroscopic image, which can then be used in the same manner as radiographic film. In the future, it is thought, the conventional simulator will be integrated onto an image and data network within the radiation therapy department. Those departments that are large enough, or can afford to, will probably also have a virtual simulator for more complicated treatment plans.

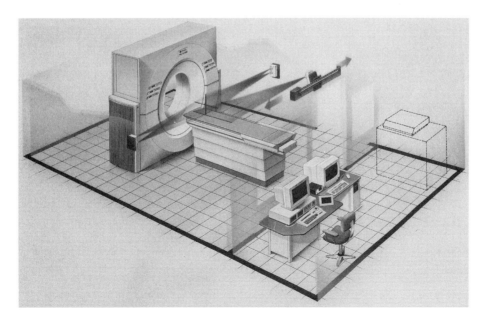

Fig. 6-19 Virtual simulation. This technique uses a CT-based simulator linked into a treatment planning computer. The laser light system delineates field borders once a plan has been completed. (Used by permission from Picker International, Cleveland, OH.)

Review Questions

Multiple Choice

1. The device that projects a scale onto the patient's skin, corresponding to the SSD, is called a(n):
   a. PSA
   b. Gantry
   c. ODI
   d. Collimator assembly

2. To control scatter radiation during fluoroscopy, the_____ should be adjusted.
   a. Isocenter
   b. PSA
   c. Field defining wires
   d. Beam restricting diaphragms

3. All of the following are optical devices used during the simulation process **except**:
   a. Patient table top
   b. ODI
   c. Light field
   d. Lasers

4. The accessory holder on the simulator may serve which of the following purposes?
   I.   Function as an electron cone adapter
   II. Simulate custom block verification
   III. Absorb scatter radiation from thicker body parts
   IV. Provide scanning movements for the imaging system
   a. I and II only
   b. I and III only
   c. II and IV only
   d. I, II, III and IV

5. Which of the following factors are **not** taken into consideration when determining shielding requirements for a simulator?
   a. Use factor (U)
   b. Occupancy factor (T)
   c. Workload (W)
   d. Inverse scattering intensity (I)

6. Which of the following involve three-dimensional treatment planning?
   I.   Virtual simulation
   II. AP radiographs
   III. CT simulators
   IV. Portal radiographs
   a. I and II only
   b. I and III only
   c. II and III only
   d. II and IV only

Questions to Ponder

1. Discuss the importance of tumor localization.
2. Describe, as though you were educating an interested patient, the purpose of the isocenter.
3. Explain the purpose of each of the components within the head of the gantry.
4. How do the PSA and the additional movements of the simulator provide an accurate representation of the treatment plan?
5. List and describe five of the functional performance values of the simulator found in Table 6-2.

REFERENCES

1. American College of Radiology: *ACR standards for radiation oncology*, Reston, VA, 1990, ACR, p 1-3.
2. Bentel GC, Nelson CE, and Noell KT: *Treatment planning and dose calculation in radiation oncology*, ed 4. New York, 1989, Pergamon Press.
3. Bomford CK: Do simulators simulate? *Brit J Rad* 43:583, 1970.
4. Bomford CK, Craig LM, and Hanna FA, et al: Treatment simulators, special report No 10, *Brit J Rad*, 1976.
5. Bomford CK, Craig LM, and Hanna FA, et al: Treatment simulators, Supplement 16, *Brit J Rad*, 1981.
6. Bomford CK, Dawes PJDK, and Lillicrap SC, et al: Treatment simulators, *Brit J Rad* Supplement 23, 1989.
7. Boring CC, Squires TS, and Tong T, et al: Cancer statistics, 1994. *Ca Cancer J Clin* 44:7-26, 1994.
8. Bleehen NM, Glastein E, and Haybittle JL, editors: *Radiation therapy planning*. New York, 1983, Marcel Dekker Inc.
9. British Standard Institution: Medical electrical equipment; part 3. Particular requirements for performance, section 3.129. *Methods of declaring functional performance characteristics of radiotherapy simulators*, Supplement 1. Guide to functional performance values. London, 1994, 1-14.

10. Bushong S: *Radiologic science for the technologist: physics, biology and protection*, ed 5. St. Louis, 1993, Mosby.
11. Carlton R and McKenna-Adler A: *Principles of radiographic imaging*, Albany, NY, 1992, Delmar Publishers, Inc.
12. Conners SG, Battista JJ, and Bertin RJ: On technical specifications of radiotherapy simulators, *Med Phys* 11:341-343, 1984.
13. Day MJ and Harrison RM: Crossectional information/treatment simulation. In Bleehen NM, Glatstein E, and Haybittle JL, editors: *Radiation therapy planning*, New York, 1983, Marcel Dekker, Inc.
14. Dritschilo A, Sherman D, and Emami B, et al: The cost effectiveness of a radiation therapy simulator: A model for determination of need. *Int J Rad Oncol Biol Phys* 5:243, 1979.
15. Glasgow GP and Purdy JA: External beam dosimetry and treatment planning. In DeVita, Jr VT, Hellman SE, and Rosenberg SA, editors: *Cancer: principles and practice of oncology*, Philadelphia, 1985, JB Lippincott.
16. Farmer ET, Fowler JF, and Haggith JW: Megavoltage treatment planning and the use of xeroradiography. *Brit J Rad* 36, 426-435, 1963.
17. Hendrickson FR and Ovadia J: Radiation treatment simulators. *Radiology* 100:701, 1971.
18. Hufton AP, Crosthwaite CM, and Davies JM, et al: Low attenuation material for table tops, cassettes, and grids: a review, *Radiography* 53:17-18, 1987.
19. International Electrotechnical Commission: *CEI/IEC 976 Medical electron accelerators in the range 1-50 MeV—Functional performance characteristics*, Geneva, 1989.
20. Jung B, Larsson B, and Rosengren B, et al: Roentgen stand for field positioning in high-energy radiotherapy, *Acta Radiologica (Therapy, Physics, Biology)* 7:282, 1968.
21. Karzmark CJ: Radiotherapy simulators—a case for special v. general purpose designs, *Brit J Rad* 44:558, 1971.
22. Karzmark CJ, Nunan CS, and Tanabe E: *Medical linear accelerators*, Princeton, NJ, 1993, McGraw-Hill Inc.
23. Karzmark CJ and Rust DC: Radiotherapy treatment simulators and automation, *Radiology* 105:157, 1972.
24. Kereiakes JG, Elson HR, and Born CG, editors: *Radiation oncology physics—1986*, New York, 1987, American Institute of Physics.
25. McCullough E: Radiotherapy treatment simulators. In Purdy JA, editor: *Advances in radiation oncology, physics, dosimetry, treatment planning, and brachytherapy*, New York, 1992, American Institute of Physics.
26. McCullough EC, and Earle JD: The selection, acceptance, testing, and quality control of radiotherapy treatment simulators, *Radiology* 131:226, 1979.
27. Meetens H, Bijhold J, and Strachee J: A method for the measurement of field placement errors in digital portal images, *Phys Med Biol* 35:299, 1990.
28. Mizer S, Scheller RR, and Deye JA: *Radiation therapy simulation workbook*. New York, 1986, Pergammon Press.
29. Myles J: Personal communication, Varian Oncology Systems, March, 1994.
30. NCRP: NCRP Report #16: *Limitation of exposure to ionizing radiation*, Bethesda, MD, 1993, NCRP.
31. Owen J, Coia L, and Hanks G: *Recent patterns of growth in radiation therapy facilities*. Poster presentation at the meeting of the American Society of Therapeutic Radiology and Oncology, Washington, DC, November, 1991.
32. Parker RG, Bogardus CR, and Hanks GE, et al: *Radiation oncology in integrated cancer management*, Philadelphia, PA, 1991, American College of Radiology.
33. Smith L, Picker International, Inc.: Personal communication, April, 1995.
34. Stanton R, Stinson D, and Shahabi S: *An introduction to radiation oncology physics*, Madison, WI, 1992, Medical Physics Publishing.
35. Taylor J: *Imaging in radiotherapy*. Kent, England, 1988, Croom Helm.
36. Van Dyk J and Mah K: Simulators and CT scanners. In Williams JR and Thaites DI, editors: *Radiotherapy physics in practice*. Oxford, 1993, Oxford University Press.

BIBLIOGRAPHY

American College of Radiology: *ACR standards for radiation oncology.* Reston, VA, 1990, ACR.
Bleehen NM, Glastein E, Haybittle JL, editors: *Radiation therapy planning.* New York, 1983, Marcel Dekker.
Bomford CK et al: Treatment simulators. Special report No 10. *Brit J Rad* 1976.
Bomford CK et al: Treatment simulators. *Brit J Rad* Suppl 16, 1981.
Conners SG, Battista JJ, Bertin RJ: On technical specifications of radiotherapy simulators. *Med Phys* 11:341-343, 1984.
Kereiakes JG, Elson HR, Born CG, editors: *Radiation oncology physics—1986*. New York, 1987, American Institute of Physics.
Meetens H, Bijhold J, Strachee J: A method for the measurement of field placement errors in digital portal images. *Phys Med Biol* 35:299, 1990.

Immobilization Devices

Rosann Keller

The practice of radiation therapy has always required accuracy in the delivery of treatment. However, the technical advances that have occurred within the past decade have placed further demands on practitioners to provide precision radiation therapy treatment. The use of sophisticated computed tomography (CT) and magnetic resonance imaging (MRI) tumor localization and simulation and the development of three-dimensional and beam's eye view treatment planning allow accurate delivery of treatment to the tumor volume while minimizing the dose to normal surrounding tissues. But the most intricately planned treatment is useless without the ability to hit the target area consistently during the treatment course. "To miss the tumor once or twice during a treatment course or to have the tumor moved out of the treatment beam during an individual treatment could well provide a 10% or greater reduction in dose below that believed to be delivered."[4] For some patients this could mean the difference between a complete cure or a recurrence or treatment failure. Thus the importance of daily reproduction of the prescribed, planned, and simulated treatment is essential to treatment outcome, as is prohibiting patient movement during simulation, treatment setup, and treatment delivery.

Patient positioning and **immobilization** tools must be used to achieve true reproducibility and accuracy in setup. In a study conducted by Byhardt et al, field placement errors occurred in 15% of the patients treated. The most common sites of field placement error were the pelvis, chest, and abdominal areas.[3] These are sites where immobilization has traditionally not been considered as important as the head and neck area.

A later study by Soffen et al evaluated the use of rigid immobilization for the pelvic regions of early stage prostate cancer patients. The 10% of daily positioning errors representing the greatest movements (anterior/posterior and superior/inferior) were eliminated by the use of immobilization.[9] It was reported that for these patients, daily setup variation could be diminished by 67%.

Accuracy and reproducibility of daily setup are essential to reducing possible treatment complications as well. "Once the threshold dose for tumor response has been reached, small increases in the absorbed dose of radiation may make large differences in tumor control. In a similar manner, once the threshold for normal tissue injury has been reached, small increases in dose may greatly increase the risk of complications."[6] Thus the need for accurate patient positioning and the maintenance of that positioning by immobilization is evident.

While the need for immobilization is apparent, achieving it is not always simple or easy. Effective immobilization devices constrain the patient from moving during treatment and[7]:

- Aid in daily treatment setup and provide reproducibility.
- Assure that immobilization of the patient or treatment area is done with a minimum of discomfort to the patient.
- Achieve the conditions prescribed in the treatment plan.
- Enhance precision of treatment with minimal additional setup time.

It is also important that immobilization devices:

- Are rigid and durable enough to withstand an entire course of treatment.
- Take into consideration the patient's condition and treatment unit limitations.

Additionally, immobilization and positioning aids that can be adapted for many patients with minimal modification and that are cost-effective are desirable.

Specific immobilization devices

Many positioning and immobilization devices are commercially available or easily created at the clinical site. They can usually be broadly divided into three categories: positioning aids, simple immobilization, and complex immobilization.[11] **Patient positioning aids** are devices designed to place the patient in a particular position for treatment. There is generally very little structure in these devices to ensure that the patient does not move. **Simple immobilization devices** restrict some movement but usually require the patient's voluntary cooperation. **Complex immobilization devices** are individualized immobilizers that restrict patient movement and ensure reproducibility in positioning.

Patient positioning devices

Positioning aids are the most commonly used devices in patient setup. Generally speaking, they are widely available, are easy to use, and may be used for more than one patient, thus making them convenient and inexpensive. Head holders are probably the most widely used positioning aids. There are typically two types used for patients in supine position: the so-called dog dish concave head holder (Fig. 7-1) and the head and neck support (Fig. 7-2). The dog dish head holders position the head but do not provide neck support. They are usually made of formed plastic. Head and neck supports may be made of molded polyurethane foam or thin translucent plastic. They come in various heights and neck contours and are typically labeled with a letter (A to F) for identification. The different heights and contours allow for the desired head and neck angulation to achieve the best treatment position. Patients who must be treated in prone position may use different versions of a support device that elevates the face from the table

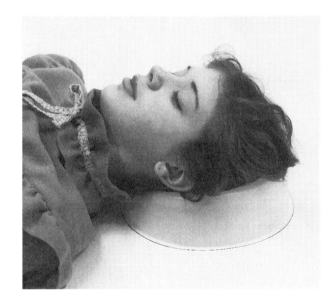

Fig. 7-1 Concave head holder. (Courtesy Radiation Products Design Inc, Albertville, MN.)

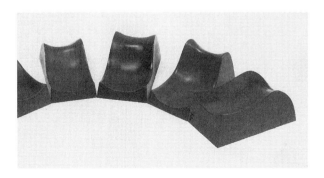

Fig. 7-2 Head and neck supports. (Courtesy Radiation Products Design Inc, Albertville, MN.)

top and is cut out in the eyes, nose, and mouth areas (Fig. 7-3). The patient's head is supported, allowing him or her to breathe normally while in treatment position. Depending on the make or design of this device, support for the chest and shoulders may or may not be available. There are also devices that support the patient's chin while in the prone position (Fig. 7-4). This device typically may be angled to have the patient in the desired position, but the face and forehead are left virtually free from pressure. Because only the chin is supported, the chest is flat on the table, making this device especially useful in the treatment of the central nervous system.

Various sponge pillows and foam cushions are available. Different sizes and shapes are useful for the various treatment positions. Foam neck rolls assist in proper chin extension, and other shapes and sizes are particularly useful in positioning extremities. Foam cushions and pillows also tend to make patients more comfortable on hard treatment and simulation tables. Comfortable patients are more likely to be cooperative and are better able to maintain treatment position, both of which contribute to setup reproducibility and treatment accuracy.

Sandbags are another commonly used positioning device. A well-placed sandbag helps to prevent movement or rotation of a body part during treatment. They are especially helpful in treating extremities. For example, placing a sandbag on each side of the foot will prevent the rotation of the patient's femur during treatment. Sandbags on either side of a patient's head help prevent head turning during treatment of the cervical spine.

To position the arm, particularly for breast treatment, the L-shaped arm board is still used in some radiation oncology centers. The horizontal portion of the board slips under the patient's back. The perpendicular support has an adjustable handgrip. The handgrip may be positioned at the proper height to ensure the patient's arm is not in the treatment field (Fig. 7-5). More recent styles of arm boards are contoured to the shape of the arm and allow the arm to rest comfortably above the patient's head. They also tend to allow for more flexibility in achieving greater arm tilt and extension (Fig. 7-6).

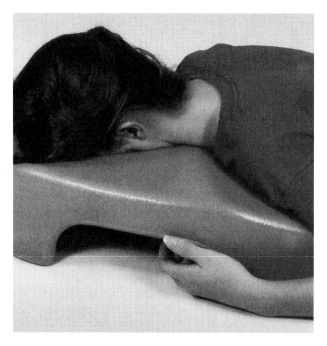

Fig. 7-3 Prone pillow. (Courtesy Radiation Products Design, Inc., Albertville, MN.)

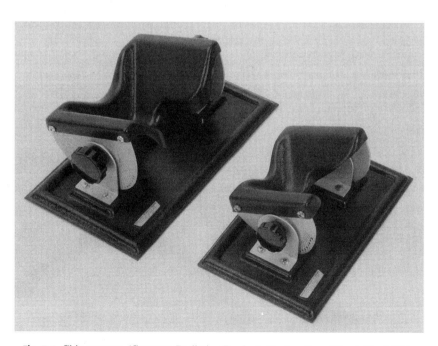

Fig. 7-4 Chin support. (Courtesy Radiation Products Design, Inc., Albertville, MN.)

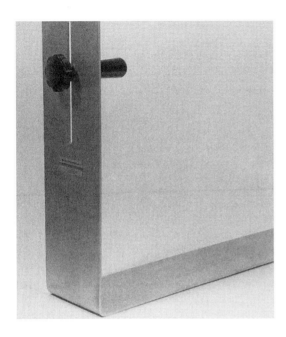

Fig. 7-5 L-shaped arm board. (Courtesy Radiation Products Design, Inc., Albertville, MN.)

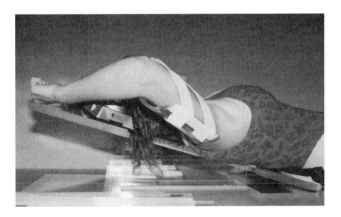

Fig. 7-6 Arm positioning board. (Courtesy Smithers Medical Products, Inc., Akron, OH.)

The positioning devices mentioned in this chapter are widely used in radiation oncology departments in all parts of the country. They assist the therapist in positioning the patient for treatment. Most are designed to be comfortable for the patient, which encourages him or her to maintain proper treatment position. These devices will not, however, prevent patient movement during treatment. The patient must be cooperative and fully understand the importance of not moving during setup or treatment so that the devices are effective.

Simple immobilization devices

Simple immobilization devices are commonly used in addition to positioning aids. They typically provide some restric-

tion of movement and stability of treatment position in cooperative patients. However, patients who insist on moving will not be entirely deterred by these devices.

The least complex and most readily available simple immobilization tool is tape. Masking tape or paper tape is a standard supply in almost every treatment room. Tape is commonly used for head and chin positioning for setups such as whole brain treatment. It can be used across the patient's forehead and over or under the chin. Using tape under the chin allows the therapist to achieve appropriate head tilt and encourages the patient to maintain that chin elevation. Tape can also be used to bind a patient's feet together to ensure proper positioning for treatment to the pelvis. It is also frequently used to position anatomy out of the treatment field, such as taping the arm or the contralateral breast out of a tangential port. Plastic or cloth straps with Velcro at the ends can sometimes be substituted for tape, especially under the chin.

Another very simple and accessible immobilization device is the rubber band. Large rubber bands, approximately 2 cm in thickness, can be used to bind the patient's feet together when he or she is in supine position. This helps to ensure that the legs and feet are consistently in a reproducible position. This enables more accurate setup of pelvic ports and assists the radiation therapist in leveling and positioning the patient for treatment.

For patients not receiving treatment to the pelvis, the rubber band prevents them from moving or shaking their feet or crossing their ankles during treatment. When patients are alone in the treatment room, they may become restless and begin moving their feet or try to become more comfortable by crossing their ankles. Movement at the inferior aspect of the patient will affect treatment position, even superiorly. The rubber band is a gentle reminder to the patient to remain still, as well as a more restrictive immobilizer of the feet and legs. Additionally, the rubber band may be used to provide passive restraint for the patient's hands and arms. Some patients request that they be allowed to hold a rubber band between their hands to steady them during treatment. For those patients who have concerns of falling off the narrow treatment table or who are unable to keep their extremities in treatment or stable position, a standard safety belt is another effective immobilization device.

A number of devices are available to restrict patient movement for treatment of the head and neck area. With some slight variation, most consist of a head frame and a **bite block** (Fig. 7-7). The head frame can be used for many different patients. Some of these systems allow for the use of a nose bridge device. After the patient's head is positioned, the nose bridge locks into place. Each patient will require his or her own bite block. The bite block serves two purposes. It helps the patient maintain the position of the chin, and it moves the tongue out of the treatment area. These can be made of cork, Aquaplast* pellets, or dental wax.

*WFR/Aquaplast Corp.

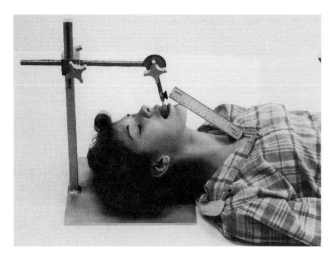

Fig. 7-7 Bit block system. (Courtesy Radiation Products Design, Inc., Albertville, MN.)

Dental wax becomes pliable when placed in warm water. When the patient bites down on the wax, impressions of the teeth are made on the bite block, thus the patient can place the bite block between his or her teeth in exactly the same position daily. The bite block is then secured to the head piece. The individual arms of the head piece are adjustable and calibrated so that they can accommodate different patient positions. With the bite block between the patient's teeth and secured in the head piece, treatment position is maintained. In using this type of device, the therapist must be careful to accurately measure the distance between the tip of the patient's chin and suprasternal notch (**chin to SSN measurement**) and to reproduce the same settings on the calibrated arms of the head holder device as were used in simulation to ensure setup accuracy.

Immobilization of the shoulders, arms, and legs can be accomplished using arm to foot straps. There are several versions of these (Fig. 7-8) commercially available. The primary purpose is to pull the patient's shoulders out of lateral head and neck fields. As the patient grasps the straps, the tension of the straps running the length of the patient's body and around the soles of the feet provides traction to move the shoulders inferiorly and out of the lateral treatment field. These devices also restrict movement of the arms, shoulders, legs, and feet.

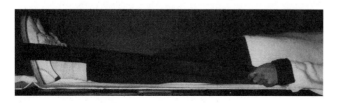

Fig. 7-8 Arm to foot straps.

Simple immobilization devices are easy to use and generally cost-effective. Items such as tape and rubber bands are quite inexpensive. Some devices may be used by several patients over time, which reduces costs. In choosing to use any simple immobilization device, the radiation therapist must keep the patient in mind. Patients must understand the importance of holding still during treatment and must cooperate with the radiation therapist, or any simple immobilization device will be ineffective.

Complex immobilization devices

Complex immobilization devices are becoming more and more popular because there are many new products available to quickly produce immobilization for individual patients. Because each device is individualized, they tend to be more costly. However, the advantages are that unusual patient positions can be achieved and, in many cases, portal markings can be made on the device, thus alleviating the need for patients to keep skin markings. Complex immobilization devices can be made of a number of different products, such as plaster, plastic, and Styrofoam. The materials used will depend on the treatment area, availability of materials, and individual practitioner preference.

The earliest complex immobilization devices were constructed of plaster of Paris. Plaster is still used today in some radiation oncology centers. The plaster is used to make a cast of the body part to be treated. If necessary, a whole body cast can be made. Preparing a plaster cast is fairly easy. A thin piece of cloth or plastic wrap is placed over the part to be immobilized. Plaster of Paris strips are prepared and applied. A number of strips must be used for the cast to be thick and strong enough so that it will maintain its shape and not break during the course of treatment. Care must also be taken to allow the strips to dry thoroughly before removing the cast because failure to do so will jeopardize the cast's integrity. Plaster masks of the head and neck area can be secured to a head frame placed on the treatment table. This device must be used when the mask is made. Once the cast is thoroughly dry, the treatment portal can be cut out if necessary. Field markings may also be made on the cast.

Light cast is another material that can be used and is often preferred by practitioners because it is lighter, quicker, and cleaner to use than plaster. Light cast is fiberglass tape that has resin in it. It comes in an airtight sealed package and is flexible enough to mold around patients. Ultraviolet light causes the resin in the tape to harden, thus creating a rigid immobilization device. Light cast is particularly useful for immobilizing the head and neck area. Carefully placing the strips of material over the patient's forehead and over and around the chin provides effective stability, especially if the light cast can be secured to a head frame that is placed on the table. The one drawback to light cast material is that it has a rather pungent odor before it dries.[1]

Another effective, yet somewhat time consuming method for making individualized immobilization, especially in the head and neck area, is the **vacuum-formed plastic shell**. The patient is prepared for the cast by being positioned on the appropriate headrest and secured by masking tape. The patient's hair is covered by a rubber swimming cap or stockinette. Straws may need to be placed in the patient's nostrils to maintain an airway. Petroleum jelly or plastic wrap should cover the area to be molded so that the cast can be removed easily and to avoid inadvertent painful removal of the patient's facial hair.

The initial impression will be a negative impression, which is made by using plaster bandage carefully shaped around the patient's anatomy. In the head and neck area, it is especially important to get an accurate impression of the chin, nose, and forehead. This usually requires several thicknesses of bandages overlapped to ensure rigidity. Once the impression has hardened, it is carefully removed from the patient. A plaster positive impression is then created by filling the negative mold with plaster. Once the plaster hardens, a perfect replica of the patient's features is complete. This mold is then ready for the vacuum-forming unit.[2]

A sheet of thin plastic is placed down the vacuum-forming unit. It is heated until it is pliable. A bubble is made in the plastic sheet using a small amount of compressed air. The plaster mold is placed into the bubble, and the vacuum pulls the plastic over the cast. When the vacuum is released and a small amount of compressed air is applied, the shell is released from the plaster.[10] The treatment portal may be cut from the plastic shell. Daily use of the shell requires an appropriate means of securing it to the patient and to the table. Thus a head frame of some type is required for use of this device.

The **Alpha Cradle*** is now becoming a widely used immobilization device (Fig. 7-9). It is becoming popular because it can be used to immobilize practically any anatomical part, such as the head and neck area, the thorax, and the extremities. Before being made for the individualized patient, the Alpha Cradle consists of a Styrofoam shell with a plastic bag or other protective sheeting and a set of foaming agents. When the foaming agents are combined and placed in the plastic-covered Styrofoam shell, they begin to expand. When a patient is positioned in the Styrofoam shell, the foam molds around the patient. After approximately 10 minutes the foam will have hardened and the cradle is complete and ready to use (see applied technology section for complete instructions). Making the cradle takes very little time on the therapist's part. The chemical reaction of the foaming agents produces a small amount of heat, which most patients do not find uncomfortable. One concern in the making of an Alpha Cradle is the safe use of the foaming agents. Inappropriate use of the agents and inaccurate disposal of their containers after use could lead to hazardous situations (see applied technology section).[8]

Another immobilization device that is currently available is called **Vac-lok**† (Fig. 7-10). This device consists of a cush-

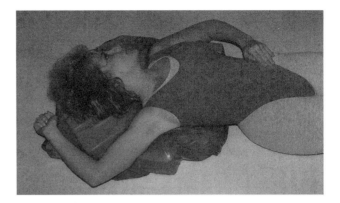

Fig. 7-9 Alpha Cradle. (Courtesy Smithers Medical Products, Inc, Akron, OH.)

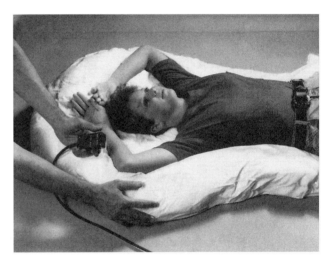

Fig. 7-10 Vac-lok. (Courtesy Med-Tec, Inc, Orange City, IA.)

ion and a vacuum compression pump. The patient is placed into the treatment position on a partially inflated cushion. The cushion is partially evacuated until it is semi-rigid, and then the therapist molds it around the area to be immobilized. Once the shape is established, the vacuum procedure is completed until the cushion is completely rigid. Cushions are available in several shapes and sizes to accommodate most anatomical sites. The advantage to using this system is that the cushions can be deflated, cleaned, and reused after a patient has completed his or her treatment course.[5]

Aquaplast is yet another commonly used immobilization device (Fig. 7-11). It is a thermoplastic that becomes pliable when warmed in a hot water bath. When pliable, it can be molded around the patient. The material comes in sheets, perforated or unperforated, in four different thicknesses ranging from 1.6 to 4.8 mm. It is lightweight and easy to use in making immobilization devices (see applied technology section) and is very popular for immobilization for head and neck treatment. Using an Aquaplast mask requires the addition of a head rest and some type of frame to secure the mask

---

*Smithers Medical Products, Inc.
†Med-Tec, Inc.

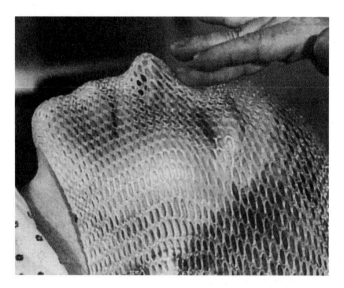

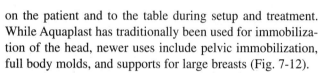

Fig. 7-11 Aquaplast mask. (Courtesy WFR/Aquaplast Corp, Wyckoff, NJ.)

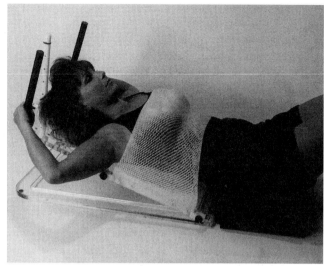

Fig. 7-12 Aquaplast immobilization for large breasts. (Courtesy WFR/Aquaplast Corp, Wyckoff, NJ.)

on the patient and to the table during setup and treatment. While Aquaplast has traditionally been used for immobilization of the head, newer uses include pelvic immobilization, full body molds, and supports for large breasts (Fig. 7-12).

There are several advantages to using this immobilizer. Patient markings can be made right on the mask. The perforated plastic also helps patients feel more comfortable because they can breathe and see through the perforations.[12] The casts may be cut to further increase patient comfort, especially if the mask is tight around the eyes and forehead, or if a patient feels claustrophobic. The treatment field may also be cut out to reduce beam attenuation, thus minimizing the possibility of skin reactions. It should be noted, however, that excessive cutting reduces the integrity of this immobilizer. Additionally, modifications in the mask to accommodate weight loss or reduction in swelling can be made on a completed mask at any time during the course of treatment. A heat gun may be used to heat the problem area until it is pliable, and then changes may be made.

While complex immobilization devices are somewhat time consuming and costly to make, they allow for unique patient positioning options. They typically provide more stability, prevent more patient movement, and are usually time-saving in daily treatment procedures, thus justifying the cost for many practitioners.

Over the years a number of immobilization devices have been developed and used to improve the treatment outcome for radiation therapy patients. Some of the devices are simple, yet effective in immobilizing the patient. Others are more complex and are made individually for the particular patient. The choice of immobilization devices depends on many considerations, including the condition of the patient, the area to be treated, and the availability and cost of materials. Radiation therapists must be prepared to recommend and use the appropriate device for a particular patient to ensure the best possible treatment outcome for that patient.

APPLIED TECHNOLOGY

The following discussions illustrate the manufacture of two commonly used complex immobilization devices. The instructions and photographs presented here are provided courtesy of the manufacturers. Users are *strongly advised to read all product instructions before using them.*

Safety Issues in Making Alpha Cradles

1. Always use care in handling foaming agents.
2. NEVER RECAP BOTTLES.
3. Avoid getting foaming agents on skin or clothing.
4. Always read product instructions carefully before use.
5. Refer to product instructions regarding handling of spills.

Alpha Cradle

Alpha Cradles are frequently used to immobilize the thorax, abdomen, and extremities. They are usually quick and easy to make, but care must be taken in handling the foaming agents.

1. Gather materials for use: foaming agents (bottles 1 and 2), polystyrene shell, large plastic bag (Fig. 7-13, *A*).
2. Place polystyrene shell inside plastic bag.
3. Pour entire contents of bottle 1 into bottle 2 (Fig. 7-13, *B*).
4. Recap bottle 2 and shake mixture vigorously for 10 seconds, holding bottle with cap pointing and down away from everyone (Fig. 7-13, *C*).
5. Pour mixture along the edge of the inside of the shell. Remove as much air from the bag as possible and fold open end of bag under the shell (Fig. 7-13, *D*).
6. Discard both empty bottles in a leakproof container. DO NOT RECAP.
7. Position patient in the shell. Have patient remain motionless for approximately 10 minutes until mold is cooled to room temperature. If foam rises above the mold, apply pressure directly to rising foam with your hand (Fig. 7-13, *E*).
8. When mold is cooled, remove patient from the form and check the part of the cradle that was under the patient. If the foam feels soft, let the cradle set for an additional 10 minutes.
9. Tape plastic bag to the back of the mold. Patient name and treatment information can be written on the cradle.

Aquaplast

Aquaplast is frequently used to make masks to immobilize the head and neck area; however, it can be used for pelvic immobilization, to make full body molds, and to support large breasts. One advantage to its use is that patient markings can be made directly on the immobilization device.

1. Preheat water bath between 160° and 180° F (70° and 80° C). A flexible mesh pan liner must be placed at the bottom of the heating unit (Fig. 7-14, *A*).
2. Position the patient on head rest and head frame.
3. Immerse the Aquaplast sheet in the hot water on top of the mesh pan liner. After about a minute the Aquaplast will turn from opaque to transparent—indicating that it is pliable and ready to mold.
4. Use the mesh pan liner as a transfer sheet to remove the softened Aquaplast from the water bath.
5. Place the Aquaplast on an absorbent towel and thoroughly blot dry with another towel.
6. Position Aquaplast over patient and mold around area to be immobilized. In the head and neck area, molding around the chin will increase head stability and treatment accuracy. Secure edges of plastic to head frame (Fig. 7-14, *B*).
7. Finish molding with fingers to gain additional patient contours. As Aquaplast cools, it becomes opaque (Fig. 7-14, *C*).
8. Allow approximately 10 minutes for mask to cool and set completely before removing from the patient.

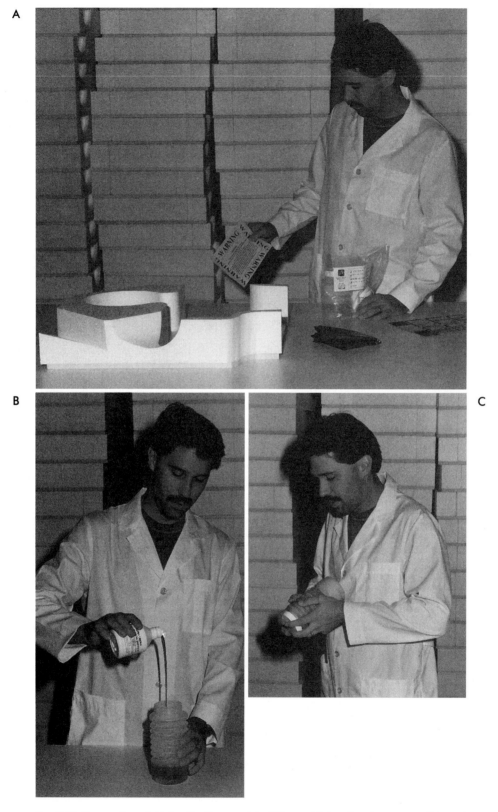

Fig. 7-13 Preparation of Alpha Cradle materials (**A**), combining foaming agents (**B**), and shaking vigorously (**C**) before pouring into styrofoam cast. (Courtesy Smithers Medical Products, Inc, Akron, OH.)

D

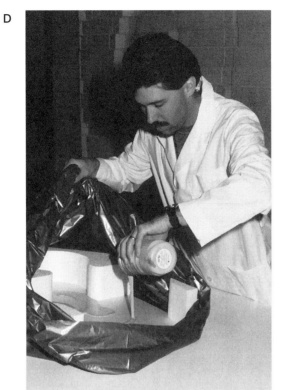

E

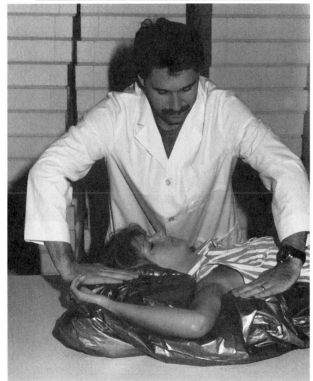

Fig. 7-13 cont'd Pouring mixture evenly (**D**), and shaping the expanding foam as Alpha Cradle hardens (**E**). (Courtesy Smithers Medical Products, Inc, Akron, OH.)

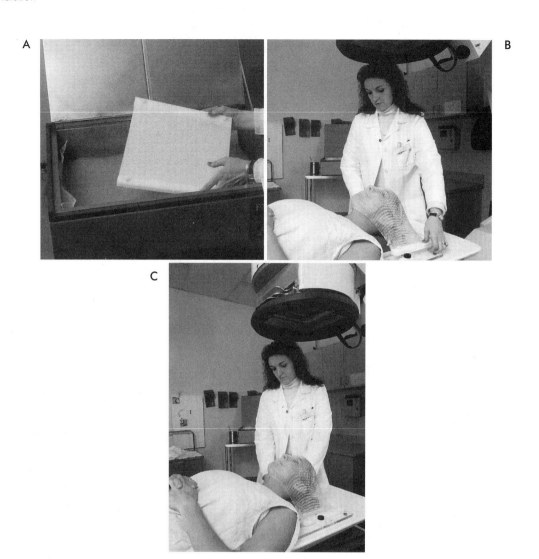

Fig. 7-14 Preparation of thermoplastic material in hot water bath (**A**), placing mask over patient's face (**B**), and shaping Aquaplast to patient's facial contour (**C**). (Courtesy WFR/Aquaplast Corp, Wyckoff, NJ.)

Review Questions

Multiple Choice

1. Which of the following is **not** a desirable quality of an effective and useful immobilization device?
   a. Ensures immobilization with minimal patient discomfort.
   b. Requires additional setup time.
   c. Is durable enough to withstand the entire treatment plan.
   d. Achieves conditions prescribed in treatment plan.
   e. Is reasonably priced.
   f. None of the above.
2. Positioning aids are:
   a. Extremely effective in immobilizing patients.
   b. Widely available and easy to use.
   c. Frequently designed for single patient use.
   d. Usually very expensive.
   e. Often uncomfortable for patients to use.
   f. All of the above.
3. Patient immobilization is important because:
   a. Sophisticated treatment planning techniques allow more accurate delivery of treatment.
   b. Missing the tumor once or twice in a treatment course can reduce the planned dose by 10% or more.
   c. Daily reproduction of the planned treatment is essential to treatment outcomes.
   d. a and b only.
   e. All of the above
   f. None of the above

True or False

4. A 10% or greater reduction in dose below that which is believed to be delivered could mean the difference between a complete cure and a recurrence or treatment failure.
   True _____ False _____
5. In a study conducted by Byhardt et al, field placement errors occurred in 5% of patients treated.
   True _____ False _____
6. Accuracy and reproducibility in daily setup could reduce possible treatment complications.
   True _____ False _____

7. Comfortable patients are more likely to be cooperative and better able to maintain treatment position.
   True _____ False _____
8. Patient cooperation is needed for effective use of positioning devices and simple immobilization devices.
   True _____ False _____
9. Manufacturing a vacuum-formed shell for patient immobilization is very simple and only takes a few minutes.
   True _____ False _____
10. The radiation therapist has no role in recommending or using appropriate immobilization devices for patients.
    True _____ False _____

Questions to Ponder

1. Describe the importance of immobilization devices in radiation therapy.
2. Compare and contrast the differences between patient positioning and immobilization devices.
3. Describe criteria for selecting effective immobilization devices.

4. Name some commonly used immobilization devices and provide examples of their uses.
5. Describe how complex immobilization devices such as vacuum-formed shells, Alpha Cradles, and Aquaplast are made.

REFERENCES

1. Bentel GC, Nelson CE, Noell KT: *Treatment planning and dose calculation in radiation oncology*, ed 4. New York, 1989, Pergamon.
2. Bomford CK, Sherriff SB, Kunkler IH: *Walter and Miller's textbook of radiotherapy: radiation physics, therapy and oncology*, ed 5. Edinburgh, 1993, Churchill Livingstone.
3. Byhart RW, et al: Weekly localization films and detection of field placement errors. *Int J Radiat Oncol Biol Phys* 4:881-887, 1978.
4. Hendrickson FR: Precision in radiation oncology. *Int J Radiat Oncol Biol Phys* 8:311-312, 1982.
5. Med-Tec, Inc., Orange City, IA.
6. O'Connor-Hartsell S, Hartsell W: Minimizing errors in patient positioning. *Radiation Therapist* 3:15-19, 1994.
7. Sampiere VA, Khan FM, Delclos L: Treatment aids for external-beam radiotherapy. In Levitt SH, Tapley N: *Technological basis of radiation therapy: practical clinical applications*. Philadelphia, 1984, Lea & Febiger.

8. Smithers Medical Products, Inc., Tallmadge, OH.
9. Soffen EM, et al: Conformal static field therapy for low volume low grade prostrate cancer with rigid immobilization. *Int J Radiat Oncol Biol Phys* 20:141-146, 1991.
10. Van Arsdale ED, Greenlaw RH: Formalized immobilization and localization in radiotherapy. *Radiology* 99:697-698, 1971.
11. Van Dyk J, Mah K: Simulators and CT scanners. In Williams JR, Thwaites DI, editors: *Radiotherapy physics in practice*. Oxford, 1993, Oxford University Press.
12. WFR/Aquaplast Corp, Wyckoff, NJ.

CHAPTER 8

Surface and Sectional Anatomy

Charles M. Washington

Outline

Key terms

Radiation therapy today is a well-established science that requires its practitioners to demonstrate a keen knowledge of human anatomy and physiology. The radiation therapist learns early in the educational curriculum that he or she must have a comprehensive understanding of surface and cross-sectional anatomy. Knowledge of human anatomy is essential in simulation, treatment planning, and daily checks of accurate treatment portal placement. This chapter will focus on the surface and sectional anatomy used in simulation and radiation therapy management of diseases commonly encountered by the radiation therapist. Surface anatomy will be related to deep-seated structures within the human body. An overview of the diagnostic tools used to visualize internal structures will be presented along with a review of lymphatic physiology. This is included because the lymphatics play a major role in treatment field delineation and disease management. A review of pertinent skeletal anatomy is presented to ensure a common basis of spatial relationships to enhance understanding. With this foundation laid, surface anatomy, sectional anatomy, and topographical landmarks are presented in practical radiation therapy scenarios.

PERSPECTIVE

The primary objective in managing cancer with ionizing radiation is to deposit enough radiation to result in the death of cancer cells while minimizing the effect on the surrounding normal tissues. The challenge is to define a patient-specific therapy plan that entails localizing the tumor and surrounding dose-limiting tissues, such as the spinal cord, kidney, and eyes. In addition, the therapist must maintain the integrity of the plan throughout its administration. The particulars of surface anatomy available to the therapist have changed little during the last 30 years. Clinical application is essential in facilitating the understanding of a disease process on anatomical grounds, corresponding surface location of internal structures, and the appearance of internal imaged structures.[8] The therapist bridges surface and sectional anatomy with the practical clinical application of patient treatment.

Visual, palpable, and imaged anatomy forms the basis of clinical examination.[9] This is the case in radiation therapy. Surface and sectional anatomy forms the road atlas the therapist needs to be effective in simulation, treatment planning, and the daily administration of therapy treatments. Without this atlas, it would be like driving from Texas to Maine for the first time, without any mapping or planning. We know the general direction of where we want to go, but we would not know the most efficient way to get there. The therapist must embrace a comprehensive knowledge of imaging modalities that enable tumor visualization, pertinent lymphatic anatomy, and the site by site relationship of surface and sectional anatomy. A systematic approach to this information will allow the therapist to link vital didactic information to its clinical application.

RELATED IMAGING MODALITIES USED IN SIMULATION AND TUMOR LOCALIZATION

More than any other innovation, the ability to painlessly visualize the interior of the living human body has governed the practice of medicine during the 20th century.[2] In recent years the explosion of medical imaging techniques allowed for effective ways to diagnose and localize pathological disorders. The medical imaging modalities used in simulation and tumor localization fit into two categories: ionizing and nonionizing imaging studies. Ionizing imaging studies use ionizing radiation to produce latent images that demonstrate anatomy. Examples of ionizing imaging studies include conventional radiography, computed tomography, and nuclear medicine imaging. Nonionizing imaging studies use alternative means of imaging the body, such as magnetic fields in magnetic resonance imaging and echoed sound waves in ultrasonography.

Conventional radiography

The branch of anatomy that is essential for the diagnosis of disease such as cancer with the use of x-rays is radiographic

anatomy or radiology. The most basic type of radiographic anatomy uses a single exposure of x-rays. These x-rays pass through the patient's body and expose a film, producing an image called a radiograph. A radiograph provides a two-dimensional image of the interior of the body. While the latent images produced delineate the obvious differences in tissue densities of the body, x-rays do not always distinguish subtle differences in tissue density. Fig. 8-1 demonstrates a conventional chest radiograph produced by a therapy simulator. The pertinent anatomy can be distinguished and outlined for practical application. Any anomaly, a variation from the standard, is recognizable on the image as well as any structure considered to be dose limiting.

Radiation therapy uses an extensive amount of diagnostic imaging in its daily practice. Simulators use specialized diagnostic x-ray equipment to localize the treatment area and reproduce the geometry of the therapeutic beam before treatment. Radiographic localization is the most common method used to localize tumor volumes. Other techniques also aid in visualization of human anatomy. A special technique used for many years in radiation therapy diagnosis is **lymphangiography**, a technique that uses special injected dyes to help visualize the lymphatic system. Fig. 8-2 shows a radiograph that employs lymphangiography. The lymphatic channels are the white areas of higher density. Filling defects, lymphatic channels that are not completely visible or appear frothy, can demonstrate the presence of pathological changes. These all

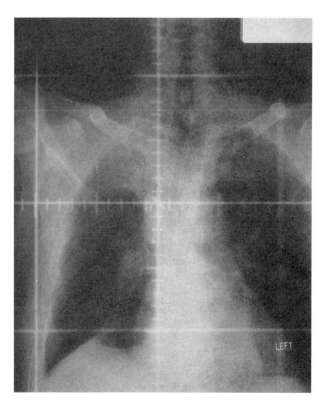

Fig. 8-1 Typical thorax simulation film. Note how bony anatomy is distinguishable from cartilage and soft tissue.

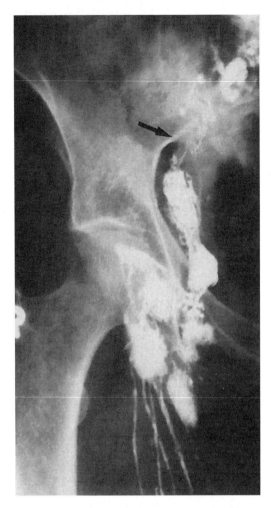

Fig. 8-2 Lymphangiogram. The lymphatic channels can be imaged and used to assess the status of the lymphatics.

provide valuable information for patient treatment planning. In all, conventional radiology is an essential component in radiation therapy.

Computed tomography

Computed tomography (CT) is an ionizing radiation–based technique in which x-ray photons interact with a scintillation crystal that is more sensitive than x-ray film.[1] CT scanning combines x-ray principles and advanced computer technologies. The x-ray source moves in an arc around the body part being scanned and continually sends out beams of radiation. As the beams pass through the body, the tissues absorb small amounts of radiation, depending on their densities. The beams are converted to signals that are projected onto a television screen. These images look like radiographs of slices through the body. They are typically perpendicular to the long axis of the patient's body. The CT scan provides important anatomical relationships at a glance. Fig. 8-3 demonstrates the spatial and anatomical orientation of a CT slice. A

series of scans allows the examination of section after section of a patient's anatomy.

The entire CT process takes only seconds for each slice, it is completely painless, and the dose of radiation to the patient is typically equal to that of many other diagnostic procedures. The detail of the images produced has about 10 to 20 times the detail of conventional radiography. Display of CT images reflects the differences among four basic densities: air (black), fat (dark/gray), water/blood (gray/light), and bone/metal (white).[1] CT demonstrates bone detail well. Radiation therapy treatment planning commonly uses CT images, particularly with three-dimensional treatment plans. CT allows for spatial relationships of human anatomy.

Nuclear medicine imaging

The branch of medicine that uses radioisotopes in the diagnosis and treatment of disease is known as nuclear medicine. Nuclear medicine imaging uses ionizing radiation to provide information about physiology as well as anatomical structure. This is typically useful in noted abnormalities secondary to tumor activity, specifically metastatic disease.[14] Sensitive radiation detection devices display images of radioactive drugs taken through the body and their uptake in tissues. While this imaging technique plays an important role in tumor imaging, it detects metastatic disease more than primary tumors. Bone and liver metastases are localized using nuclear medicine scans. These scans are relatively safe and can yield very valuable information. The radionuclide bone scan is the procedure of choice for skeletal scanning. Fig. 8-4 shows a bone scan. Areas of increased uptake, the dark spots, demonstrate high activity areas that correspond to pathological changes (uptake in the urinary bladder is normal). The radionuclide liver scan is the initial scan of choice for liver metastasis. Gallium scans localize areas of inflammation and tumor activity in lymphoma patients. They are useful in monitoring changes in tumor size. Radiation safety procedures are important in nuclear medicine scanning. In both intravenous application and ingestion of radioactive isotopes, care in monitoring patient exposure to ionizing radiation is important. The elimination of isotopes that have run through the body (through urination) also requires careful monitoring and precautions.

Positron emission tomography (PET) scanning employs short-lived radioisotopes such as carbon 11, nitrogen 13, or oxygen 15 in a solution commonly injected into a patient. The radioisotope circulates through the body and emits positively charged electrons, called positrons. These positrons collide with conventional electrons in body tissues, causing the release of gamma rays. These rays are detected and recorded. The computer creates a colored PET scan that demonstrates function rather than structure. It can detect blood flow through organs like the brain and heart, diagnose coronary artery disease, and identify the extent of stroke or heart attack damage. PET is useful in diagnosing two types of breast cancer (those with and without estrogen receptors).

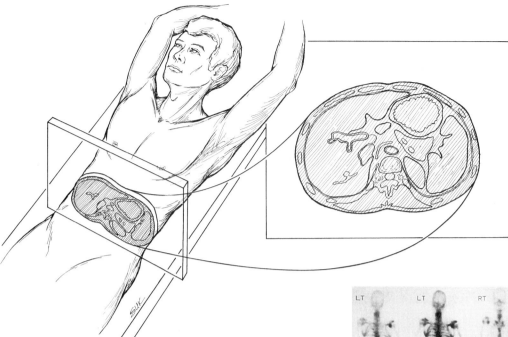

Fig. 8-3 Spatial and anatomical orientation of a CT and/or MR slice. Internal anatomy can be referenced to surface location and contour.

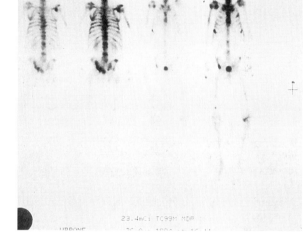

Fig. 8-4 Radionuclide bone scan. Multiple focal lesions in bone of patient with prostate cancer.

Thus the physician can prescribe the appropriate treatment regimen early.

Magnetic resonance imaging

Magnetic resonance (MR) imaging records data based on the magnetic properties of the hydrogen nuclei, which can be thought of as tiny magnets spinning in random directions. These hydrogen nuclei (magnets) interact with neighboring atoms and with all applied magnetic fields.[1] In this imaging modality a strong uniform magnetic energy is applied to small magnetic fields that lie parallel to the direction of the external magnet. The patient is pulsed with radiowaves, which cause the nuclei to send out a weak radio signal that is detected and reworked into a planar image of the body. The images, which indicate cellular activity, look similar to a CT scan. Fig. 8-5 shows a coronal MR scan of the head.

MR has a diagnostic advantage over CT in that it provides information about chemicals in an organ or tissue. In this way, MR can perform a noninvasive (one not involving puncture of incision of the skin or insertion of a foreign object into the body) biopsy on tumors. The disadvantages of MR are the expensive shielding requirements, low throughput (the number of patients an hour a machine can serve) when compared to CT, and increased cost in comparison to CT. This imaging technique is expanding to become one of the diagnostic standards in radiation therapy.

Ultrasound

Ultrasound (US) uses high frequency sound waves, which are not heard by the human ear. These waves travel forward and continue to move until they make contact with an object; at that point, a certain amount of the sound bounces back. Submarines use this principle to find other underwater vessels as well as the depth of the ocean floor. Ultrasound remains a less expensive and less hazardous alternative to the earlier studies.[14] A transducer, a hand-held instrument, generates high frequency sound waves. It moves over the body part being examined. The transducer also picks up the returning sound waves. Normal and abnormal tissues exhibit varying densities that reflect sound differently. The resultant image is processed onto a screen and is called a sonogram. The images can be a still two-dimensional, cross-sectioned image or a moving image, like the heart of a fetus.

Ultrasound offers no exposure to ionizing radiation, is noninvasive and painless, and requires no contrast media. However, it does not effectively penetrate bone or air-filled spaces. It is therefore not useful in imaging the skull, lungs, or intestines. In radiation therapy the poor quality images do

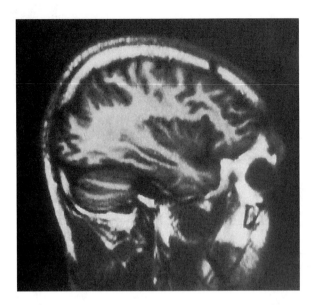

Fig. 8-5 Coronal magnetic resonance image section through the head. (From Haaga JR: *Computed tomography and magnetic resonance imaging of the whole body*, St. Louis, 1995, Mosby.)

not adequately define specific localization information for conventional treatment planning. However, it is very helpful in noninvasively determining internal organ location. This is evident in the increasing use of ultrasound to locate and guide brachytherapy implants in the prostate as well as locating tumors within the eye.

Modern imaging modalities provide essential information to the radiation therapy team for tumor localization and anatomical patient mapping. Cross-sectional images are very valuable. They provide views within the patient and display organs with their normal shape and orientation, typically in treatment position. The direct relationships allow for accurate treatment planning. We can spatially relate the patient's surface anatomy to the inner structure. In addition to displaying organs with their normal living shape, normal anatomical relationships can be observed. In particular, the study of sectional images allows the radiation therapy practitioner to develop an excellent three-dimensional concept of anatomy.[10] These modalities provide the basic information necessary to develop critical thinking skills in surface and sectional anatomy that is essential in the role of the radiation therapist.

ANATOMICAL POSITIONING

Radiation therapy requires daily reproducible positioning for effective treatment delivery. The radiation therapist uses various terms to describe the relationship of body parts, planes, and sections. These terms serve as the foundation in understanding the body's structural plan.[17]

Definition of terms

When using terms that reference human body position, it is assumed that the body is in the anatomical position; this allows for clear reference of directional relationships. The **anatomical position** is one in which the subject stands upright, with feet together flat on the floor, toes pointed forward, eyes looking forward, arms straight down by the sides of the body with palms facing forward, fingers extended, and thumbs pointing away from the body.[9,17] Fig. 8-6 demonstrates this position.

Directional terms explain the location of various body structures in relation to each other. These terms are precise and avoid the use of unnecessary words and paint a clear picture for the radiation therapist.[17] *Superior* means toward the head; *inferior*, toward the feet; *medial*, toward the midline of the body; and *lateral*, toward one side or the other. *Anterior* relates to anatomy nearer to the front of the body; *posterior*, nearer to or at the back of the body. *Ipsilateral* refers to a body component on the same side of the body, whereas *contralateral* refers to the opposite side of the body. *Supine* means lying face up; *prone*, lying face down. Table 8-1 outlines the directional terms commonly used by the radiation therapy team.

Planes and sections

The human body may also be examined with respect to planes, which are imaginary flat surfaces, that pass through it. Fig. 8-7 illustrates the standard anatomical planes. The *sagittal plane* divides the body vertically into right or left

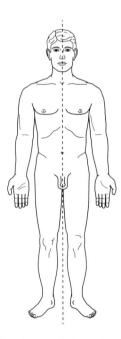

Fig. 8-6 Anatomical position and bilateral symmetry. In the anatomical position the body is in an erect, or standing, posture with the arms at the sides and palms forward. The head and feet are also pointing forward. The dotted line shows the body's bilateral symmetry. As a result of this organizational feature, the right and left sides of the body are mirror images of each other. (From Thibodeau GA, Patton KT, editors: Anatomy and physiology, ed 2. *The body as a whole*. St Louis, 1993, Mosby.)

Table 8-1	Directional terms	
Term	**Definition**	**Example**
Superior	Toward the head or upper part of a structure	The manubrium is superior to the body of the sternum
Inferior	Away from the head or lower part of the structure	The stomach is inferior to the lung
Anterior	Toward or nearer to the front	The trachea is anterior to the esophagus, which is anterior to the spinal cord
Posterior	Nearer to the back	The esophagus is posterior to the trachea
Medial	Nearer to the midline; the midline is an imaginary vertical line that divides the body into equal right and left components	The ulna is on the medial side of the forearm
Lateral	Farther from the midline or to the side	The pleural cavities are lateral to the pericardial cavity
Ipsilateral	On the same side	The ascending colon and appendix are ipsilateral
Contralateral	On the opposite side	The ascending colon and descending colon are contralateral
Proximal	Nearer to the point of origin or attachment	The humerus is proximal to the radius
Distal	Farther from the point of origin or attachment	The phalanges are distal to the carpals
Superficial	On or near the body surface	The skin is superficial to the thoracic viscera
Deep	Away from the body surface	The ribs are deep to the skin of the chest

Adapted from Tortora G, Anagnostakos N, editors: *Principles of anatomy and physiology*, ed 6. Copyright © 1990 by Biological Sciences Textbooks, Inc., A & P Textbooks, Inc., and Elia-Sparta, Inc. Reprinted by permission of Harper Collins Publishers, Inc.

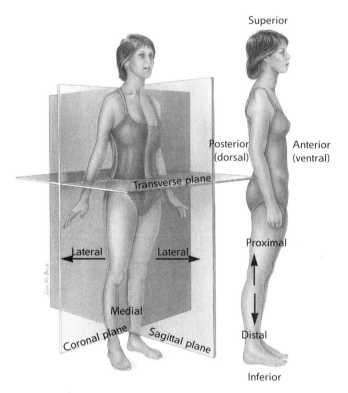

Fig. 8-7 Directions and planes of the body. These planes provide a standardized reference for the radiation therapist. (From Thibodeau GA, Patton KT, editors: Anatomy and physiology, ed 2. *Organization of the body*. St Louis, 1993, Mosby.)

sides. The *median sagittal plane*, also called the midsagittal plane, divides the body into two symmetrical right and left sides. There is only one median sagittal plane. A *parasagittal plane* is a vertical plane that is parallel to the median sagittal plane and divides the body into unequal components, both right and left. A *coronal* or *frontal plane* is perpendicular (at right angles) to the sagittal plane and vertically divides the body into anterior and posterior sections. A *horizontal* or *transverse plane* is perpendicular to the midsagittal, parasagittal, and coronal planes and divides the human body into superior and inferior parts. When a health care professional views a body structure, it is often seen in a sectional view. A sectional view looks at a flat surface resulting from a cut made through the three-dimensional structure.

Surface and cross-sectional anatomy in radiation therapy are not solely a set of definitions or a listing of body parts. The practitioner must relate the body's physical perspective to its overall function. The standardized anatomical nomenclature presented will assist in accurately realizing those relationships.

BODY HABITUS

Roentgen's discovery of the x-ray allowed scientists at the turn of the 19th century to revolutionize the medical field, both diagnostically and therapeutically.[2] These early radiographs demonstrated that there were great differences in the location of internal anatomy from one person to the next. While everyone had the same organs, they were not necessarily in the exact same place. It was agreed that man is a variable species with regard to structural characteristics. It is evident that variety in general physique corresponds to great variation in visceral form, position, and motility. There is consistency between certain physiques and certain types of visceral form and arrangement. It is obvious that a thorax of certain dimensions can only house lungs of a certain form. The same is true for the abdomen. Knowing this can greatly assist the radiation therapist in relating internal anatomy to varying types.

The physique, or **body habitus**, of an individual can be classified into four groups. The *hypersthenic habitus* represents about 5% of the population. This body type exhibits a short, wide trunk, great body weight, and a heavy skeletal framework. The abdomen is long with great capacity, the alimentary tract is high, and the stomach is almost thoracic. The pelvic cavity is small. When taking a chest film of this body type, it may be necessary to turn the cassette sideways to image the entire chest.

The *sthenic habitus* resembles the hypersthenic habitus. These individuals make up close to half (~48%) of the population. They are of considerable weight with a heavy skeletal framework. The alimentary tract is high but not as high as in the hypersthenic habitus. Most stout, well-built persons are sthenics.

The *hyposthenic habitus*, entailing about 35% of the population, has a slender physique. This habitus demonstrates many of the sthenic characteristics but appears to be more frail. The abdominal cavity falls between the sthenic and the asthenic.

The *asthenic habitus* demonstrates a more slender physique, light body weight, and a lighter skeletal framework. It is found in 10% to 12% of the population. The thorax has long, narrow lung fields with its widest portion in the upper zones. The heart is commonly pendant in form. The asthenic has an abdomen longer than the hypersthenic and is typically accompanied by a pelvis with great capacity. The alimentary tract is lowest of all types mentioned. Fig. 8-8 compares the various body habiti. While the internal components are the same in all body types, the locations vary. These categories can help standardize the variances demonstrated from person to person.

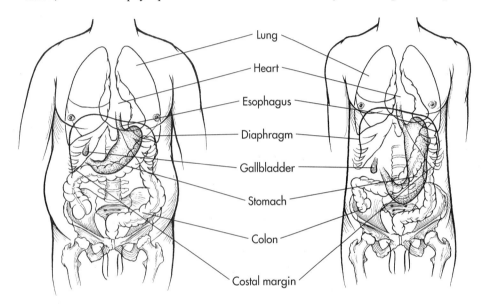

Hypersthenic   **Hyposthenic**

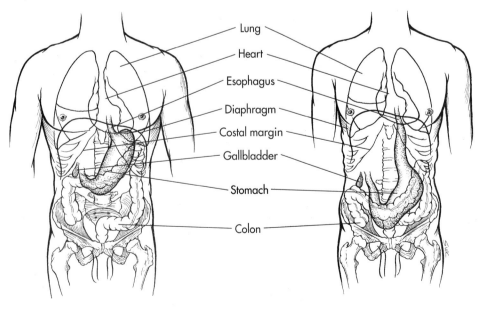

Sthenic   **Asthenic**

Fig. 8-8 Comparison of the four body habiti. Note that all feature the same structures. However, the internal viscera vary in position from one physique to another.

Body cavities

The spaces within the body that contain internal organs are called body cavities (Fig. 8-9). The two main cavities are the posterior, or dorsal, and the anterior, or ventral, cavities. The dorsal cavity can be further divided into the spinal or vertebral cavity, protected by the vertebrae, which contains the spinal cord, and the cranial cavity, which contains the brain.

The anterior cavity is subdivided by a horizontal muscle called the diaphragm into the thoracic cavity and the abdominopelvic cavity. The thoracic cavity is further divided into a pericardial cavity, which contains the heart and two pleural cavities, including the right and left lungs.

The abdominopelvic cavity has two sections: the upper abdominal cavity and the lower pelvic cavity. There is no intervening partition between the two. The principal structures located in the abdominal cavity are the peritoneum, liver, gallbladder, pancreas, spleen, stomach, and most of the large and small intestines. The pelvic section contains the rest of the large intestine, rectum, urinary bladder, and internal reproductive system.

The abdominopelvic cavity is large and is divided into four quadrants by placing a transverse plane across the midsagittal plane at the point of the umbilicus (navel). The four quadrants are the right upper, left upper, right lower, and left lower. The abdominal cavity can also be sectioned into a number of regions. Fig. 8-10 shows the quadrants and regions of the abdomen and pelvis. Table 8-2 outlines the regions of the abdominal cavity.

The surface markings and locations of all structures are approximations and generalizations.[8] However, knowledge of the varying body types will provide the radiation therapist with practical information. If the therapist has an idea of where the internal structures are, especially during a simulation, he or she can locate the placement of the treatment portal sooner and more accurately. This equates to less time on the simulation table for the patient and lower fluoroscopic exposure times, since it will not require as much location time.

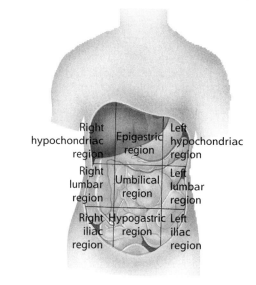

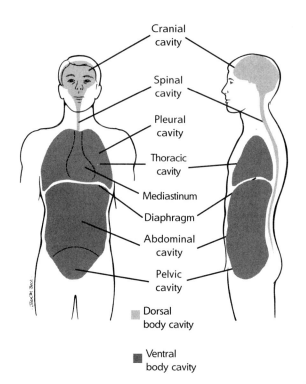

Fig. 8-9 Major body cavities. (From Thibodeau GA, Patton KT, editors: Anatomy and physiology, ed 2. *Organization of the body*. St Louis, 1993, Mosby.)

Fig. 8-10 Abdomen. **A**, Division of the abdomen into four quarters. Diagram shows relationship of internal organs to the abdominopelvic quadrants; **1**, right upper quadrant (RUQ); **2**, left upper quadrant (LUQ); **3**, right lower quadrant (RLQ); **4**, left lower quadrant (LLQ). **B**, Nine regions of abdominopelvic cavity showing the most superficial organs. (From Seeley RR, Stephens TD, Tate P, editors: *Essentials of anatomy and physiology*, ed 2. St Louis, 1996, Mosby.)

Table 8-2	Regions of the abdominal cavity

Region	Description
Umbilical	Centrally located around the navel
Lumbar	Regions to the right and left of the navel; lumbar refers to the lower back, which occurs here
Epigastric	Central region superior to the umbilical region
Hypochondriac	Regions to the right and left of the epigastric region and inferior to the cartilage of the rib cage
Hypogastric	Central region inferior to the umbilical region
Iliac	Regions to the right and left of the hypogastric region; iliac refers to the hip bones, which occur here

LYMPHATIC SYSTEM

Knowledge of the **lymphatic system** is paramount in the therapeutic administration of ionizing radiation. In an effort to achieve local and regional control of malignant disease processes, the anatomy of the lymphatic system must be considered. Many tumors spread through this system; quite often, areas of tumor spread are predicted based solely on that knowledge. For example, in a three-field head and neck treatment plan the supraclavicular fossa (SCF) is commonly treated even if there is no clinical evidence of tumor present because the lymphatic drainage of the head and neck eventually drains to that area. Treatment that provides radiation dosage in a body site in anticipation of possible future involvement is called prophylactic treatment. In any examination of surface and cross-sectional anatomy specific to radiation therapy, the lymphatic system must not be overlooked.

The lymphatic system consists of lymphatic vessels, lymphatic organs, and the fluid that circulates through it, called *lymph*. The system is closely associated with the cardiovascular system and is composed of specialized connective tissue that contains a large quantity of lymphocytes. Lymphatic tissue occurs throughout the body.

The lymphatic system has three main functions. First, lymphatic vessels drain tissue spaces of interstitial fluid that escapes from blood capillaries and loose connective tissues, filters it, and returns it to the bloodstream. This is important in maintaining the overall fluid levels in the body. Second, the lymphatic system absorbs fats and transports them to the bloodstream. Third, this intricate system plays a major role in the body's defense and immunity. **Immunity** is the ability of the body to defend itself against infectious organisms, foreign bodies, and cancer cells. Specifically, lymphocytes and macrophages protect the body by recognizing and responding to the foreign matter.

Lymphatic vessels

Lymphatic vessels contain lymph. Lymph is excessive tissue fluid consisting mostly of water and plasma proteins from capillaries. It differs from blood by the absence of formed elements in it. Lymphatic vessels start in spaces between cells; at that point they are referred to as lymphatic capillaries. These lymphatic vessels are quite extensive; virtually every region of the body that is vascularized is richly supplied with these capillaries. It stands to reason that those areas that are avascular do not demonstrate the same abundance. Examples of these avascular areas are the central nervous system and bone marrow. These lymphatic capillaries are more permeable than associated blood capillaries for substances to enter. Cellular debris, sloughed off cells, and foreign substances that occur in the intercellular spaces are more readily collected through these lymphatic pathways and transported away for filtration. They start blindly in the interstitial spaces and flow in only one direction.

The lymphatic capillaries join to form larger lymphatic vessels. Lymphatic vessels resemble veins in structure but have thinner walls and more valves that promote the one-way flow. These larger vessels follow veins and arteries and eventually empty into one of two ducts in the upper thorax—the **thoracic duct** or the **right lymphatic duct**—which then flow into the subclavian veins.

Fluid movement in the lymphatic system depends on hydrostatic and osmotic pressures that increase through skeletal muscular contraction. As the muscles around the vessels contract, the lymph is moved past a one-way valve that closes. This prevents the lymph from flowing backward. Respiratory movements create a pressure gradient between two ends of the lymphatic system. Fluid flows from high pressure areas, like the abdomen, to low pressure areas, like the thorax where pressure falls as each inhalation occurs.[17]

Lymph nodes

Along the paths of the lymph vessels are lymph nodes. These nodes vary in size from 1 to 25 mm in length, and they often occur in groups. A lymph node contains both afferent and efferent lymphatic vessels. **Afferent lymphatic vessels** enter the lymph node at several points along the convex surface. They contain one-way valves that open into the node, bringing the lymph into it. On the other side of the node are efferent vessels. The **efferent lymphatic vessels** are typically wider than the afferent vessels; their valves open away from the node, again facilitating one-way flow. There are more afferent vessels coming into a node than efferent vessels coming out of it, slowing the flow through the nodes. Fig. 8-11 demonstrates the components of a typical lymph node. This is similar to driving along a four-lane highway during rush hour and getting to a point of road construction that restricts traffic flow to one lane. You can only go in one direction and must wait your turn to move through the area. This slowing of the lymph through the node permits the nodes to effectively filter the lymph, and, through phagocytosis, the endothelial cells of the node engulf, devitalize, and remove even the bacterial contaminants.

The substances are trapped inside the reticular fibers and pathways throughout the node. Edema is an excessive accu-

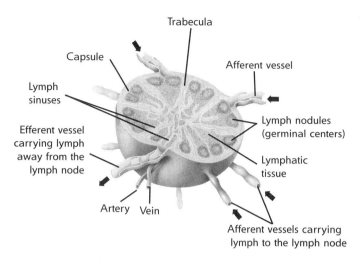

Fig. 8-11 Lymph node. *Arrows* indicate the direction of lymph flow. The germinal centers are sites of lymphocyte production. As lymph moves through the lymph sinuses, macrophages remove foreign substances. (From Seely RR, Stephens TD, Tate P, editors: Essentials of anatomy and physiology. *The lymphatic system and immunity*. St Louis, 1991, Mosby.)

mulation of fluid in a tissue, producing swelling. This can occur when excessive foreign bodies, lymph, and debris are being engulfed in the node. This is evident when a person has a cold or the flu. The subdigastric nodes, located in the neck just below the angle of the mandible, become swollen and tender because of the heightened phagocytic activity in that area to rid the body of the trapped contaminants. The swelling goes down as the pathogen is devitalized. Edema also occurs when altered lymphatic pathways cause more than normal amounts of lymph filtration. This is commonly seen in postmastectomy patients. The arm on the side of the surgery is often swollen because of the alteration of the natural lymphatic pathways secondary to the operation. The same amount of lymph is redirected through alternate routes, causing the slowdown of lymphatic flow.

Lymphatic organs

The spleen is the largest mass of lymphatic tissue in the body. It is located posterior and to the left of the stomach in the abdominal cavity, between the fundus of the stomach and the diaphragm. It is roughly 12 cm in length and actively filters blood, removes old red blood cells, manufactures lymphocytes (particularly B-cells, which develop into antibody-producing plasma cells) for immunity surveillance, and stores blood. Since the spleen has no afferent lymphatic vessels, it does not filter lymph. However, the spleen is often thought of as a large lymph node for the blood. During a *laparotomy*, which is surgical inspection of the abdominal cavity, in patients with lymphoma, this organ is often removed for biopsy and staging purposes. In this case the functions of the spleen are then assumed by the bone marrow and liver.

The thymus is located along the trachea superior to the heart and posterior to the sternum in the upper thorax. This gland is larger in children than adults and more active in pediatric immunity. The gland serves as a site where T-lymphocytes can mature.

The tonsils are series of lymphatic nodules embedded in a mucous membrane.[17] They are located at the junction of the oral cavity and pharynx. These collections of lymphoid tissue protect against foreign body infiltration by producing lymphocytes. The *pharyngeal tonsils*, or *adenoids*, are in the nasopharynx; the *palatine tonsils* are in the posterior lateral wall of the oropharynx; and the *lingual tonsils* are at the base of the tongue in the oropharynx.

The *thoracic duct* is on the left side of the body and is typically larger than the right lymphatic duct. It serves the lower extremities, abdomen, left arm, and left side of the head and neck and drains into the left subclavian vein. This duct is about 35 to 45 cm in length and begins in front of the second lumbar vertebra (L2) called the *cisterna chyli*. As lymph travels through the lower extremities to the cisterna chyli, it continues its upward trek to the thoracic duct. As it passes through the mediastinum, it bypasses many of the mediastinal node stations. Because of this anatomical fact, pedal lymphangiography, a technique used to visualize nodal status by injecting dye into lymphatic outlets in the feet, cannot be used to visualize mediastinal disease. The *right lymphatic duct* serves only the right arm and right side of the head and neck and drains into the right subclavian vein. This duct is about 1 to 2 cm in length. These ducts drain into the right and left subclavian veins, which in turn drain to the heart by way of the superior vena cava. The box below reviews the flow of lymph through the lymphatic system.

Knowledge of the location of the lymph nodes and direction of lymph flow is important in the diagnosis and prognosis of the spread of metastatic disease. Cancer cells often spread through the lymphatic system. Metastatic disease sites are predictable by their lymphatic flow from the primary site.[15] Inadequate knowledge of the lymphatic system often translates into ineffective treatment delivery.

Lymphatic Flow Overview

Tissue fluid leaves the cellular interstitial spaces and becomes
Lymph; as it enters a
Lymphatic capillary, it merges with other capillaries to form an
Afferent lymphatic vessel, which enters a
Lymph node where lymph is filtered. It then leaves the node via an
Efferent lymphatic vessel, which travels to other nodes, then merges with other vessels to form a
Lymphatic trunk, which merges with other trunks and joins a
Collecting duct, either the right lymphatic or the thoracic, which empties into a
Subclavian vein where lymph is returned to the bloodstream.

AXIAL SKELETON—SKULL, VERTEBRAL COLUMN, AND THORAX

The vast majority of imaging modalities provide valuable information through visualization of differences in anatomical densities. The denser a component, the "whiter" it appears on a radiograph. The axial skeleton provides the radiation therapist with a wealth of information used to reference the location of internal anatomy. The following sections will review axial skeleton anatomy and provide the reader with a reference necessary in relating internal structures to surface anatomy.

Skull

There are about 29 bones in the skull, and these are for the most part joined by sutures, joints held together by connective tissue, which limits movement (Fig. 8-12). The mandible and ossicles, which are bones in the middle ear, are the only bones in the skull not joined by sutures.

The lateral aspect of the skull vault is formed by the frontal, parietal, and occipital bones. The first two meet in the midline at the *bregma*, the roof of the skull often referred to as the "soft spot," and the last two meet at the *lambda*.

The facial skeleton, or visceral cranium, includes the 14 bones of the face. It consists of two maxillary bones, two zygomatic bones, two nasal bones, two lacrimal bones, two palatine bones, two inferior conchae (which make up the vomer), and one mandible.

Sutures

There are four prominent sutures in the skull. The *coronal suture* lies between the frontal bone and the two parietal bones. On either side of the skull, it begins at the bregma and

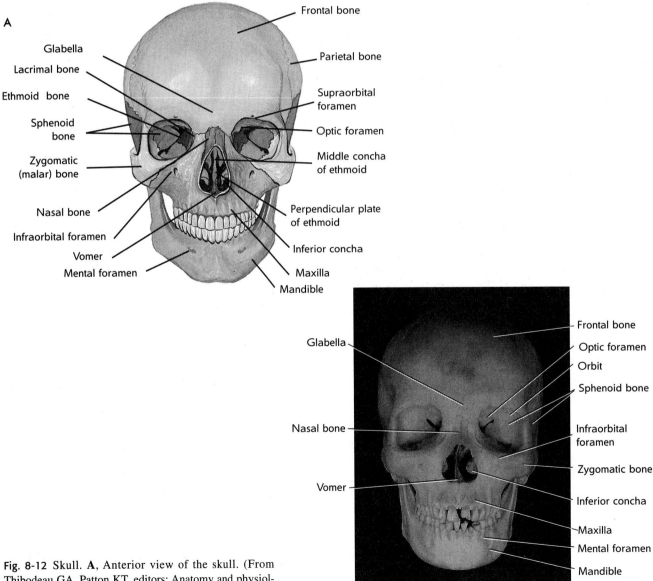

Fig. 8-12 Skull. **A**, Anterior view of the skull. (From Thibodeau GA, Patton KT, editors: Anatomy and physiology, ed 2. *Support and movement*. St Louis, 1993, Mosby.)

ends at the temporal bone. The *sagittal suture* lies between the two parietal bones and runs from the bregma to the lambda. The *lambdoidal suture* is in the posterior portion of the skull and lies between the parietal and occipital bones. Finally, the *squamosal suture*, one on each side of the skull, is located near the ear and lies between the parietal and temporal bones. Identification of these sutures radiographically can assist the radiation therapist in locating corresponding underlying structures.

Bones of the skull

The *calvaria* is the part of the skull that protects the brain. It is made up of one frontal bone, two parietal bones, one occipital bone, two temporal bones, one sphenoid bone, and one ethmoid bone. The *frontal bone* forms the forehead, part of the nose, and the superior portions of each orbit, called the superior orbital margin (SOM). The frontal sinuses are located within this bone. The *parietal bones* are posterior to the frontal bones and form the roof of the cranium as well as

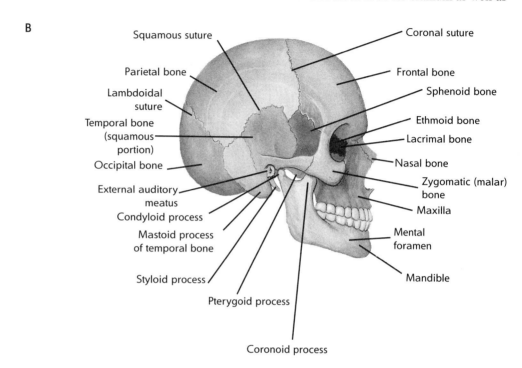

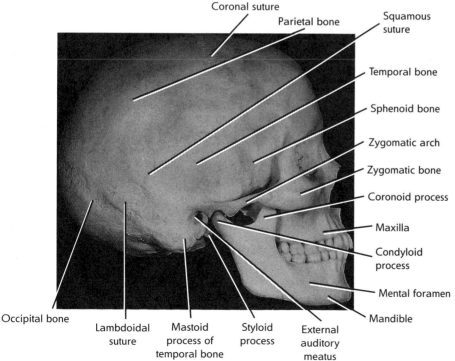

Fig. 8-12 Skull. **B**, Skull viewed from the right side. (From Thibodeau GA, Patton KT, editors: Anatomy and physiology, ed 2. *Support and movement.* St Louis, 1993, Mosby.)

the sides of the skull. The *occipital bone* forms the most posterior portion of the skull and base of the cranium along with the sphenoid bone. There are two *occipital condyles*, round bony prominences that articulate with the first cervical spine, the *atlas*. Also in the occipital bone is the external occipital protuberance, which is a prominence on the outer surface. It is also known as the *inion*.

The *temporal bones* are immediately inferior to the parietal bones on the cranial sides. Each temporal bone demonstrates the following:

- *Zygomatic process*, the slender portion of the temporal bone that extends on the side of the cheek.
- *Mastoid process*, a portion of the temporal bone that extends out at the base of the ear. This serves as a point of attachment for several neck muscles. Within the mastoid process are the mastoid air cells. These are small cavities in the mastoid bones that are easily seen radiographically.
- *Styloid process*, a sharp pointed process that extends down from the base of the temporal bone. Lateral skull radiographs demonstrate this structure behind the ramus of the mandible. This structure provides points of muscular attachment for the tongue and pharynx.
- *External auditory meatus* (EAM) is a tubelike passage that extends into the petrous part of the temporal bone. It ends at the tympanic membrane (eardrum).
- *Internal auditory meatus* (IAM) lies in the middle or inner ear. At the inner end of the IAM is an opening where the facial and auditory nerves leave the cranial cavity and enter the internal meatus.
- *Mandibular fossa*, a depression on the temporal bone that is anterior to the EAM. It forms the *temporomandibular joint* (TMJ), an articulation with the mandible.

The *sphenoid bone* forms part of the sides and base of the cranium, as well as the floor and sides of the orbits. The body of the sphenoid lies in the midline of the floor of the skull, anterior to the occipital bone. The *sella turcica*, or Turkish saddle, is a depression in the upper surface of the sphenoid body that houses the pituitary gland. It is roughly 2 cm anterior and 2 cm superior to the EAM.

The *ethmoid bone* is situated between the orbits and forms part of the anterior cranial fossa as well as part of the nasal and orbital walls. The *maxillary bones* form the upper jaw, and each has an alveolar process that houses the teeth. The *palatine process* extends from the maxillary bones and forms the anterior aspect of the roof of the mouth, the *hard palate*. The *infraorbital margin (IOM)*, the inferior part of the orbit, is formed by these bones. The *zygomatic bones* form the sides of the orbit and the cheekbone. The zygomatic process of these bones articulates with the zygomatic arch. The *lacrimal bones* are small bones located on the medial orbit walls. The orbital wall has an opening that holds the tear duct, which carries tears into the nasal cavities. If these ducts become blocked by infection or fibrotic changes secondary to radiation, a watery eye syndrome can occur.

The mandible, or lower jaw, is the only movable bone in the skull. The following are components of the mandible:

- *Angle*, located on each side of the mandible. It lies anterior and inferior to the ear.
- *Ramus*, the flat parts of the bone that extend up to the temporal bone. Each ramus has a *coronoid process* on its anterior surface that serves as a point of muscular attachment for muscles of mastication and a *condyloid* or *mandibular process* on the posterior ramus that articulates with the temporal bone at the TMJ.
- *Mental protuberance*, which forms the chin.
- *Alveolar border*, located on the upper part of the mandibular body, which houses the lower teeth.[9]

Paranasal sinuses

The bones of the skull and face contain the **paranasal sinuses**, which are air spaces, lined by mucous membranes, that reduce the weight of the skull and give a resonant sound to the voice. When a person has sinusitis, an inflammation and blockage of the sinus cavities, the voice often has a "stuffed up" tone (loss of resonance). The paired sinuses are formed from each nasal cavity within the frontal, maxillary, sphenoid, and ethmoid bones. They are lined with mucous membranes and are relatively small at birth. They enlarge during development of the permanent teeth and reach adult size shortly after puberty.[8] The paranasal sinuses are easily seen on plain x-ray, CT, and MRI. Cross-sections are an excellent tool to study the surface relations in these areas.[13] Fig. 8-13 demonstrates the paranasal sinuses in cross-section.

The maxillary sinus is a pyramidal-shaped cavity that is enclosed in the maxilla. It is the largest of the paranasal sinuses. The roof of the sinus forms the floor of the orbit. The *frontal sinus* lies in the frontal bone above the orbit. It may be located on the surface by a triangle between the following three points: the nasion, a point 3 cm above the nasion, and the junction of the medial and middle thirds of the SOM. The *sphenoid sinus* lies posterior and superior to the nasopharynx enclosed in the body of the sphenoid bone at the level of the zygomatic arch. Superiorly the sinus is related to the sella turcica and the pituitary. It is possible to have surgical removal of the pituitary through a trans-sphenoidal approach, one that goes through the nasal cavity. The *ethmoid sinus* is bilateral but consists of a honeycomb of air cells lying between the middle wall of the orbit and the upper lateral wall of the nose.

Vertebral column

The vertebral column, located in the midsagittal plane of the posterior cavity, extends from the skull to the pelvis. It consists of separate bones, the vertebrae, which appear as rectangles on radiographs.[8] There are 33 bones in the adult ver-

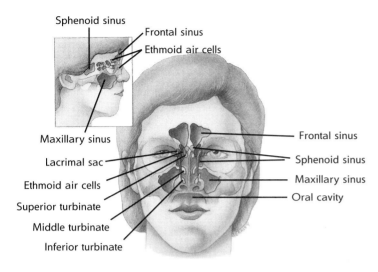

tebral column, as shown in Fig. 8-14, which also indicates the number of bones in each section. There are 7 cervical, 12 thoracic, 5 lumbar, 5 sacral, and 4 coccygeal vertebrae. At the inferior aspect of the column, the sacrum has 5 fused bones, whereas the coccyx is composed of 4 fused bones.

The sacrum supports the rest of the vertebral column and thus provides the support necessary for the human body's erectness. The vertebrae are separated by radiolucent fibrocartilage called intervertebral disks. In the cervical and thoracic spine the disks are of similar height. In the lumbar spine their height increases progressively down the column.[8,11,12]

The vertebral column is also very flexible. There is an additive effect of the limited motion between any two vertebrae, and, as a whole, the vertebral column is capable of substantial motion. The column also protects the spinal cord and provides points of attachment for the skull, thorax, and extremities.

Vertebral characteristics

Most vertebrae share several common characteristics. They have a body that is attached to a posterior vertebral arch. These two components border the *vertebral foramen*, the passage that the spinal cord passes through. There are typi-

Fig. 8-13 The paranasal sinuses. The anterior view shows the anatomical relationship of the paranasal sinuses to each other and to the nasal cavity. The inset is a lateral view of the position of the sinuses. (From Thibodeau GA, Patton KT, editors: Anatomy and physiology, ed 2. *Anatomy of the respiratory system.* St Louis, 1993, Mosby.)

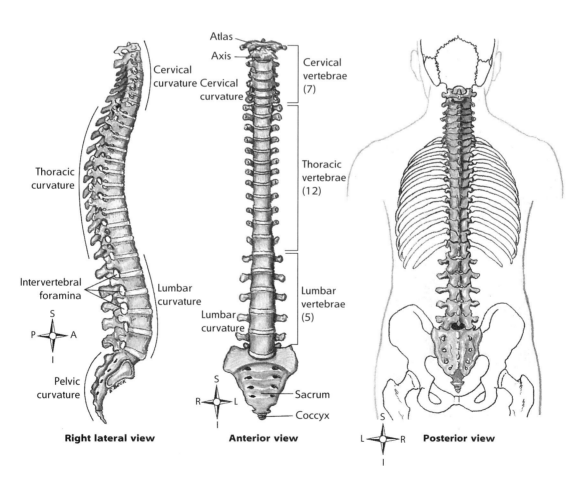

Fig. 8-14 The vertebral column (three views). (From Thibodeau GA, Patton KT, editors: Anatomy and physiology, ed 2. *Support and movement.* St Louis, 1993, Mosby.)

cally spinous and transverse processes that allow for muscle attachments. The *spinous process* is posterior and forms where two laminae meet. These laminae are typically palpated in aligning spinal treatment fields. The *transverse processes* are lateral projections where a pedicle joins a lamina. Fig. 8-15 exhibits a typical vertebra with its prominent features labeled.

The first two vertebrae, C1 and C2, are atypical from all others. *C1*, the *atlas*, serves the specialized function of supporting the skull and allowing it to turn. It has no vertebral body. *C2*, the *axis*, has an odontoid process that extends into the ring of the atlas. When the head turns from side to side, it pivots on this process. These two vertebrae are shown in Fig. 8-16.

Vertebral column curvatures

The vertebral column demonstrates several curvatures that develop at different intervals.[8] These curvatures can be classified as either primary or compensatory (secondary) curvatures. **Primary vertebral curves** are developed in utero as the fetus develops in the C-shaped fetal position, and they are present at birth. **Compensatory** or **secondary vertebral curves** develop after birth as the child learns to sit up and walk. Muscular development and coordination influence the rate of secondary curvature development.

The *cervical curve* extends from the first cervical to the second thoracic vertebrae (C1 to T2). It is convex anteriorly and develops as the child learns to hold his or her head up and sits alone at about 4 months of age. This curve is a secondary curvature. The *thoracic curve* extends from T2 to T12 and is concave anteriorly. This is one of the primary curves of the vertebral column. The *lumbar curve* runs from T12 to the anterior surface of L5. This convex forward curve develops when the child learns to walk at about 1 year of age. The *pelvic curve* is concave anteriorly and inferiorly and extends

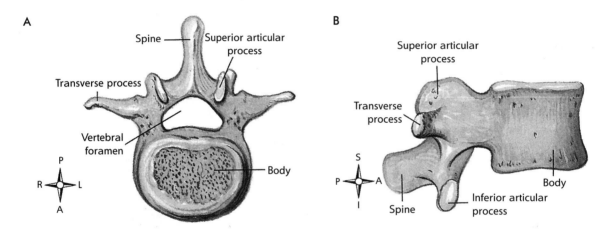

Fig. 8-15 Lumbar vertebrae. **A**, Third lumbar vertebra viewed from above (superior). **B**, Third lumbar vertebra viewed from the side (lateral). (From Thibodeau GA, Patton KT, editors: Anatomy and physiology, ed 2. *The skeletal system.* St Louis, 1993, Mosby.)

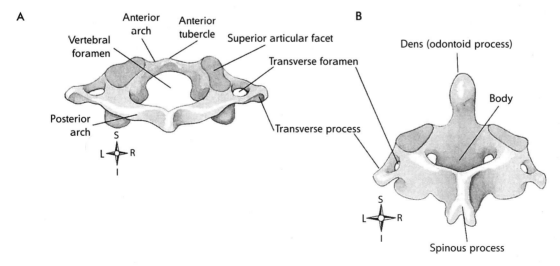

Fig. 8-16 Cervical vertebrae. **A**, First cervical vertebra (atlas) viewed from behind (posterior). **B**, Second cervical vertebra (axis) viewed from behind (posterior). (From Thibodeau GA, Patton KT, editors: Anatomy and physiology, ed 2. *The skeletal system.* St Louis, 1993, Mosby.)

from the anterior surfaces of the sacrum and coccyx. This is the other primary curve.

The aforementioned curvatures are normal curves demonstrated in the human vertebral column. There are also three abnormal curvatures that are present both clinically and radiographically. *Kyphosis* is an excessive curvature of the vertebral column that is convex posteriorly. These curves can develop with degenerative vertebral changes. Those afflicted with this are referred to as hunchbacks. *Scoliosis* is an abnormal lateral curvature of the vertebral column with excessive right or left curvature in the thoracic region. This abnormal curvature can develop if only one side (half) of the vertebral bodies are irradiated in pediatric patients, as in the case of early Wilms' tumor treatments. The radiation retards vertebral body growth on one side while the contralateral side grows at a normal rate, thus creating scoliotic changes. *Lordosis* is an excessive convexity of the lumbar curve of the spine.

Thorax

The final part of the axial skeleton is the thorax, which is illustrated in Fig. 8-17. The illustration shows the full *thorax* made up of the bony cage formed by the sternum, costal cartilage, ribs, and the thoracic vertebrae to which they are attached.[9,15] The thorax encloses and protects the organs in the thoracic cavity and upper abdomen. It also provides support for the pectoral girdle and upper extremities.

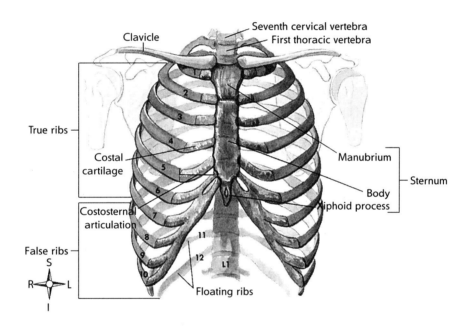

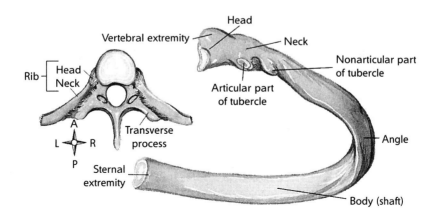

Fig. 8-17 The bony framework of the thorax provides many useful landmarks. (From Thibodeau GA, Patton KT, editors: Anatomy and physiology, ed 2. *Support and movement*. St Louis, 1993, Mosby.)

Sternum and ribs

The sternum, or breastbone, comprises three parts: the *manubrium*, which is the superior portion; the *body*, the middle and largest portion; and the *xiphoid process*, which is the inferior projection that serves as ligament and muscle attachments. The manubrium has a depression called the **suprasternal notch** (SSN), which occurs at the level of T2 and articulates with the medial ends of the clavicles. This point is commonly used in measuring the angle of chin tilt in head and neck patients. It also serves as a palpable landmark when setting up a supraclavicular fossa field. The manubrium also articulates with the first two ribs. The junction of the manubrium and the body form the *sternal angle*, also called the angle of Louis; it occurs at the level of T4.

The body of the sternum articulates with the second through tenth ribs. There are 12 pairs of ribs, of which the superior 7 pairs are considered true ribs. They are easily seen in the asthenic body habitus and palpable in most others.[9] They articulate posteriorly with the vertebrae and anteriorly with the sternum directly through a cartilaginous joint. These are known as the vertebrosternal ribs. The next three pairs join with the vertebrae posteriorly and anteriorly with the cartilage of the immediately anterior rib. These ribs are classified as vertebrochondral ribs. The next (last) pairs only articulate with the vertebrae and do not connect with the sternum in any way; they are called floating ribs.

The axial skeleton is easily demonstrated with most imaging techniques employed in radiation therapy. A thorough working knowledge of these components serves the radiation therapist in overall daily operations. This information is the basis, the road map, that will be used in relating the surface and cross-sectional anatomy as well as the palpable bony landmarks that are used in field placement and treatment planning. The next series of sections in this chapter will outline this anatomy.

SURFACE AND SECTIONAL ANATOMY AND LANDMARKS OF THE HEAD AND NECK

The human head demonstrates various anatomical features that are both interesting and useful to the radiation therapist. These structures are rich in bony and fleshy (moveable, soft tissue) landmarks and lymphatics commonly used in field placement, position locations, etc. The bony landmarks are very stable and are typically used as reference points, as in the case of locating a positioning or central axis tattoo. Fleshy landmarks can also be extremely useful. However, they tend to be more mobile and provide a less reliable reference than the bony landmarks.

Bony landmarks—anterior and lateral skull

Figs. 8-18 and 8-19 outline the locations of the following anterior and lateral bony structures.

The *frontal bone* is the area of maximum convexity on the forehead and articulates with the frontal process of the max-

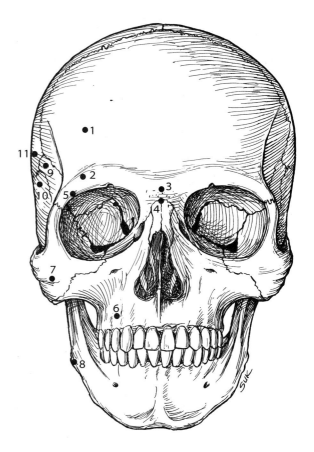

Fig. 8-18 Bony landmarks of the anterior skull. *1.* Frontal bone; *2.* superciliary arch; *3.* glabella; *4.* nasion; *5.* superior orbital margin (SOM); *6.* maxilla; *7.* zygomatic bone; *8.* angle of mandible; *9.* sphenoid bone (greater wing); *10.* temporal bone; *11.* parietal bone.

illary bone on the medial side of the orbit.[8,9] Together with the lacrimal bones, it protects the lacrimal duct and glands.

The *glabella* is the slight elevation directly between the two orbits in the frontal bone. It is just above the base of the nose. This palpable landmark is more prominent in some individuals than in others.

The *nasion* is the central depression at the base of the nose. It is formed by the point of joining of the frontal and nasal bones.

The *superciliary arch* starts at the glabella and moves superiorly and laterally above the central portion of the eyebrow. The central part lies superficially to the frontal sinuses on either side.

The *superior orbital margin* rests just inferior to the eyebrow and is more pronounced on its lateral aspect. The SOM forms the roof of the orbit and serves as one of the points used to delineate the inferior border of whole brain fields (along with the tragus and mastoid tip). By ensuring that part of the SOM is in the treatment field, the frontal part of the brain will also be in the field.

The *maxilla* is the bone felt between the ala (lateral soft tissue prominence) of the nose and the prominence of the

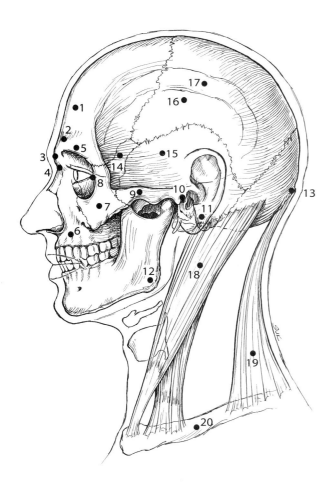

Fig. 8-19 Bony landmarks of the lateral skull. *1.* Frontal bone; *2.* superciliary arch; *3.* glabella; *4.* nasion; *5.* superior orbital margin (SOM); *6.* maxilla; *7.* zygomatic bone; *8.* lateral canthus; *9.* mid-zygoma point; *10.* external acoustic meatus (EAM); *11.* mastoid process; *12.* angle of mandible; *13.* external occipital protuberance (EOP) or inion; *14.* greater wing of sphenoid; *15.* temporal bone; *16.* parietal bone; *17.* parietal eminence; *18.* sternocleidomastoid muscle; *19.* trapezius muscle; *20.* clavicle.

cheek. This bone houses the largest of the paranasal sinuses. The inferior alveolar ridge of the maxilla houses the teeth sockets.

The *zygomatic bone* forms part of the lateral aspect of the orbit and the prominence of the cheek. The articulation between the frontal process of the zygomatic bone and the zygomatic process of the frontal bone can be palpated in the lateral orbital margin. The *mid-zygoma point*, a point midway between the EAM and the lateral canthus, lies roughly at the floor of the sphenoid sinus and roof of the nasopharynx. One centimeter superior to that point corresponds to the floor of the sella turcica, and 1.5 cm superior to the point corresponds to the pituitary gland.

The *mastoid process* is an extension of the mastoid temporal bone at the level of the ear lobe. It is commonly used to delineate the posterior point of the inferior whole brain

border (imaginary line that extends from the SOM to the mastoid tip, commonly going through the tragus of the ear).

The *external occipital protuberance* (EOP or inion) is the prominence in the posterolateral aspect of the occipital bone of the skull.

The *angle of the mandible* is the point at which the muscles of mastication are attached. Also, there are several lymph node groups located inferior and medial to that point and is also a classic landmark for the tonsils.

Landmarks around the eye

Whenever practical, the landmarks used around the eye should be the bony landmarks. They are radiographically visible and are easily checked if a second course of treatment is necessary in the same or neighboring area. The soft tissue landmarks often change with age, weight, and surgical changes. They are open to variable interpretation and misinterpretation because of the extreme flexibility of the skin. Fig. 8-20 illustrates these landmarks. The following outlines the landmarks about the eye, some being reiterated from previous sections.

The *superior orbital margin* is a bony landmark that forms the superior margin of the orbit.

The *inferior orbital margin* (IOM) is another bony landmark that forms the inferior margin of the bony orbit.

The *lateral orbital margin* (LOM) is a bony landmark that forms the lateral margin of the bony orbit.

The *medial orbital margin* is extremely difficult to palpate and is therefore not clinically useful as an anatomical landmark. It does have some usefulness radiographically.

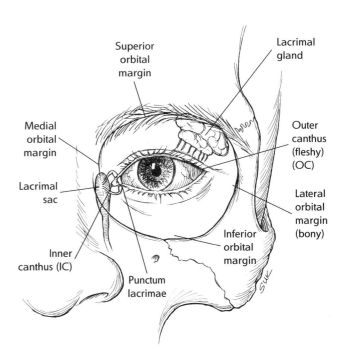

Fig. 8-20 Landmarks around the eye and orbit.

The *inner canthus* (IC) is a soft tissue landmark that is formed at the junction of the upper and lower eyelid at the medial aspect of the eye.

The *outer canthus* (OC) is a soft tissue landmark that is formed at the junction of the upper and lower eyelid at the lateral aspect of the eye.

The *punctum lacrimae* is a soft tissue landmark that can be used as a point of reference in the surface anatomy of the eye. This white-appearing section of the eye lies just lateral to the inner canthus on the lower eyelid. Tears are drained through this duct into the lacrimal duct. This opening can become blocked by fibrotic changes secondary to ionizing radiation administered to the area, causing constant tearing.

Landmarks around the nose

As in the case of the eye, the landmarks used around the nose should be the bony landmarks. Soft tissue landmarks often change with age, weight, and surgical changes and are open to variable interpretation and misinterpretation because of the extreme flexibility of the skin. Fig. 8-21 illustrates these landmarks. The following outlines the landmarks about the nose, some being reiterated from previous sections.

The *lateral ala nasi* (LAN) is a soft tissue landmark formed by the lateral attachment of the ala nasi with the cheek. The *inferior ala nasi* (IAN) is a soft tissue landmark formed by the inferior attachment of the ala nasi with the cheek. Both of these landmarks are prominent in most people and can be very useful landmarks when measuring in any direction, such as superior to inferior, medial to lateral, and anterior to posterior.

The *nasion* is the depression of the nose where it joins the forehead at the level of the SOM. It is a very useful landmark if it is deep and pronounced and coincides with the crease of the nose. If it is shallow, it is more open to variable interpretation.

The *glabella* is the bony prominence in the forehead at the level just superior to the SOM. As in the case of the nasion, it is useful if it is prominent and sharp. It is not very useful if it is flat or extremely curved, where it, too, would be open to misinterpretation.

The ala nasi, dorsum of the nose, and external nares are useful as checkpoints in the surface anatomy of the nose. Mainly used in positional definition of superficial skin lesions, these structures are useful in the positioning of radiation treatment portals.

Landmarks around the mouth

Landmarks around the mouth are generally not very accurate because of the extreme flexibility in the area. Every effort should be made to document these landmarks with reference to more stable anatomical points, if possible. If these landmarks are used, it is important to note the position of the mouth as well as any positioning or immobilization devices used, such as a cork, oral stent, or similar devices. Fig. 8-22 illustrates the landmarks around the mouth.

The *commissure of the mouth* is formed at the junction of the upper and lower lip. This landmark is extremely mobile.

The *mucocutaneous junction* (MCJ) is located at the junction of the vermilion border of the lip with the skin of the face.

The *columella* is located at the junction of the skin of the nose with the skin of the face at the superior end of the philtrum.

Landmarks around the ear

The external ear consists of the auricle or pinna, which is formed from a number of irregularly shaped pieces of fibrocartilage covered by skin. It has a dependent lobule, or ear lobe, and an anterior tragus, commonly used as anatomical references.[7,9,14] Parts of the ear are labeled in Fig. 8-23.

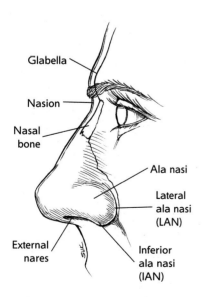

Fig. 8-21 Landmarks around the nose.

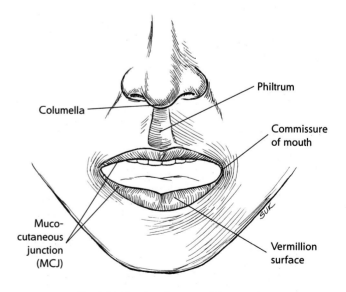

Fig. 8-22 Landmarks around the mouth.

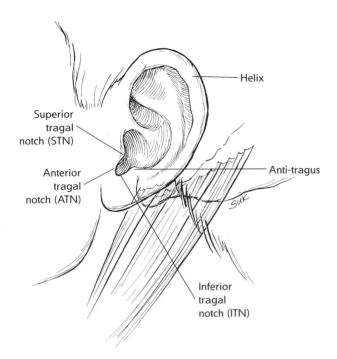

Fig. 8-23 Landmarks around the ear.

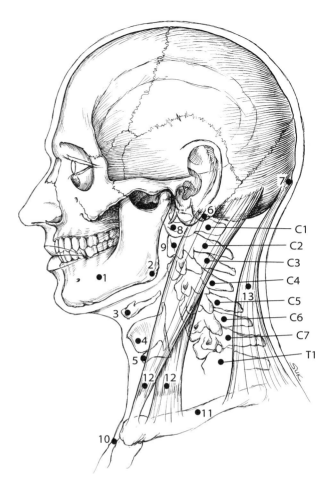

Fig. 8-24 The neck demonstrates many useful anatomical landmarks that can assist the radiation therapist. Relating surface structures to deeper anatomy is essential in the practice of radiation therapy. *1.* Body of mandible; *2.* angle of mandible; *3.* hyoid bone; *4.* thyroid cartilage; *5.* cricoid cartilage; *6.* mastoid process; *7.* external occipital protuberance (EOP); *8.* atlas; *9.* axis; *10.* suprasternal notch; *11.* clavicle; *12.* sternocleidomastoid muscle; *13.* trapezius muscle.

The *tragus* is made up of a fairly stable cartilage that partially covers the external auditory meatus in the external ear. The tragus is relatively stable and is often used in radiation therapy during initial positioning. A pair of optical lasers, coincident with each other, can be focused on the tragus on both sides of the patient. Doing this places the patient's head in a relatively nontilted position, as their locations are typically symmetrical. Just anterior to the tragus corresponds to the posterior wall of the nasopharynx. The posterior limit of many head and neck off cord fields lies at this point.

The *tragal notch* is the semicircular notch in the ear immediately inferior to the tragus. The *superior tragal notch* (STN) makes up the superior margin of the tragal notch. The *inferior tragal notch* (ITN) defines the inferior margin of the tragal notch. The *anterior tragal notch* (ATN) makes up the anterior margin of the tragal notch.

Landmarks and anatomy around the neck

The boundaries of the anterior aspect of the neck are the body and angles of the mandible superiorly, and the superior border and suprasternal notch of the sternum and the clavicles. The posterior aspect of the neck is bound superiorly by the external occipital protuberance and laterally by the mastoid processes. The posterior inferior border ends at roughly the level of cervical vertebra seven to thoracic vertebra one (C7-T1).[8] Fig. 8-24 illustrates the features of the neck anatomy.

The upper cervical vertebrae are not easily palpated; the last cervical and first thoracic vertebrae are the most obvious. The hyoid bone lies opposite the superior border of C4.

When the head is in the anatomical position, the hyoid bone may be moved from side to side between the thumb and middle finger, about 1 cm below the level of the angle of the mandible, C2. Table 8-3 relates the location of the cervical bony landmarks to other associated anatomical features.

Pharynx

The pharynx is a membranous tube that extends from the base of the skull to the esophagus. It connects the nasal and oral cavities with the larynx and esophagus. It is divided into the following sections, which are illustrated through coronal and transverse CT and MRI slices in Fig. 8-25. Note that in looking at the low neck in a sectional view, the therapist can easily remember how to distinguish the order of the spinal cord, esophagus, and trachea. If looking from a posterior to anterior perspective, the order is always **SET** up: **S**—spinal cord, **E**—esophagus, and **T**—trachea.

Table 8-3	Cervical neck landmarks and associated anatomy
Cervical spine	**Associated anatomy and nodes**
C1	Transverse process lies just inferior to the mastoid process; may be palpated in the hollow inferior to the ear
C2	Level with the angle of the mandible; lies 5 to 7 cm below the external occipital protuberance
C3	Located just superior to the hyoid bone of the neck; serves as a point of muscle attachment
C4	Level with the superior portion of the thyroid cartilage and marks the beginning of the larynx
C6	Level with the cricoid cartilage; location of the junction of the larynx to trachea and pharynx to esophagus
C7	First prominent spinous process in the posterior neck

- The *nasopharynx*, or *epipharynx*, communicates with the nasal cavity and provides a passageway for air during breathing.
- The *oropharynx*, or *mesopharynx*, opens behind the soft palate into the nasopharynx and functions as a passageway for food moving down from the mouth as well as for air moving in and out of the nasal cavity.
- The *laryngopharynx*, or *hypopharynx*, is located inferior to the oropharynx and opens into the larynx and esophagus.

Larynx

The larynx is contiguous with the lower portion of the pharynx above it and is connected with the trachea below it. It extends from the tip of the epiglottis at the level of the junction of C3 and C4 to the lower portion of the cricoid cartilage at the level of the C6 vertebra.[7] The larynx is subdivided into three anatomical regions: the supraglottis, glottis, and subglottis. Fig. 8-26 illustrates sectional views of the larynx. The larynx is actually an enlargement in the airway at the top of the trachea and below the pharynx. It serves as a passageway for air moving in and out of the trachea and functions to prevent foreign objects from entering the trachea.

The *thyroid cartilage* forms a midline prominence, the laryngeal prominence or Adam's apple, which is more obvious in the adult male. The vocal cords are attached to the posterior part of this prominence. The *cricoid cartilage* serves as the lower border of the larynx and is the only complete ring of cartilage in the respiratory passage; the others are open posteriorly. It is palpable as a narrow horizontal bar inferior to the thyroid cartilage and is at the level of the C6 vertebra.

Nasal and oral cavities

The nasal cavity opens to the external environment through the nostrils, and posteriorly the nostrils are continuous with the nasopharynx and lined with a ciliated mucous membrane. The oral cavity has a vestibule, which is the space between the cheeks and teeth and the oral cavity proper that opens posteriorly into the oropharynx and houses the soft palate, hard palate, uvula, anterior tongue, and floor of mouth.

Surface anatomy of the neck

Anatomical landmarks around the neck are mainly used as checkpoints and reference points that can establish the patient's position or the anatomical position of the treatment field. The most frequently used landmarks of the neck are as follows:

- Skin profile
- Sternocleidomastoid muscle—attached to the mastoid and occipital bones superiorly and sternal and clavicular heads inferiorly. These muscles form the V shape in the neck and are associated with a great number of lymph nodes.
- Clavicle
- Thyroid notch
- Mastoid tip
- External occipital protuberance
- Spinous processes

These surface neck landmarks assist the radiation therapist in referencing locations of treatment fields and dose-limiting structures. They are illustrated in Fig. 8-27.

Lymphatic drainage of the head and neck

The lymphatic drainage of the head and neck is through deep and superficial lymphatic rings, around the base of the skull, and deep and superficial lymph chains. The head and neck area is very rich in lymphatics. Enlarged cervical lymph nodes are the most common lumps seen in clinical practice.[9] They are typically associated with upper respiratory tract infections but may also be the site of metastatic disease from the head and neck, lungs, or breast or primary lymphoreticular disease such as Hodgkin's disease. The lymph nodes of the head and neck are outlined in the following section. Figs. 8-28 and 8-29 demonstrate the lymphatic chains and nodes in the head and neck.

The *occipital lymph nodes*, typically one to three in number, are located on the back of the head, close to the margin of the trapezius muscle attachment on the occipital bone. These nodes provide efferent flow to the superior deep cervical nodes.

The *retroauricular lymph nodes*, usually two in number, are situated on the mastoid insertion of the sternocleidomastoid muscle deep to the posterior auricular muscle. They drain the posterior temporooccipital region of the scalp, auricle, and external auditory meatus. They provide efferent drainage to the superior deep cervical nodes.

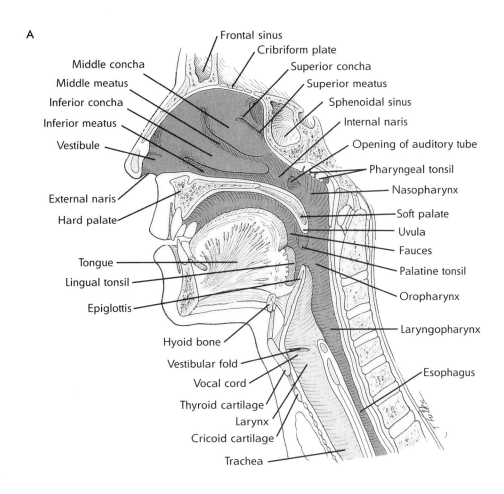

A

Middle concha
Middle meatus
Inferior concha
Inferior meatus
Vestibule

Frontal sinus
Cribriform plate
Superior concha
Superior meatus
Sphenoidal sinus
Internal naris
Opening of auditory tube
Pharyngeal tonsil
Nasopharynx

External naris
Hard palate

Tongue
Lingual tonsil
Epiglottis

Hyoid bone
Vestibular fold
Vocal cord
Thyroid cartilage
Larynx
Cricoid cartilage
Trachea

Soft palate
Uvula
Fauces
Palatine tonsil
Oropharynx
Laryngopharynx
Esophagus

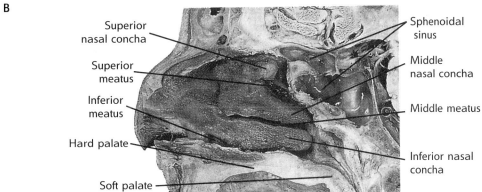

B

Superior
nasal concha
Superior
meatus
Inferior
meatus
Hard palate
Soft palate

Sphenoidal
sinus
Middle
nasal concha
Middle meatus
Inferior nasal
concha

Fig. 8-25 Nasal cavity and pharynx. **A,** Sagittal section through the nasal cavity and pharynx viewed from the medial side. **B,** Photograph of a sagittal section of the nasal cavity. (From Seely RR, Stephens TD, Tate P, editors: Essentials of anatomy and physiology. *The lymphatic system and immunity.* St Louis, 1991, Mosby.)

The *deep parotid lymph nodes* are arranged into two groups. The first group is embedded in the parotid gland, whose superior border is the TMJ; posterior border, the mastoid process; inferior border, the angle of the mandible; anterior border, the anterior ramus. The second group—the subparotid nodes—are located deep to the gland and lie on the lateral wall of the pharynx. Both drain the nose, eyelid, fron-

totemporal scalp, EAM, and palate. They provide efferent flow to the superior deep cervical nodes.

The *submaxillary lymph nodes* are facial nodes that are scattered over the infraorbital region. They span from the groove between the nose and cheek to the zygomatic arch. The *buccal lymph nodes* are scattered over the buccinator muscle. These nodes drain the eyelids, nose, and cheek and

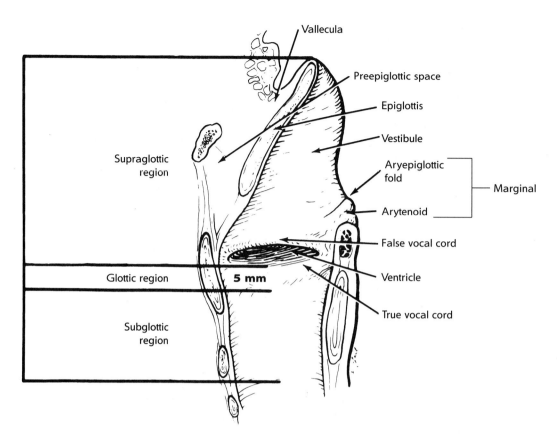

Fig. 8-26 Posterior view of the base of the tongue, larynx, and hypopharynx. Note the pyriform sinus, pharyngeal wall, and postcricoid area. (From Cox JD, editor: *Moss' radiation oncology: rationale, technique, results*, ed 7. St Louis, 1994, Mosby.)

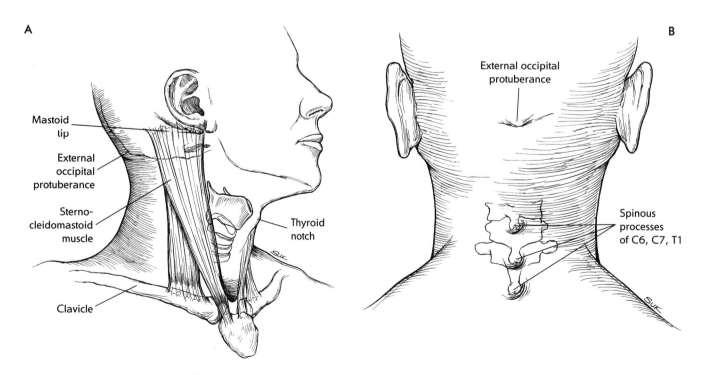

Fig. 8-27 Surface anatomy of the neck. **A,** Anteriolateral view. **B,** Posterior view.

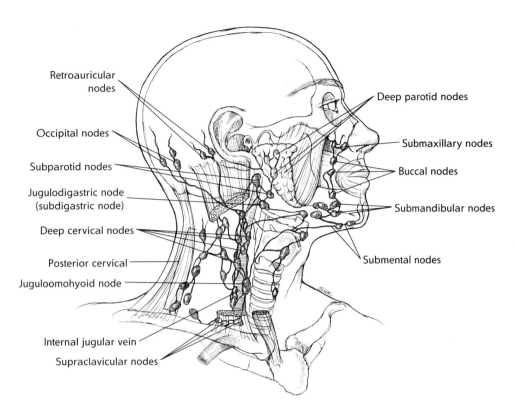

Retroauricular nodes

Occipital nodes

Subparotid nodes

Jugulodigastric node (subdigastric node)

Deep cervical nodes

Posterior cervical

Juguloomohyoid node

Internal jugular vein

Supraclavicular nodes

Deep parotid nodes

Submaxillary nodes

Buccal nodes

Submandibular nodes

Submental nodes

Fig. 8-28 Topographic view of head and neck lymph nodes.

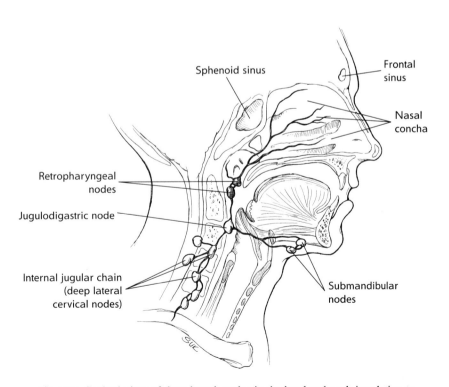

Sphenoid sinus

Frontal sinus

Nasal concha

Retropharyngeal nodes

Jugulodigastric node

Internal jugular chain (deep lateral cervical nodes)

Submandibular nodes

Fig. 8-29 Sagittal view of deep lymph nodes in the head and neck in relation to underlying structures.

supply efferent flow to the submandibular nodes. The *sub-mandibular lymph nodes* lie on the outer surface of the mandible. They drain the scalp, nose, cheek, floor of mouth, anterior two thirds of the tongue, gums, teeth, lips, and the frontal, ethmoid, and maxillary sinuses. They provide efferent drainage to the superior deep cervical nodes.

The *retropharyngeal lymph nodes*, one to three in number, lie in the buccopharyngeal fossa, behind the upper part of the pharynx and anterior to the arch of the atlas. These nodes are commonly involved in nasopharyngeal tumors and subsequently are included in the treatment fields.

The *submental lymph nodes* are found in the submental triangle of the digastric muscles, lower gums and lips, tongue, central floor of mouth, and skin of the chin. These nodes provide efferent drainage to the submandibular nodes.

The *superficial cervical lymph nodes* form a group of nodes located below the hyoid bone and in front of the larynx, trachea, and thyroid gland.

The *deep cervical lymph nodes* form a chain of 20 to 30 nodes along the carotid sheath and around the internal jugular chain along the sternocleidomastoid muscle. The *jugulodigastric lymph node*, at times called the *subdigastric node*, is typically located superior to the angle of the mandible and drains the tonsils and the tongue. Inferiorly, the chain spreads out into the subclavian triangle. One of the nodes in this group lies in the omohyoid tendon and is known as the jugulo-omohyoid lymph node.[8,9] When these two nodes are enlarged, it may signal carcinoma of the tongue, since enlarged neck nodes may be the only sign of the disease. These vessels supply efferent flow to form the jugular trunk, which drains to the thoracic or right lymphatic duct,

both in the supraclavicular fossa. The cervical lymph nodes are typically included in the treatment fields of most head and neck cancers that spread through the lymphatics, which include most of them. The fields that encompass the group are commonly called *posterior cervical strips*.

SURFACE AND SECTIONAL ANATOMY AND LANDMARKS OF THE THORAX AND BREAST

Various malignant diseases manifest themselves in the human thorax. Cancers of the lung, breast, and mediastinal lymphatics require the radiation therapist to have a working knowledge of the surface and sectional anatomy of the thorax. The human thorax demonstrates various anatomical features that are commonly used in field placement, position locations, etc. The thorax extends from the clavicles superiorly to the costal margin inferiorly.

Anterior thoracic landmarks

The chest and anterior thorax are formed by the ribs, sternum, and associated muscles. Figs. 8-30 and 8-31 demonstrate the bony and muscular anatomical features of the anterior chest wall.

The sternum is a midline structure that is composed of the manubrium, the body, and the xiphoid process. The *suprasternal notch* (SSN) is a palpable structure found on the superior aspect of the manubrium between the clavicles.[8,9] This structure, located at the level of T2, is commonly used by the radiation therapist as a point of measurement because of its stability. The manubrium and body of the sternum are palpable landmarks in the anterior chest wall. The sternal angle, or angle of Louis, is formed at the junction of these

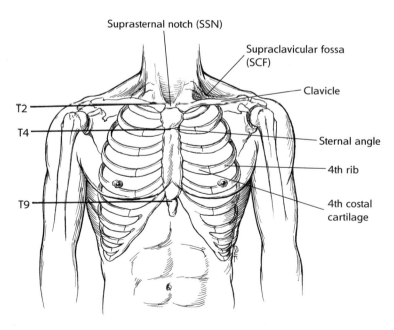

Fig. 8-30 Topographic anatomy of the anterior chest wall. Note relationships to underlying bony anatomy.

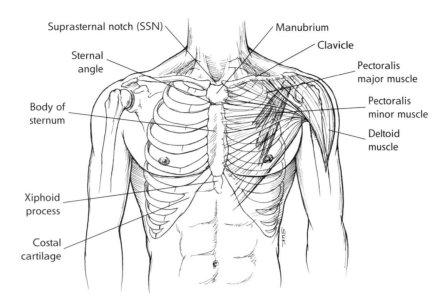

Fig. 8-31 Muscularity of the anterior chest wall.

two sternal structures at the level of T4. This widely used point of reference is very stable and is used by radiation therapists to locate many internal thoracic features. For example, this point is often used to start counting ribs (the second rib articulates with the sternal angle) and thoracic vertebrae. The xiphoid process is a palpable bony feature at the inferior portion of the sternum. It is typically located at the level of T9.

The clavicles are visible throughout their entire length, especially in the asthenic body habitus. In more obese individuals, only the medial aspect may be visible. In any case, the clavicles are easily palpable. The radiation therapist uses the clavicles when outlining a supraclavicular fossa (SCF) field to treat the lower neck and upper chest lymphatics. The supraclavicular lymph nodes are located superior to the clavicles; they are often treated prophylactically in head and neck as well as lung cancers. Also, the brachial plexus, a network of nerves located at the medial section of the clavicle and often involved in superior sulcus (Pancoast) tumors of the lung, can be referenced to this point.

The musculature of the anterior chest wall includes the pectoralis major, pectoralis minor, and the deltoid. The pectoralis major is medially attached to the clavicle and superior five costal cartilages. It passes laterally to the axilla. The inferior border of the muscle is not as visible in the female, since it is masked by the breast.[8,9] The pectoralis minor is overlapped by the pectoralis major. The deltoid muscle forms the rounded portion of the shoulder.

The breast and its landmarks

The male breast remains poorly developed throughout life, while the female breast develops to a variable degree during puberty. While the sizes of the female breasts vary, they typically lie between the second rib superiorly and the sixth rib inferiorly. The female breast is shown in Fig. 8-32. The medial border is the lateral aspect of the sternum, and the lateral border would correspond to the midaxilla. The breast tissue is teardrop shaped; the round, drop portion is situated medially, while the upper outer portion, called the tail of Spence, extends into the axilla. The upper limits of tangential treatment fields are typically high near the suprasternal notch, to include the entire breast and tail of Spence when the supraclavicular fossa is not treated.

The breast can be divided into quadrants: upper outer, upper inner, lower outer, and lower inner. Most tumors are located in the upper outer quadrant of the breast. Tumor location is important in associating the tumor spread patterns. If the breast tumor is located in an inner quadrant, the medially located nodes, such as the internal mammary nodes, may be involved. If the tumor is located in an outer quadrant, the axillary nodes need to be examined for possible involvement. This information is particularly important to the therapist because field parameters are dictated by tumor location and extension.

Other surface anatomy of the breast includes the nipple, areola, and inframammary sulcus. The nipple projects just below the center of the breast. In the male the nipple lies over the fourth intercostal space; the location varies in the female. The areola is the area that surrounds the nipple. Its coloration changes with varying hormonal levels, as seen in pregnancy. The inframammary sulcus, the inferior point of breast attachment, varies from person to person. In females with large breasts, the breast overhangs this point of attachment and causes considerable concern during its external beam treatment because the breast can bolus itself in these cases.

Radiographically, the breast produces shadows that are easily seen on conventional radiographs. Fig. 8-33 shows a CT slice through a section of the thorax and breast. Note how the patient's internal anatomy can be related to the contour of the breast. This information is very useful in treatment planning.

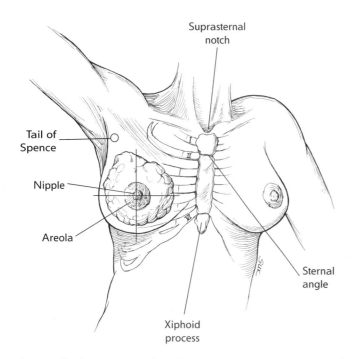

Fig. 8-32 Surface anatomy of the female breast. This gland is teardrop shaped with a portion extending from the anterior chest wall into the axilla.

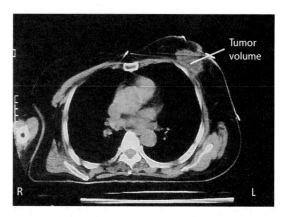

Fig. 8-33 Computed tomography view of the female breast and thorax. The contour of the breast and chest wall from images like this greatly enhance accuracy of treatment planning. Note how tumor volume can easily be related to other internal anatomy.

Posterior thoracic landmarks

The posterior thorax is formed by the structures commonly referred to as the back. On initial inspection, the back is made up of various muscles and bony landmarks. The major musculature includes the trapezius, teres major, and latissimus dorsi. The *trapezius* muscle is a flat triangular muscle that produces a trapezoid shape with the lateral angles at the shoulders and the superior angle at the EOP. The inferior angle is at the level of T12. The *teres major* is a band of muscle between the inferior angle of the scapula and the humerus and forms the posterior wall of the axilla. The *latissimus dorsi* is the broad muscle on either side of the back that spans from the iliac crest of the pelvic bones to the posterior axilla.[4,8,9] Fig. 8-34 demonstrates the surface anatomy of the posterior thorax.

The spines of the thoracic vertebrae slope inferiorly; the tips lie more inferior than the corresponding vertebral bodies and are easily palpable. The scapula, the large posterior bone associated with the pectoral girdle, is easily palpated on the back. The spine of the scapula is located at the level of T3. The inferior angle of the scapula is located at the level of T7.

The lower back has a few bony landmarks that serve the radiation therapist well. The *crest of the ilium* is located at the level of L4. This point is important in locating the subarachnoid space, the point at which lumbar punctures are commonly made. The *posterior superior iliac spine* (PSIS) is roughly 5 cm from midline, is easily palpable, and lies at the level of S2.

Internal and sectional anatomy of the thorax

Bone detail can be visualized sectionally with CT quite easily. MRI demonstrates soft tissue anatomy not clearly seen with conventional x-ray equipment. Fascial planes are identified, allowing separation of organ systems, vascular supply, muscles, bone, and lymphatic system.[1,3,6] The thorax provides a wealth of anatomical information that the radiation therapist uses in the daily administration of ionizing radiation.

The *trachea* is the part of the airway that begins at the inferior cricoid cartilage, at the level of C6. It is about 10 cm long and extends to a point of bifurcation, called the *carina,* at the level of T4-5. Topically, it corresponds to the angle of Louis and is demonstrated in Fig. 8-35. The bifurcation forms the beginning of the right and left main bronchi. This can assist the therapist in locating the initial location of treatment field borders, especially lung cancer fields whose inferior border commonly lies a few centimeters below this anatomical reference point.

The diaphragm is the dome-shaped muscle that separates the thorax and abdomen. It is important in respiration and lies between T10-11. The esophagus and inferior vena cava pass through the diaphragm at the level of T8-9, whereas the descending aorta goes through at the level of T11-12. These features are shown in cross-section in Fig. 8-36.

The pleural cavity extends superiorly 3 cm above the middle third of the clavicle. The anterior border of the

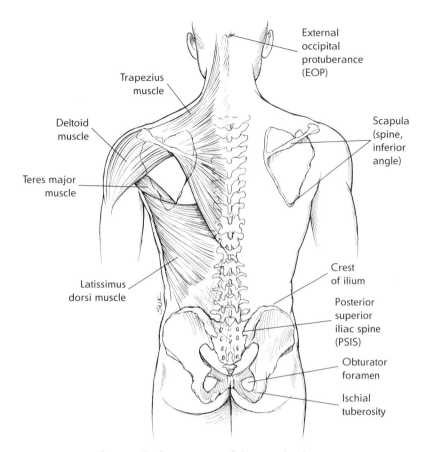

Fig. 8-34 Surface anatomy of the posterior thorax.

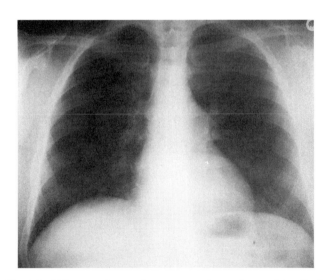

Fig. 8-35 This x-ray image demonstrates the trachea and its distal bifurcation, the carina. The branching typically occurs at T3-T4.

pleural cavity reaches the midline of the sternal angle. The pleura is more extensive in the peripheral regions around the outer chest wall. The diaphragm bulges up into each pleural cavity from below. The pleura marks the limit of expansion of the lungs.[8,9]

The lungs correspond closely with the pleura, except in the inferior aspect where they do not extend down into the lateral recesses. The anterior border of the right lung corresponds to the right junction of the costal and mediastinal pleura down to the level of the sixth chondrosternal joint. The anterior border of the left lung curves away laterally from the line of pleural reflection. The surface projection of the lung and pleura is noted in Fig. 8-37.

The heart rests directly on the diaphragm in the pericardial cavity and is covered anteriorly by the body of the sternum. The base of the heart lies at the level of T4. A cardiac shadow can clearly be seen in a plain radiograph of the chest.

Associated with the thorax and heart are an abundance of arteries and veins—the great vessels. The aorta has ascending and descending components. The ascending aorta runs from the aortic orifice at the medial end of the third left intercostal space up to the second right chondrosternal joint. This arch continues above the right side of the sternal angle and then turns down behind the second left costal cartilage. The descending aorta runs down behind this cartilage, gradually moving across to reach a point just to the left of midline, about 9 cm below the xiphisternal joint where it enters the abdomen. This aortic arch has the innominate, left common carotid, and left subclavian arteries extending from it. The superior vena cava is located at the level of T4. It runs down

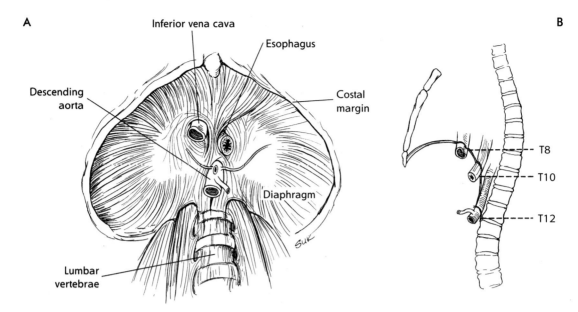

Fig. 8-36 Cross-section of the lower thorax showing esophagus and inferior vena cava passing through the diaphragm. **A,** Inferior surface of the diaphragm. **B,** Sagittal view of the diaphragm.

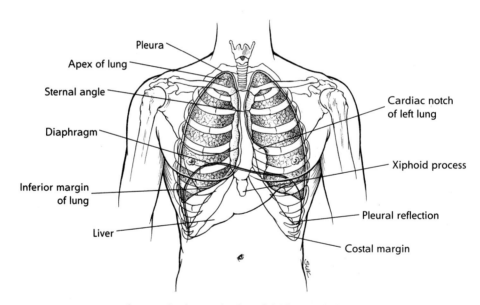

Fig. 8-37 Surface projection of the lung and pleura.

through the pericardium, where it enters the heart. The inferior vena cava does not extend a great distance in the thorax; it lies in the right cardiodiaphragmatic angle and enters the heart behind the sixth right costal cartilage.

Lymphatics of the breast and thorax

The lymphatic drainage of the thorax and breast is very important to the radiation therapist. The thorax is very rich in lymphatic vessels. The lymphatics of the axilla, supraclavicular fossa, and mediastinum play a major role in radiation therapy field arrangement of breast, head and neck, lung, and

lymphatic cancers. The lymph nodes of the thorax are divided into nodes that drain the thoracic wall and breast and those that drain the thoracic viscera.

There are three lymphatic pathways associated with the breast: the axillary, transpectoral, and internal mammary pathways. These pathways are the major routes of lymphatic drainage for the breast. There are specific lymph node groups associated with each pathway that are shown in Fig. 8-38.

The **axillary lymphatic pathway** comes from trunks of the upper and lower half of the breast. Lymph is collected in lobules that follow ducts, which anastomose behind the

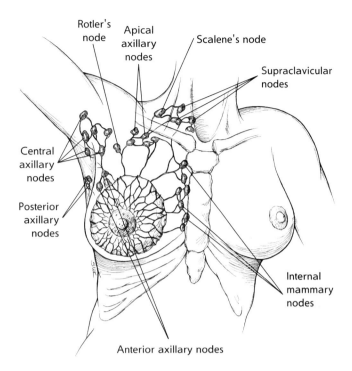

Fig. 8-38 The lymphatic pathways associated with the breast: axillary, transpectoral, and internal mammary.

areola of the breast; from that point they drain to the axilla. This pathway is also referred to as the principal pathway. The nodes of this pathway drain the lateral half of the breast. It is important to note these nodes in the case of invasive breast cancers: axillary nodes are commonly biopsied to assess disease spread. The axillary lymph nodes are commonly at the level of the second to third intercostal spaces and can be divided into low, mid-, and apical axillary nodes.

The **transpectoral lymphatic pathway** passes through the pectoralis major muscle and provides efferent drainage to the supraclavicular and infraclavicular fossa nodes. One of the intermediate nodes in the infraclavicular fossa worth noting is Rotter's node. Nodes of the supraclavicular fossa and low neck, generally 1 to 3 cm deep, are often treated when there is involvement of the transpectoral pathway. The scalene node, found in the low neck/supraclavicular fossa, is often biopsied in lung cancers to note disease spread.

The **internal mammary lymphatic pathway** runs toward the midline and passes through the pectoralis major and intercostal muscles close to the body of the sternum (T4 to T9). Associated with this pathway are the *internal mammary nodes*. These nodes are more frequently involved with primary breast cancers that are located in the inner breast quadrants and when there are positive axillary nodes. These nodes are generally 2.5 cm from midline (with variations from 0 to 5 cm) and about 2.5 cm deep (with variations from 1 to 5 cm). CT scans are extremely helpful to the radiation oncology team in assessing the location of these nodes. The

lateral location and depth assist in determining the field width and treatment energy, respectively.

Breast lymphatic flow is also important from a surgical standpoint. With radical breast surgery, lymphatic flow is often compromised. As the channels of flow are altered because of surgical intervention, the lymph has fewer drainage paths back to the cardiovascular system. This slowed drainage causes edema that is sometimes seen in the arm of patients who have received radical breast surgery. Exercise and elevation of the limb help drain stagnant lymph. This complication has led the cancer management team to use less radical surgery when possible, along with other modalities.

The mediastinum demonstrates a rich intercommunicating network of lymphatics. The most important nodes to note are the lymphatics of the thoracic viscera and pulmonary veins. They are commonly involved in Hodgkin's disease as well as lung cancers, where they can be radiographically demonstrated as a widened mediastinum. The lymphatics of the lung and mediastinum are shown in Fig. 8-39.

The *superior mediastinal nodes* are located in the superior mediastinum. They lie anterior to the brachiocephalic veins, the aortic arch, and the large arterial trunks that arise from the aorta. They receive lymphatic vessels from the thymus, heart, pericardium, mediastinal pleura, and anterior hilum. The *tracheal nodes* extend along both sides of the thoracic trachea. They are also called the *paratracheal nodes*. The *superior tracheobronchial nodes* are located on each side of the trachea. They are superior and lateral to the angle at which the trachea bifurcates into the two primary bronchi.

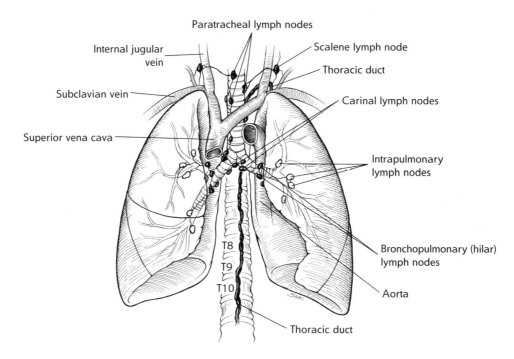

Fig. 8-39 The mediastinum demonstrates a large number of lymph nodes.

The *inferior mediastinal nodes* are located in the inferior mediastinum. The *inferior tracheobronchial nodes* lie in the angle below the bifurcation of the trachea. They are also called the *carinal nodes*. The *bronchopulmonary nodes*, often called the hilar nodes, are found at the hilus of each lung, at the site of the division of the main bronchi and pulmonary vessels into the lobular bronchi and vessels. These nodes are involved in a majority of lung cancer cases. The *pulmonary nodes*, also known as the intrapulmonary nodes, are found in the lung parenchyma along the secondary and tertiary bronchi.

In the right lung, all three lobes drain to the intrapulmonary and hilar nodes. They then flow to the carinal nodes and then to the paratracheal nodes before they reach the brachiocephalic vein through the scalene node and right lymphatic duct. In the left lung the upper lobe drains to the pulmonary and hilar nodes, carinal nodes, left superior paratracheal nodes, and then the brachiocephalic vein through the thoracic duct. The lower lobe drains to the pulmonary and hilar nodes, but then the right paratracheal nodes, where it follows the path of the right lung. This is important when designing the treatment field of a lung cancer patient. The therapist will need to assess whether or not a supraclavicular fossa field will need to be included and, if so, which side should be treated.

SURFACE AND SECTIONAL ANATOMY AND LANDMARKS OF THE ABDOMEN AND PELVIS

The abdomen and pelvis house many organs that are treated for malignant disease. Their management presents treatment planning challenges for the radiation therapist because there are an abundance of radiosensitive structures within the abdominal and pelvic cavities. Treating a colorectal cancer to a dose of 60+ Gy can be difficult when the neighboring anatomy tolerates much less. Knowledge of surface and cross-sectional anatomy of the abdomen and pelvis is essential in radiation therapy. The radiation therapist must be able to bridge knowledge of surface and sectional anatomy with various body habiti to visualize internal anatomy. However, relating internal structures to the topography of the area is not without certain challenges, particularly in the anterior abdomen. When compared to the head, neck, and thorax, the anterior abdomen does not demonstrate as many bony landmarks to reference. There are stable bony landmarks in the pelvis that are commonly referenced. This section will focus on the anatomy of the anterior and posterior abdominal wall along with the anterior and posterior pelvis.

Anterior abdominal wall

The *anterior abdominal wall* is bordered superiorly by the inferior costal margin and inferiorly by the symphysis pubis, inguinal ligament, anterior superior iliac spine, and iliac crest. The anterior aspect of the wall is formed by sheets of interlacing muscles that provide stability and form to the abdomen. The major muscles that help form the anterior abdominal wall include the rectus abdominis, transverse abdominis, internal oblique, and external oblique.

The *external oblique muscle* extends from the lower eight ribs to an insertion point that spans from the iliac crest to the midline aponeurosis, a sheetlike tendon that joins one muscle to another. It extends from the outer lateral body to the midline.

The *internal oblique muscle* spans from the iliac crest and inguinal ligament to the cartilage of the last four ribs. It runs in a midline to an outer, lateral perspective.

The *transverse abdominis muscle* runs from the iliac crest, inguinal ligament, and last six rib cartilages to the xiphoid process, linea alba (a tough fibrous band that extends from the xiphoid process to the pubic symphysis), and pubis on both sides. Thus, this muscle runs from side to side.

The *rectus abdominis muscle* is commonly called the "six pack" by sports buffs. This muscle runs from the symphysis pubis to the xiphoid process and has three transverse fibrous bands that separate the muscle into six sections that are prominent in individuals with pronounced muscular tone.

These muscles work together in providing structure to the anterior abdominal wall. Fig. 8-40 shows the interrelated nature of these muscles.

A number of structures can be palpated in the abdomen. The xiphoid process lies in the epigastric fossa at the level of T9. This bony landmark is very stable. The radiation therapist typically uses this structure and the SSN in making sure that a patient is lying straight on the treatment couch. If both landmarks are in line with the projection of a sagittal laser, the thorax is usually straight. The xiphoid can also be used in conjunction with the pubic symphysis or associated soft tissue landmarks to ensure that the lower body is straight. The *costal margin* is formed by the cartilages of the seventh to tenth ribs. This forms the inferior border of the rib cage. The *umbilicus*, also known as the navel or belly button, is an inconsistent, mobile landmark on the anterior abdomen. It is typically at the level of L4 when an individual is in a recumbent position. When standing, in the infant, and in the pendulous abdomen, it lies at a lower level. If measurements are taken from it, it should be stated whether they are taken from the center, the upper level, or the lower level. However, it may be used as an arbitrary check measurement.

Posterior abdominal wall (trunk)

In the posterior wall the lower ribs, lumbar spines, posterior superior iliac spine, and iliac crest are palpable. A line, called the *intercristal line*, can be drawn between the iliac crests.[9] This line will typically pass between the spines of the third and fourth lumbar vertebrae, a location important when performing lumbar punctures.

Landmarks of the anterior pelvis

The anterior pelvis exhibits several bony and fleshy landmarks that are useful to the radiation therapist. They are outlined below and demonstrated in Fig. 8-41.

The *iliac crest* extends from the anterior superior iliac spine to the posterior superior iliac spine. The *anterior superior iliac spine (ASIS)* is palpable, and measurements may be taken from it in the superoinferior or mediolateral direction. It is frequently used in referencing the location of the femur. The *lateral iliac crest* is also easily palpable and, being on the lateral pelvic wall, may be used as a transverse level on either the anterior or the posterior pelvis. The *lateral iliac crest level* is the line joining the right and left lateral iliac crests. These crests are the most superior margin of the ilium on the lateral pelvic wall. Measurements may be taken from this level in the superoinferior direction.

The head of the femur and greater trochanter, although not direct components of the true pelvis, are important to note when considering the lateral pelvic anatomy. The *head of the femur* articulates with the hip at the acetabulum. If irradiated beyond tolerance, fibrotic changes can occur, causing painful and/or limited motion of the joint. Usually this joint is

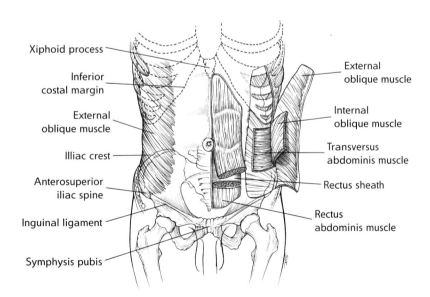

Fig. 8-40 The muscles of the anterior and lateral abdominal wall work in unison to provide structure and stability to the torso.

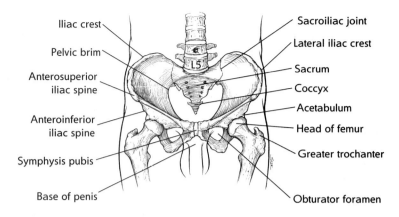

Fig. 8-41 Bony landmarks about the anterior pelvis.

shielded in moderate to large anteroposterior/posteroanterior pelvic portals to limit this occurrence. The *greater trochanter* is the only part of the proximal femur that can be palpated; therefore its relationship to bony points of the hip bone is important.[8] The radiation therapist uses the greater trochanter when aligning patients during simulation to alleviate pelvis rotation. The patient should be horizontally level when the greater trochanters are at the same height from the table top. The radiation therapist can measure this using a ruler and optical lasers.

The pubis symphysis appears as the 5 mm midline gap between the inferior parts of the pelvic bones.[8] The *upper border pubis* is the palpable upper border of the midline pubic bone. It is generally fairly easy to palpate, except in extremely obese patients. When palpating it, care should be taken to allow for overlying tissue. The *lower border pubis* is the palpable lower border of the pubic bone in midline. It is not as easily palpable as the upper border pubis, since it lies more inferiorly and posteriorly. All of these can be accurately located radiographically. These components are used by the radiation therapist when setting the anterior border of lateral prostate fields (the prostate lies immediately posterior to the pubis symphysis).

The ischial tuberosities are located in the inferior portion of the pelvis. This corresponds to the lower region of the buttock. When a person sits down, the ischial tuberosities bear the weight of the body. Many radiation oncologists use the ischial tuberosities as the inferior border of the anterior and posterior prostate treatment portals.

When pelvic irradiation is indicated, the radiation therapist can use the anatomy of the perineum, the diamond-shaped area bounded laterally by the ischial tuberosities, anteriorly by the pubic symphysis, and posteriorly by the coccyx, to assist in portal location. Treatment lines in these areas commonly fade because of perspiration and garment rubbing.[8] Knowledge of the area can thus provide a practical means of field verification. Both male and female anatomy demonstrates useful landmarks.

The *anterior commissure of the labia majora* is easily distinguishable in the female. It is an important soft tissue landmark, since it is used as a reference point from which the upper or lower border pubis is measured. Thus variations in the palpation of the pubic bone may be eliminated by checking back to this soft tissue landmark.

The *base of the penis* is taken as being the line joining the anterior skin of the penis with the skin of the anterior pelvic wall. This level is used as a reference point from which the upper or lower border pubis is measured in the male. A therapist may measure changes in the lateral position of prostate fields by referencing appropriate measurements from the base of the penis.

Landmarks of the posterior pelvis

The most commonly used bony surface landmarks of the posterior pelvis are the posterior superior iliac spines, the coccyx, the iliac crests, and the lateral iliac crests. Since the latter two were also mentioned in the previous section, only the posterior superior iliac spine will be discussed. The *posterior superior iliac spines* (*PSIS*) are indicated by dimples above and medial to the buttock, about 5 to 6 cm from the midline. They are palpable, and measurements may be taken in the superoinferior or mediolateral direction. The *coccyx* lies deep to the natal cleft with its inferior end roughly 1 cm from the anus.

Abdominopelvic viscera

The organs of the abdomen and pelvis can be visualized by various means. Plain x-ray, CT, MRI, and ultrasound are commonly employed to provide information concerning organ location. It is worth noting that the location of any organ in the abdomen and pelvis can vary with respiration, anatomical position, and level of fullness. This is why it is extremely important to place radiation therapy patients in a reproducible position that limits movement daily. As observed earlier, body habitus affects the location of internal organs. This holds true for the abdomen and pelvis as well. This section will examine the location of the abdominal and pelvic viscera.

Location of the alimentary organs

The esophagus begins at the lower border of the cricoid cartilage in the neck and travels through the diaphragm to the cardiac sphincter, the entrance to the stomach, at the level of T10 about 2 to 3 cm to the left of midline. To visualize the esophagus radiographically the patient commonly is instructed to swallow a radiopaque substance like barium before examination.

The duodenum, a C-shaped section of the small bowel about 25 cm in length, starts to the right of midline at the edge of the epigastric region. The stomach lies between the duodenum and the distal esophagus and is of variable size and location, partly covered by the left rib cage and filling the epigastric region. The root of the small gut mesentery, made up of sections called the jejunum and ileum, extends from the duodenum to the inlet to the large bowel.[8,9]

The start of the large bowel is the cecum. It lies in the right iliac region at the level of L4. The ascending colon (15 cm in length) and hepatic flexure of the colon on the right side and the splenic flexure and descending colon (25 cm in length) on the left side are largely retroperitoneal structures, whereas the transverse and sigmoid colon have a mesentery

and vary in their position from one person to the next.[8,9] However, similarities are demonstrated within common body habiti. The rectum starts at the level of S3 and ends about 4 cm from the anus. It is one of the dose-limiting structures when outlining prostate treatment fields. Rectal visualization is thus important during the simulation process.

Fig. 8-42 delineates the surface projections of the alimentary tract in the abdomen and pelvis.

Location of nonalimentary organs

The radiation therapist benefits from a working knowledge of the nonalimentary organs of the abdomen and pelvis. Many times these organs are involved in malignant processes and must be included in the patient's treatment scheme. Fig. 8-43 demonstrates the surface projections of the organs outlined here.

The liver is an irregularly shaped organ located in the right hypochondriac region of the abdomen above the costal margin. The superior margin of the liver, which bulges into the diaphragm, is at the level of T7-8. The liver is commonly imaged by CT scan, ultrasound, and nuclear medicine studies.

The gallbladder is located below the lower border of the liver and contacts the anterior abdominal wall where the right lateral border of the rectus abdominis crosses the ninth costal cartilage. This location is called the transpyloric plane.

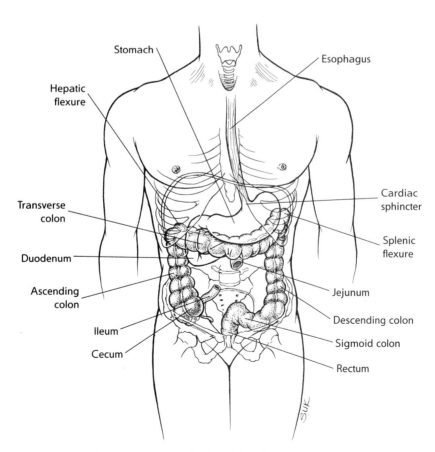

Fig. 8-42 Surface projection of the alimentary organs.

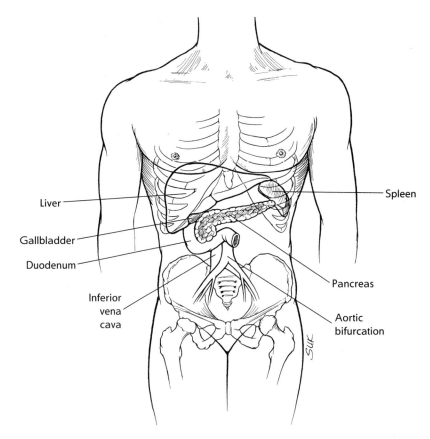

Liver

Gallbladder

Duodenum

Inferior
vena
cava

Spleen

Pancreas

Aortic
bifurcation

Fig. 8-43 Surface projection of non-alimentary organs.

Again, ultrasound is useful in distinguishing biliary obstructions as well as gallstones.

The spleen, mentioned earlier as a "lymph node for the blood," is located posteriorly about 5 cm to the left of midline at the level of T10-11. The normal organ lies beneath the ninth through eleventh ribs on the left side of the body. This organ is often examined surgically in patients with lymphoma to determine disease extension. If the organ is removed for biopsy, the splenic pedicle, the point of attachment of the organ to its vascular and lymphatic connections, is included in the inverted Y treatment portal.

The pancreas can be sectioned into three components: the head, body, and tail. The head of the pancreas is located in the "C" section of the duodenum. The body extends slightly superiorly to the left across midline, at the level of L1. The tail of the pancreas passes into the hilum, a concave point of an organ that has vascular inlets and outlets, of the spleen.

Location of the urinary tract organs

The kidneys lie on the posterior abdominal wall in the retroperitoneal space. The hilum of the right kidney is at the level of L2, whereas the hilum of the left is at the level of L1. The right kidney lies lower than the left because of the presence of the adjacent liver. Each organ measures about 12 cm long by 5 cm wide. Superior and medial to each kidney are

the adrenal glands. The kidneys are generally not fixed to the abdominal wall; they can move as much as 2 cm with respiration. When the radiation therapist outlines the location of these radiation-sensitive structures, it is important to take this into account.

The ureters are tubular structures that transport urine from the kidneys to the urinary bladder. They run anterior to the psoas muscles and enter the pelvis lateral to the sacroiliac (SI) joint. The ureters, as well as the kidneys, are commonly imaged with CT, ultrasound, and intravenous and retrograde studies.

The urinary bladder is located in the pelvis. The neck of the bladder lies posterior to the pubis symphysis and anterior to the rectum. This organ also lies immediately superior to the prostate in the male. The urinary bladder is a dose-limiting structure in the treatment of prostatic cancer. It is commonly visualized with contrast agents during the simulation process and is outlined in Chapter 9.

The topographic relations of the urinary tract organs are shown in Fig. 8-44.

Lymphatics of the abdomen and pelvis

The lymphatic drainage routes for the abdomen and pelvis are very important to the radiation therapist. There is an abundance of lymphatic vessels in this section of the body.

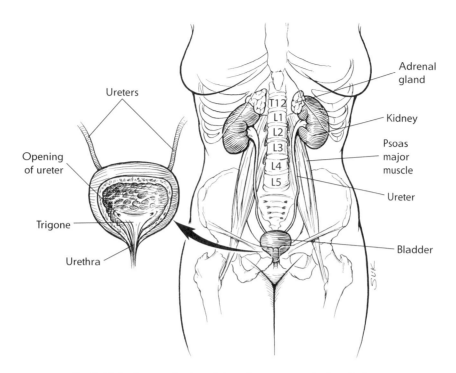

Fig. 8-44 Surface projection of the urinary tract and adrenal glands.

Those of the retroperitoneum and pelvis play a major role in radiation therapy field arrangement of gynecological, genitourinary, and lymphatic cancers. Figs. 8-45 and 8-46 show the nodes and nodal groups outlined here.

The lymphatic pathways and nodes of the abdomen are frequently referred to as the visceral nodes because they are closely associated with the abdominal organs. The three principal groups of nodes of the abdomen that drain the corresponding viscera before entering the cisterna chyli or the thoracic duct are the celiac, superior mesenteric, and inferior mesenteric groups, also called the preaortic nodes.

The *celiac nodes* include the nodes that drain the stomach, greater omentum, liver, gallbladder, and spleen, as well as most of the lymph from the pancreas and duodenum. The *superior mesenteric nodes* drain part of the head of the pancreas, a portion of the duodenum, the entire jejunum, ileum, appendix, cecum, ascending colon, and most of the transverse colon. The *inferior mesenteric nodes* drain the descending colon, the left side of the mesentery, the sigmoid colon, and the rectum.

The posterior abdominal wall demonstrates a rich intercommunicating network of lymphatic vessels. The *para-aortic nodes* provide efferent drainage to the cisterna chyli, which is the beginning of the thoracic duct. These nodes run adjacent to the abdominal aorta from T12 to L4. This major section of the lymphatic system eventually receives lymph from most of the lower regions of the body. The para-aortics directly drain the uterus, ovary, kidneys, and testicles. It is interesting to note that embryonically the

testes develop near the kidneys and descend into the scrotum after birth. As they descend, they take the vascular and lymphatic vessels with them as direct means for blood and lymph flow.

The *common iliac nodes* lie at the bifurcation of the abdominal aorta at the level of L4. These nodes directly drain the urinary bladder, prostate, cervix, and vagina. This chain moves laterally and breaks up into the external and internal iliac nodes. The external iliac nodes drain the urinary bladder, prostate, cervix, testes, vagina, and ovary. The *internal iliac nodes*, also known as the hypogastric nodes, directly drain the vagina, cervix, prostate, and urinary bladder. These nodes are more medial and posterior to the external iliac nodes previously mentioned.

The *inguinal nodes* are more superficial than the previously mentioned nodes. These nodes directly drain the vulva, uterus, ovary, and vagina. These nodes are commonly treated with electrons because of their superficial location.

APPLIED TECHNOLOGY

Practical application of the material presented in this chapter is very important. To enhance the comprehensive understanding of the relationships presented, the last section of this chapter will present diagrams that relate structures to vertebral body levels and CT scans through the head, neck, thorax, abdomen, and pelvis. The appropriate structures pertinent to the radiation oncology practitioner will be demonstrated. Figs. 8-47 through 8-52 show these diagrams and scans.

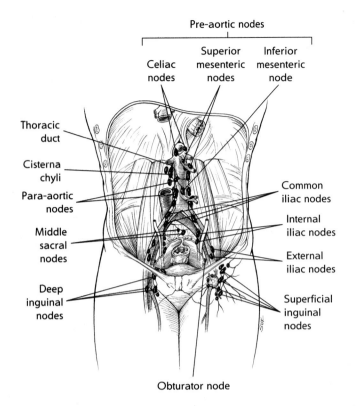

Fig. 8-45 Abdominal lymph nodes.

SUMMARY

Radiation therapy requires its practitioners to demonstrate more than a passing acquaintance with surface and sectional anatomy. The complex simulation procedures and planning used in patient treatment mandates strict attention to detail. The radiation therapist must use information provided by several imaging modalities to achieve its ultimate goal: to administer a tumoricidal dose of radiation to the tumor and tumor bed while sparing as much normal tissue as possible. Also, the lymphatic vessels play a major role in treatment field delineation and disease management. To accomplish this goal the radiation therapist must command a comprehensive knowledge of surface and sectional anatomy. The complexity of radiation therapy demands that the radiation therapist use all available means to function effectively. Without this base the therapist and the technology used are at best mediocre. Each therapist should take an honest inventory of his or her practical skills in surface and sectional anatomy. Without a strong foundation, the most beautiful and stout structure eventually falls; for radiation therapists, one of the cornerstones of their foundation is surface and sectional anatomy.

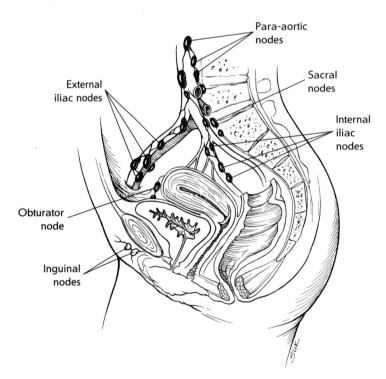

Fig. 8-46 Lymphatics of the pelvis.

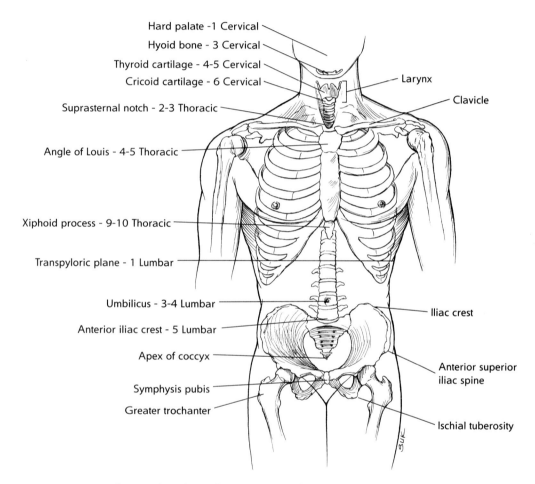

Hard palate -1 Cervical

Hyoid bone - 3 Cervical

Thyroid cartilage - 4-5 Cervical

Cricoid cartilage - 6 Cervical

Suprasternal notch - 2-3 Thoracic

Larynx

Clavicle

Angle of Louis - 4-5 Thoracic

Xiphoid process - 9-10 Thoracic

Transpyloric plane - 1 Lumbar

Umbilicus - 3-4 Lumbar

Iliac crest

Anterior iliac crest - 5 Lumbar

Apex of coccyx

Anterior superior iliac spine

Symphysis pubis

Greater trochanter

Ischial tuberosity

Fig. 8-47 Anterior surface projections of selected skeletal anatomy.

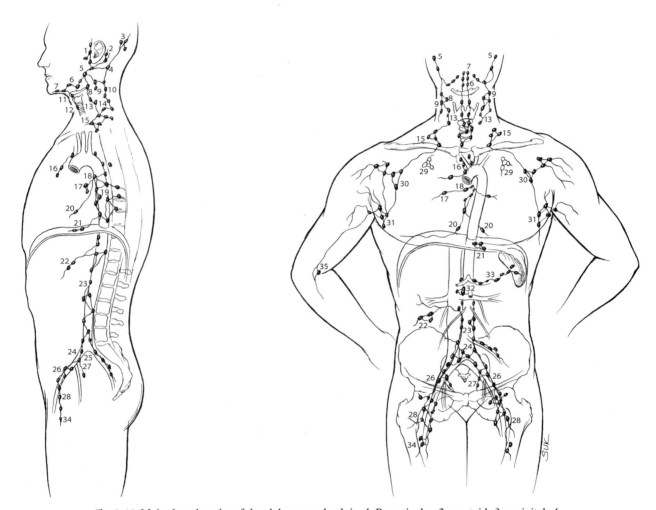

Fig. 8-48 Major lymph nodes of the abdomen and pelvis. *1*. Preauricular, *2*. mastoid, *3*. occipital, *4*. upper cervical, *5*. parotid, *6*. submaxillary, *7*. submental, *8*. jugulo-digastric, *9*. upper deep cervical, *10*. spinal accessory chain, *11*. infrahyoid, *12*. pretracheal, *13*. jugulo-omohyoid, *14*. lower deep cervical, *15*. supraclavicular, *16*. mediastinal, *17*. interlobar, *18*. intertracheal, *19*. posterior mediastinal, *20*. lateral pericardial, *21*. diaphragmatic, *22*. mesenteric, *23*. para-aortic, *24*. common iliac, *25*. lateral sacral, *26*. external iliac, *27*. interpectoral, *28*. inguinal, *29*. interpectoral, *30*. axillary apex, *31*. axillary, *32*. cisterna chyli, *33*. splenic, *34*. femoral, *35*. epitrochlear.

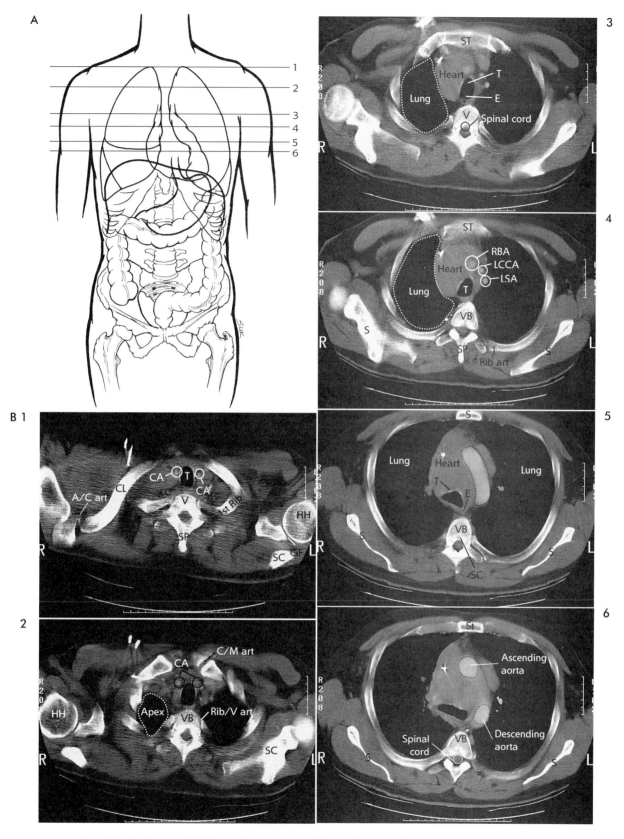

Fig. 8-49 A, Sectional CT views of the thorax with labeled anatomy. **B,** Carotid artery, *CA*; Humeral head, *HH*; Vertebral body, *VB*; Trachea, *T*; Esophagus, *E*; Acromial clavicular articulation, *A/C art*; Scapula *(S)SC*; Glenoid fossa, *GF*; Sternum, *S*; Clavicular macrobial articulator, *C/M art*, Left sub-clavian artery, *LSA*; Left common carotid artery, *LCCA*; Right bronchocephalic artery, *RBA*; *Rib/V art*; Clavicle, *C*; Vein, *V*; Ascending aorta, *ACA*; Descending aorta, *DCA*.

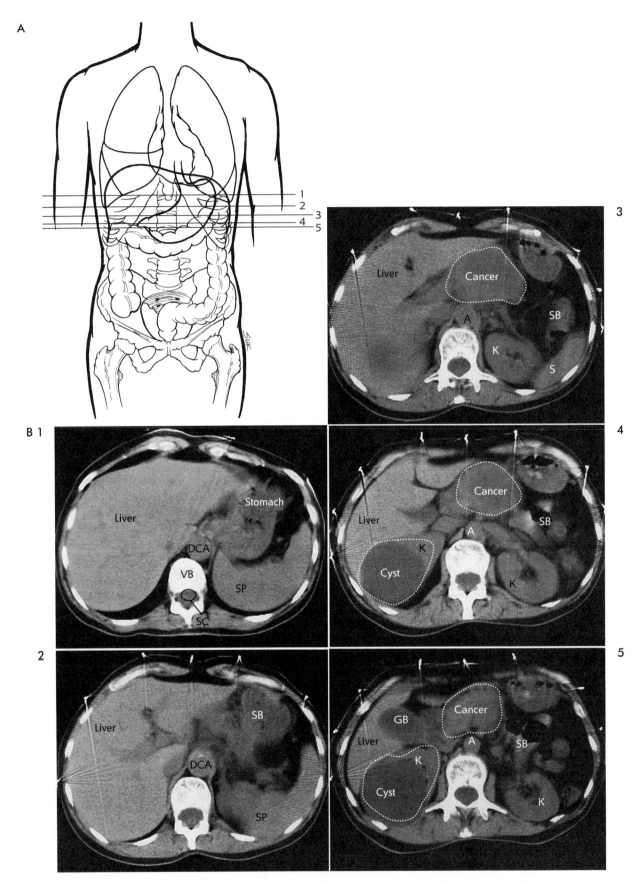

Fig. 8-50 A, Sectional CT views of the abdomen with labeled anatomy. **B**, Small bowel, *SB*; Aorta, *A*; Kidney, *K*; Liver, *L*; Spleen, *S (SP)*; Spinal cord, *SC*; Vertebral body, *VB*; Descending aorta, *DCA*; Gallbladder, *GB*.

159

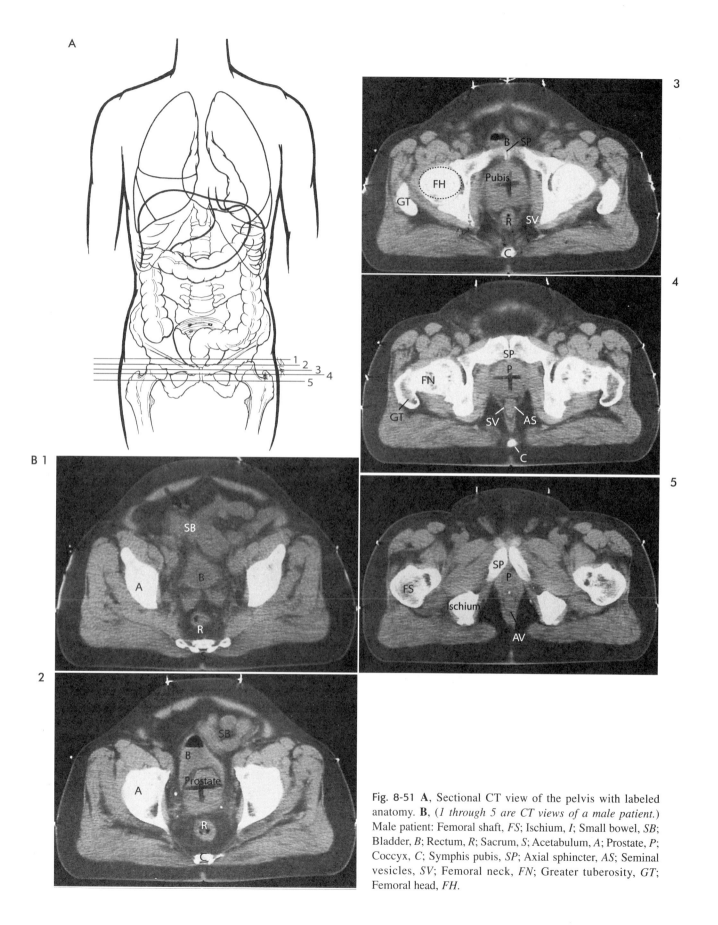

Fig. 8-51 **A**, Sectional CT view of the pelvis with labeled anatomy. **B**, (*1 through 5 are CT views of a male patient.*) Male patient: Femoral shaft, *FS*; Ischium, *I*; Small bowel, *SB*; Bladder, *B*; Rectum, *R*; Sacrum, *S*; Acetabulum, *A*; Prostate, *P*; Coccyx, *C*; Symphis pubis, *SP*; Axial sphincter, *AS*; Seminal vesicles, *SV*; Femoral neck, *FN*; Greater tuberosity, *GT*; Femoral head, *FH*.

160

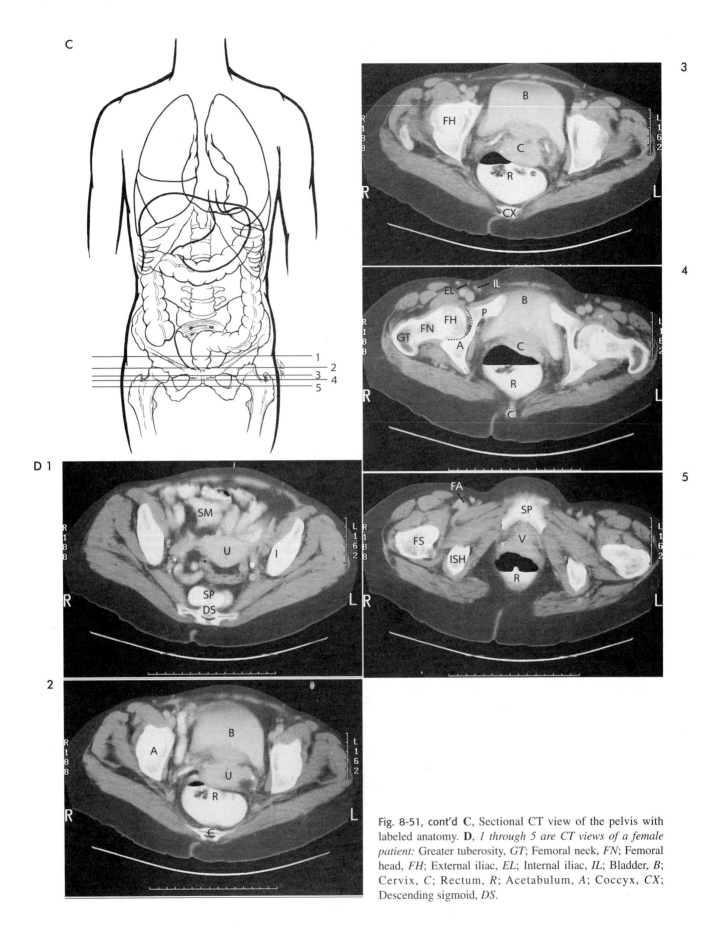

Fig. 8-51, cont'd **C**, Sectional CT view of the pelvis with labeled anatomy. **D**, *1 through 5 are CT views of a female patient:* Greater tuberosity, *GT*; Femoral neck, *FN*; Femoral head, *FH*; External iliac, *EL*; Internal iliac, *IL*; Bladder, *B*; Cervix, *C*; Rectum, *R*; Acetabulum, *A*; Coccyx, *CX*; Descending sigmoid, *DS*.

Review Questions

Fill in the Blank

1. _____ is a plane through the middle of the body from the front to back through the sagittal suture of the skull that divides the body into two equal parts.
2. The _____ is the muscle that partitions the anterior cavity into the thoracic and abdominal portions.
3. _____ returns lymph from the entire body back into the bloodstream, with the exception of the upper right limb and the right side of the thorax, head, and neck.
4. The angle of the mandible is generally located at the level of cervical vertebra number _____.
5. The _____ runs anterior to the psoas stripes (muscles) and enters the pelvis lateral to the sacroiliac joint. Tumors in these structures are very rare.

Multiple Choice

6. If the punctum lacrimae of the eye is overirradiated, fibrotic changes can occur. If this happens, what would be the clinical signs?
   a. Dry eye
   b. Constantly tearing eye
   c. Cataracts
   d. Ocular muscle atrophy

7. In the lower neck, the esophagus lies:
   a. Anterior to the trachea and posterior to the spinal cord
   b. Anterior to the spinal cord and posterior to the trachea
   c. Anterior to the trachea and inferior to the spinal cord
   d. Inferior to the spinal cord and posterior to the trachea
8. Which of the following are examples of primary curves?
   I. thoracic
   II. lateral
   III. pelvic
   a. I and II
   b. I and III
   c. II and III
   d. I, II, and III
9. The trachea is a hollow tube about 4.5 cm in length that extends from the larynx to a bifurcation called the:
   a. Bronchus
   b. Carina
   c. Bronchiole
   d. Lung
10. Which of the following are commonly used soft tissue landmarks of the anterior pelvis?
    a. Umbilicus
    b. Base of penis
    c. Both a and b
    d. Neither a nor b

Questions to Ponder

1. Examine the process of how lymph is transported through the lymphatic system.
2. Describe how the directional flow of lymph is facilitated through the lymphatic system.
3. Describe events that can occur if lymphatic channels are compromised through either surgical or radiation damage.
4. Why are landmarks about the mouth, as well as other fleshy landmarks, not very accurate? What would we have to do to use them accurately?
5. How could a therapist locate the pituitary by using only topographical landmarks?
6. How can body habitus affect abdominal organ location?
7. What is the significance of including a portion of lung tissue in the tangential fields of the patient treated for breast cancer?
8. Analyze the relationship of surface anatomy knowledge with performance of effective simulation procedures. How can this knowledge also affect daily treatment administrations?

REFERENCES

1. Barrett CP et al: *Primer of sectional anatomy with MRI and CT correlation.* Baltimore, 1990, Williams & Wilkins.
2. Bentel GC: *Radiation therapy planning.* New York, 1992, Macmillan.
3. Collins JD et al: Anatomy of the abdomen, back, and pelvis as displayed by magnetic resonance imaging: part one. *J Natl Med Assoc* 81(6):680-684, 1989.
4. Collins JD et al: Anatomy of the abdomen, back, and pelvis as displayed by magnetic resonance imaging: part two. *J Natl Med Assoc* 81(7):809-813, 1989.
5. Collins JD et al: Anatomy of the abdomen, back, and pelvis as displayed by magnetic resonance imaging: part three. *J Natl Med Assoc* 81(8):857-861, 1989.
6. Collins JD et al: Magnetic resonance imaging of chest wall lesions. *J Natl Med Assoc* 83(4):352-360, 1991.
7. Cox JD, editor: *Moss' radiation oncology: rationale, techniques, results,* ed 7. St Louis, 1994, Mosby.
8. Keogh B, Ebbs S: *Normal surface anatomy.* Philadelphia, 1984, Lippincott.
9. Lumley JSP: *Surface anatomy: the anatomical basis of clinical examination.* London, 1990, Churchill Livingstone.
10. Novelline RA, Squire LF: *Living anatomy: a working atlas using computed tomography, magnetic resonance and angiography images,* Philadelphia, 1987, Hanley & Belfus.

11. Panjabi MM et al: Thoracic human vertebrae. *Spine* 16(8):888-901, 1991.
12. Panjabi MM et al: Human lumbar vertebrae. *Spine* 17(3):299-302, 1992.
13. Philippou M et al: Cross-sectional anatomy of the nose and paranasal sinuses. *Rhinology* 28:221-230, 1990.

14. Rubin P: *Clinical oncology: a multidisciplinary approach for physicians and students*, ed 7. Philadelphia, 1993, Saunders.
15. Tortora GJ, Anagnostakos NP: *Principles of anatomy and physiology*, ed 6. New York, 1990, Harper & Row.

BIBLIOGRAPHY

Stanton R, Stinson D: *An introduction to radiation oncology physics.* Madison, WI, 1992, Medical Physics Publishing.
Stewart GS: Trends in radiation therapy for the treatment of lung cancer. *Nurs Clin North Am* 27(3):643-651, 1992.

Wechsler RJ, Steiner RM: Cross-sectional imaging of the chest wall. *J Thorac Imag* 4(1):29-40, 1989.

Simulation Procedures

Sandra Nava
Dennis T. Leaver

Outline

Key terms

Body habitus
Caliper
Contour
Contrast media
Field size
Irradiated volume
Isocentric technique
Localization
Orthogonal films

Pantograph
Phototiming
Radiopaque marker
Separation
Simulation
Target volume
Treatment volume
Verification
Verification simulation

Patients treated with radiation therapy, either for cure or for palliation, will be involved in numerous procedures ranging from diagnosis to ongoing patient follow-up. Fig. 9-1 lists the various steps a patient may experience as part of the entire process of external beam radiation therapy. The actual delivery of a prescribed dose of radiation, although important, is a small part of the whole process. Before therapy can begin, a simulation procedure is necessary. The ultimate success of treatment will be directly related to the effectiveness of the simulation procedure. This procedure helps in determining the location and extent of disease relative to adjacent critical normal tissues.[5,7] Each step in the radiation therapy process may not be needed for every patient nor will the steps occur in sequence. The process varies for each patient, depending on the patient's condition and the type and extent of disease.

The simulation process involves the participation of several team members, each with a variety of unique skills. Both simulation and treatment require a solid foundation in the theory and application of radiation oncology techniques. In addition, patient care skills are necessary. It is the team approach, involving each member, that can provide effective planning as well as localization and documentation of the patient's disease in relationship to normal tissue structures. Table 9-1 identifies key staff functions in the radiation therapy process.

A simulator can take various forms, ranging from a simple diagnostic radiographic unit attached to a treatment machine to a complicated isocentric unit with fluoroscopy

DIAGNOSIS
- tumour pathobiology
- staging

THERAPEUTIC DECISIONS
- cure/palliation
- treatment modalities

TARGET VOLUME LOCALIZATION
- tumour/normal tissue definition
- patient measurements
- field shaping

TREATMENT PLANNING
- selection of technique
- computation of dose distribution
- optimization

SIMULATION
- treatment
- confirmation of measurements
- confirmation of shields

FABRICATION OF TREATMENT AIDS
- blocks/shields
- compensators/bolus
- immobilization devices

TREATMENT
- verification of set-up
- verification of equipment performance
- dosimetry checks
- record keeping

PATIENT EVALUATION DURING TREATMENT
- treatment tolerance
- tumour response

PATIENT FOLLOW-UP
- tumour control
- normal tissue response

Fig. 9-1 The various steps involved in the process of external beam radiation therapy. (From Van Dyk J, Mah K: Simulators and CT scanners. In Williams JR, Thwaites DI, editor: *Radiotherapy physics in practice.* Oxford, 1993, Oxford University Press.)

Table 9-1	Key staff functions in the radiation therapy process
Function	**Team member(s)**
Diagnosis	Pathologist Referring physician Radiation oncologist
Therapeutic decisions	Radiation oncologist Referring physician
Target volume localization	Radiation oncologist Radiation therapist Dosimetrist Physicist
Treatment planning	Radiation oncologist Physicist Dosimetrist
Simulation	Radiation therapist Radiation oncologist Dosimetrist Physicist
Fabrication of treatment aids	Dosimetrist Radiation therapist Mold room technologist
Treatment	Radiation therapist Physicist Dosimetrist Radiation oncologist
Patient evaluation during treatment	Radiation oncologist Radiation therapist Oncology nurse
Patient follow-up	Radiation oncologist Oncology nurse Radiation therapist

and computed tomography (CT) capabilities. In each case the outcome should define the anatomical area so that it is reproducible for daily treatment. An elaborate and complicated simulation is of no value unless it is reproducible on the treatment unit.

In this chapter the complexities of simulation and target volume localization are discussed. This includes some nomenclature (definitions) and the importance of patient assessment and education before the simulation procedure. A description of tumor and normal tissue localization methods and an outline of the steps involved in the simulation procedure/treatment verification process are also included. In addition, a practical application section is presented to help provide an appreciation of the importance of the simulation process.

NOMENCLATURE

Before a discussion of exactly what simulation is, a review of several key definitions and acronyms, designed to provide a foundation in *simulation procedures*, will be helpful.

Simulation (which may be a one- or a two-step process) is carried out by the radiation therapist under the supervision of the radiation oncologist. It is the precise mockup of a patient treatment with radiographic documentation of the treatment portals.[12] The term *simulation* may take on different meanings, depending on the institution and the individual. First, it is a general term describing the mockup process, which can also include the selection of immobilization devices, radiographic documentation of treatment ports, measurement of the patient, construction of patient contours, and shaping of fields.[12] Second, it may be a more specific term where the simulator artificially duplicates the actual treatment conditions (verification) by confirming measurements, verifying treatment, and confirming shields.[7]

Localization means geometrical definition of the position and extent of the tumor or anatomical structures by reference of surface marks that can be used for treatment setup purposes.[4] The radiation oncologist and radiation therapist, along with other team members, localize the tumor volume and critical normal structures using both clinical and radiographic information.

Verification is a final check that each of the planned treatment beams does cover the tumor or target volume and does not irradiate critical normal structures.[4] This is usually done as the second part of a two-step process on the simulator. It involves taking radiographs of each of the treatment beams using external marks and other immobilization devices intended for treatment reproducibility.

Radiopaque marker refers to a material with a high atomic number. It is usually made of lead, copper, or solder wire. Frequently it is used on the surface of a patient or appropriately placed in a body cavity. This is done to delineate special points of interest for calculation purposes or marking of critical structures requiring visualization during treatment planning.

Separation refers to the measurement of the thickness of a patient along the central axis or at any other specified point within the irradiated volume. Separations are helpful in learning about the amount of tissue in front of, behind, or around a tumor. A **caliper**, which is a graduated ruled instrument with one sliding leg and one that is stationary, is used to figure out the patient's thickness. A patient's separation is also referred to as the intrafield distance, or sometimes the innerfield distance (IFD).

Field size involves the dimensions of a treatment field at the isocenter, which are represented by width × length. This measurement, determined by the field defining wires on the simulator and collimator opening on the treatment unit, defines the dimensions of the treatment portal.

There are several definitions related to the patient planning process provided by the International Commission on Radiation Units and Measurements in an effort to standardize radiation therapy terminology.[11] Fig. 9-2 illustrates three terms—target volume, treatment volume, and irradiated volume—used to describe dose specifications for patient planning. Fig. 9-3 also provides a schematic representation of the target and treatment volume surrounding the tumor.

Target volume consists of the tumor, if present, and any other tissue with presumed tumor.[16] Generally, a volume larger than the tumor itself should be irradiated to a uniform dose. This is done to account for factors such as occult microscopic disease, local invasive capacity of the tumor, potential spread to regional lymph nodes, expected motion, and variations in daily treatment setup.[7] The target volume, which contains tissues that are to be treated to a specific dose in a planned fractionation schedule, should be thought of in a three-dimensional volume.

Treatment volume, which is generally larger than the target volume, encompasses the additional margins around the target volume to allow for limitations of the treatment technique. Thus the minimum target absorbed dose should be enclosed by an isodose surface that adequately covers the target volume.[7,16] At times the treatment volume may be larger than the target volume because of the geometry of the patient and the number and complexity of the treatment beams. In other situations it is nearly the same size as the target volume. The whole process of deciding the treatment volume is tailored to meet the needs of each individual case.

Irradiated volume is the volume of tissue receiving a significant dose (e.g., > 50%) of the specified target dose.[7,16] To adequately cover the target volume, normal tissue in front of, behind, and around the target volume must be treated. During treatment planning a technique is developed to maximize the dose to the target volume and minimize the absorbed dose to the treatment and irradiated volumes.

ACRONYMS

Acronyms are commonly used in any highly technical work environment. A common language evolves in communicating thoughts and ideas between team members. An introduction to several more important acronyms used during simulation procedures will be helpful. Many of the useful acronyms are illustrated in Fig. 9-4, *A* and *B*. In trying to standardize radiation therapy terminology, the American Registry of Radiologic Technologists (ARRT) has also provided a list of terms or abbreviations listed in the ARRT Conventions Specific to Radiation Therapy Technology Examinations[1] (see Table 9-2, p. 168).

TUMOR AND NORMAL TISSUE LOCALIZATION

The primary function of the simulator is to localize the tumor volume in three dimensions. The simulator is not used exclusively or in total isolation for the localization of a majority of tumors but together with other imaging modalities such as CT and MRI.[5] However, some simulation procedures may be done exclusively on the simulator radiographically or fluoroscopically with or without the aid of contrast media. In this section, several aspects of tumor localization will be discussed. These include anatomical body planes, CT/MRI, SSD/SAD localization methods, fluoroscopy/radiography, and the use of contrast media in tumor and normal tissue localization.

Anatomical body planes

A review of the three major body planes helps in understanding the nature of three-dimensional localization. As illustrated in Fig. 9-5, the body can be described in three planes: the coronal, sagittal, and axial planes. An AP radiograph displays anatomy in the coronal plane, showing structures in the inferior/superior and left/right direction (two dimensions only). This radiographic view provides information for planning purposes in only one plane. The depth of the tumor volume cannot be found without the aid of a lateral radiograph (Fig. 9-6). This view shows anatomical information in the sagittal plane, displaying structures in the inferior/superior and AP direction. Axial images can only be obtained through CT and MRI modalities.

MRI and CT imaging

Applications and advantages of CT and MRI in radiation therapy treatment planning have been documented.[9] Radiation therapy CT planning procedures are distinctly different from conventional diagnostic procedures. For example, unlike CT scans done for diagnostic purposes, where a

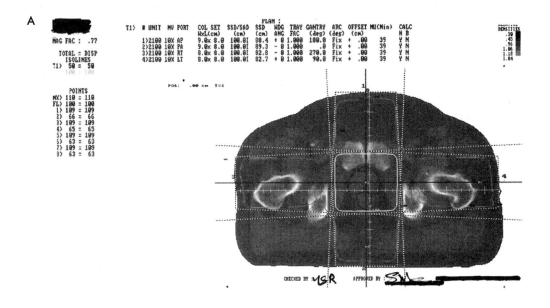

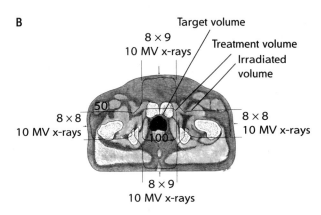

Target volume
Treatment volume
Irradiated volume

8 × 9
10 MV x-rays

8 × 8
10 MV x-rays

8 × 8
10 MV x-rays

8 × 9
10 MV x-rays

Fig. 9-2 The treatment plan using a CT image (**A**) is needed to plan this patient's course of radiation therapy. The diagram of the CT image (**B**) illustrates three terms: target volume, treatment volume (100% isodose line), and irradiated volume (50% isodose line), used to describe dose specifications for patient planning purposes.

curved couch top is used, a flat insert is required when scanning for radiation therapy planning purposes. It is important to scan the patient in the treatment position. If the treatment position is supine on a flat couch, then the patient should be scanned supine on a flat surface. In addition, positional lasers incorporated into the design of the CT scanner will aid in the reproducibility of the simulation process.[7]

Some studies have shown modifications in 30% to 80% of a select number of conventional non-CT treatment plans because of the additional information provided by CT. In addition, some 10% to 40% of all radiation therapy patients might benefit from CT scanning for radiation therapy treatment planning. Cross-sectional information provided by MRI/CT imaging contributes considerable information to the radiation oncologist in four major areas: diagnosis, tumor

and normal tissue localization, tissue density data for dose calculations, and follow-up treatment monitoring.[7]

There are two types of applications involving CT imaging in radiation therapy. One provides detailed diagnostic information used by the radiologist and radiation oncologist to evaluate the extent of the disease. This is conventional CT. The second is designed solely for radiation therapy treatment planning. Concerning the second application, some manufacturers have introduced simulators that can reconstruct information analogous to conventional CT images. Others have developed software where the radiation therapy beam can be displayed in coronal, sagittal, and axial planes. A beam's eye view allows the possibility of virtual simulation. By outlining target volumes on each image, irregular field shapes can be determined and a special laser device used to

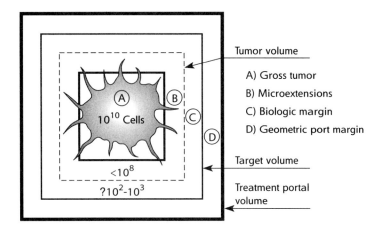

Fig. 9-3 Provides a schematic representation of the target and treatment volume surrounding the tumor. (From Perez CA, Purdy JA: Rationale for treatment planning in radiation therapy. In Levitt SH, editor: *Technological basis of radiation therapy: practical clinical applications*, ed 2. Philadelphia, Lea & Febiger.)

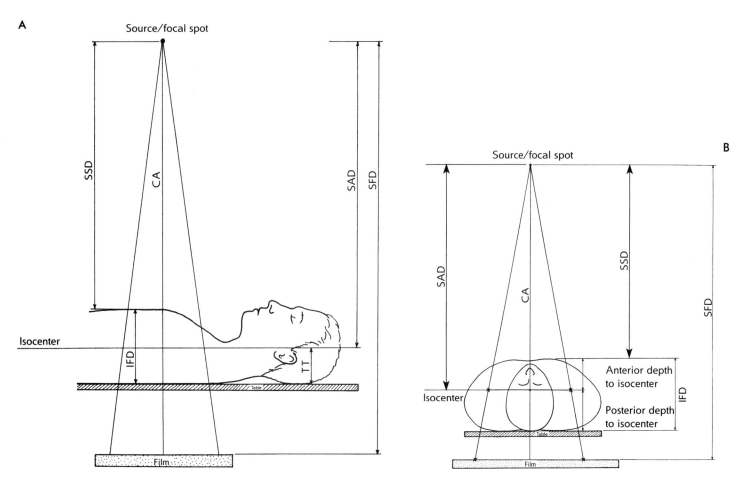

Fig. 9-4 A list of common acronyms used in radiation therapy; (**A**) a lateral view and (**B**) a superior view illustrating terms in a transverse plane.

Table 9-2	American Registry of Radiologic Technologists (ARRT) Conventions
Anteroposterior (AP)*	The central axis is directed from anterior to posterior.
Central axis (CA, CAX)	The central axis, which is an imaginary ray perpendicular to the cross-section of the simulation or treatment field.
Film*	Refer to "film" if it is truly film (i.e., unexposed); otherwise, use "radiograph."
Intrafield distance (IFD)	The measurement of the thickness of the patient along the central axis of the beam (or along a line parallel to the central axis) from the entrance point to the exit point. Also referred to as the patient's "separation."[18]
Left anterior oblique (LAO)*	The central axis is directed from the left anterior aspect of the patient.
Left posterior oblique (LPO)*	The central axis is directed from the left posterior aspect of the patient.
Parallel opposed (POP)	Two treatment fields planned 180° apart.
Patient support assembly (PSA)	Also referred to as the table or couch.
Right anterior oblique (RAO)*	The central axis is directed from the right anterior aspect of the patient.
Right posterior oblique (RPO)*	The central axis is directed from the right posterior aspect of the patient.
Optical distance indicator (ODI)	A device mounted on or near the collimator head that optically displays the SSD on the patient's skin.
Source-to-axis distance (SAD)*	The distance from the source of radiation to the axis of the radiation beam or isocenter.
Source-to-collimator distance (SCD)*	The distance between the source of radiation and the heavy metal collimators.
Source-to-diaphragm distance (SDD)*	The distance between the source of radiation and the collimators; used interchangeably with SCD.
Source-to-film distance (SFD)*	The distance from the source of radiation to the film. It replaces target-film distance (TFD) and focal-film distance (FFD).
Source-to-skin distance (SSD)*	The distance from the source of radiation to the skin or surface of the patient (either x-ray or radionuclide). It replaces target-skin distance (TSD) and focal-skin distance (FSD).
Source-to-tray distance (STD)*	The distance from the source of radiation to the blocking tray.
Table top distance (TT)	The distance from the table top to the isocenter.

*Indicates those terms or abbreviations described in the ARRT Conventions Specific to Radiation Therapy Technology Examination. Used with permission from the ARRT, St. Paul, MN.

outline this field shape directly on the patient's skin.[7,17] In the institutions where this technology is available, virtual simulation is reserved for 15% to 20% of the patients. These patients often need a second simulation process to provide verification and assurance that the treatment plan can be reproduced on the treatment unit.[17]

SSD/SAD localization methods

Most treatment planning on the simulator is divided into two types of procedures: SAD and SSD setups. Both methods may use *fluoroscopy* to scan the area. In each case, radiographs document what has been done during the simulation process. These *radiographs* are considered part of the patient's medical record. They are routinely used as "masters" when comparing subsequent port films from the treatment unit.

The decision to use one setup method over the other may be decided by many factors. They include the nature and extent of the patient's disease and the goals and expected outcome of the treatment (cure or palliation).

Other factors that are considered include the type of equipment available and the philosophy and education of the radiation therapy team.

The SSD approach positions a fixed treatment distance of 80 or 100 cm on the patient's skin for each field (Fig. 9-7, *A*). This method requires repositioning the patient for each field before treatment. Usually this approach uses a single field, two laterals or an AP/PA treatment approach (sometimes called parallel opposed [POP] fields because the central axes of each field oppose each other). This field arrangement requires tumor localization in two dimensions only, since all tissues within these fields are treated and the exact depth of the tumor is not critical.[3] Note that in Fig. 9-7, *A*, the field size is defined (at 100 cm) on the patient's skin.

The SAD approach is also called the **isocentric technique** (Fig. 9-7, *B*). It provides tumor localization in three dimensions. With the SAD strategy the isocenter is placed within the target volume with the aid of fluoroscopy and other imaging modalities. Here, as illustrated in Fig. 9-7, *B*, the field size is defined at the isocenter within the patient (100 cm). In

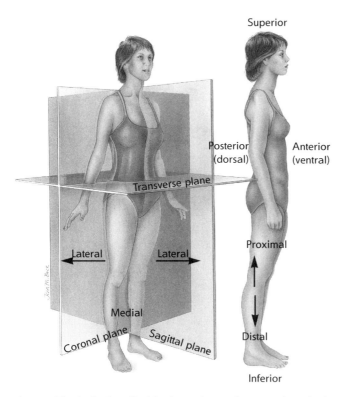

Fig. 9-5 The body described in three planes: the coronal, sagittal, and axial planes. (From Thibodeau GA, Patton KT: *Anatomy and physiology*, St Louis, 1994, Mosby.)

both situations the field size is defined at 100 cm. The only difference is where that distance is located (on the skin surface or within the patient). Once the isocenter has been located, orthogonal films may be taken. **Orthogonal films** are two radiographs taken at right angles to one another. They are often obtained to aid in the treatment planning process (see Fig. 9-6). In simulating a four-field pelvis, for example, some departments may take one radiograph to represent the anterior and posterior fields and one radiograph to represent the right and left lateral fields.

With the isocentric approach, the reading on the patient's skin varies from field to field. It depends on several factors. It will not be 80 or 100 cm, as happens with the SSD approach. Rather, the distance will vary for each field (Fig. 9-8), depending on the thickness or separation of the patient. It may also depend on the depth of the tumor from the AP, PA, oblique, or lateral skin surface.

Contrast media

To help in localizing the tumor volume and normal critical structures, contrast media may be needed during the simulation procedure. **Contrast media**, used in radiographic or fluoroscopic studies, visually enhance anatomical structures that would normally be more difficult to see. Commonly used contrast media include: barium sulfate, iodinated con-

trast materials, and negative contrast agents. Fig. 9-9, a lateral radiograph of the pelvis, illustrates both barium and iodine contrast agents used to localize the prostate.

Before the administration of any contrast medium, a careful evaluation of the patient should be performed. Severe allergic reactions to some contrast agents, requiring emergency intervention, have been observed. In addition, barium sulfate, for example, may be contraindicated with a suspected bowel perforation or obstruction. The proper selection and administration of the contrast medium should be evaluated before the simulation procedure.

Barium sulfate, which is not absorbed by the gastrointestinal (GI) tract when administered, outlines the GI tract. Before its administration either orally or rectally, it is prepared as a suspension in water to obtain the desired concentration or consistency. It is commonly used to visualize the esophagus, stomach, small bowel, colon, or oral cavity. Depending on the patient's condition, amount of barium, and its application, the patient should be advised as to the use of a laxative. Patients who had a small dab of barium paste inside the cheek to help localize a tonsillar lesion would be advised differently than someone who drank a 12-ounce cup of barium to evaluate the amount of small bowel in a pelvic treatment field.

Iodinated contrast materials used in radiation therapy are usually of two types: aqueous ionic contrast medium and nonionic contrast medium.[24] Although their actions are different, both provide positive contrast (a white area on the radiograph) of a vessel or organ. Iodinated contrast materials are commonly used to help localize the kidneys, bladder, and prostate, and they are sometimes used in the GI tract when barium is contraindicated. Except for the GI tract, sterile procedures must be followed when administering iodinated contrast material. For example, contrast medium may be used intravenously to document the location of the kidneys (for Hodgkin's disease or seminoma) or through a bladder catherization to localize the prostate.

Negative contrast agents, which include substances such as carbon dioxide, oxygen, and air, have a low atomic number and appear as dark areas on a radiograph. Examples of their use include a small amount of air introduced (with or without barium) into the rectum to help define its location or the use of normal gas exchange in the thorax, which helps define some lung tumors. Another example might include a Foley catheter balloon filled with 5 to 10 cc of air within the bladder. This is used to define the inferior extent of the bladder in reference to the prostate gland.

The primary function of the simulator is to localize the tumor volume relative to normal tissue structures. The use of contrast agents, fluoroscopy, and radiography together with other imaging modalities, such as CT and MRI, greatly enhances the ability to localize and pinpoint the tumor volume. Many of these tools are available to the radiation oncologist and radiation therapist. However, their use and applica-

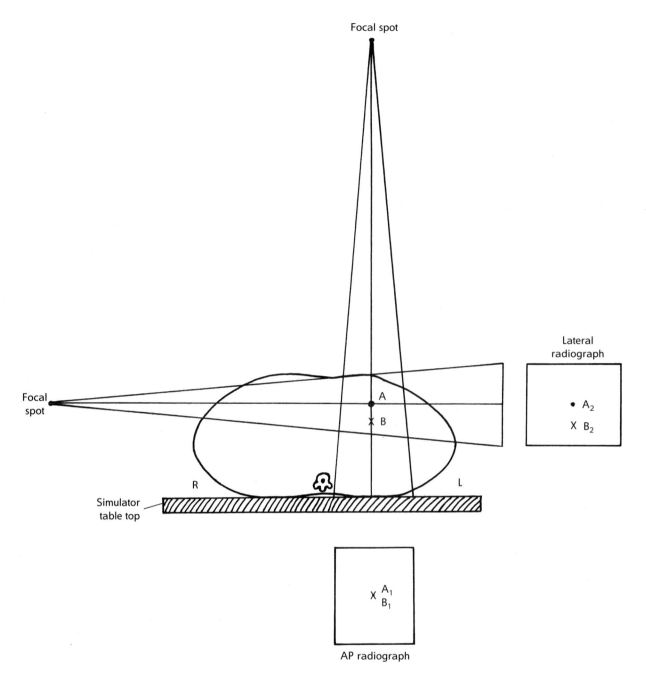

Focal spot

Lateral
radiograph

A

X B

• A₂

X B₂

Focal
spot

R

L

Simulator
table top

X A₁
B₁

AP radiograph

Fig. 9-6 Two radiographs taken at right angles to one another (orthogonal radiographs) are often obtained to aid in the treatment planning process. Note in this schematic that *points A and B* cannot be distinguished from one another, except on the lateral radiograph.

tion may vary from patient to patient and institution to institution. The actual process of simulating a patient, which will be discussed in the next section, varies less.

SIMULATION PROCEDURE

The use of treatment simulators during tumor and normal tissue localization is well documented.[*] The localization of a treatment field during simulation must reflect precisely what

*References 4, 7, 8, 14, 18, 21.

will happen in the treatment room. Patient position, beam alignment, and field size must be the same at the end of simulation and the beginning of treatment.[21] In this section the simulation procedure will be discussed in detail. The box on p. 174 outlines the common components involved in a simulation procedure.

Presimulation planning

An assessment of all relevant patient information and an evaluation of possible treatment approaches before the

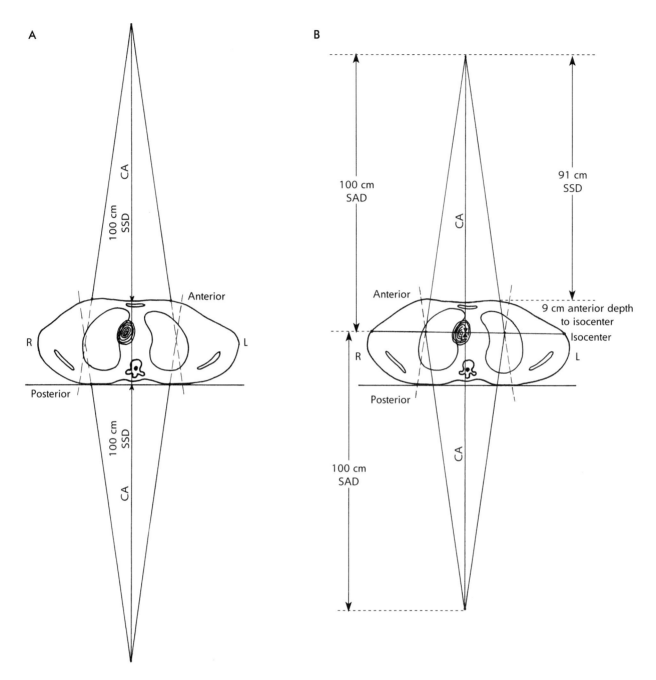

Fig. 9-7 Differences between an SSD approach (**A**), where the field size is defined on the surface, and SAD (**B**) approach, where the field size is defined at a depth calculated within the patient, are demonstrated. Both methods used in the planning and delivery of a prescribed course of radiation therapy require careful documentation.

patient arrives are ideal. This is especially true for difficult cases, involving patients who have had previous treatment or have extensive disease.[8] In many institutions this may be done as part of a morning conference, where the discussion of specific cases occurs among the radiation therapy team members. The discussion during these meetings should relate to treatment planning, simulation, and concerns for those patients under treatment, although, because of busy schedules or a late addition to the day's schedule, this is not always

possible. Minimally, the patient's history and physical examination notes should be reviewed by the radiation oncologist and radiation therapist, using other available pertinent information such as radiographs, CT/MRI scans, pathology reports, and operating reports.

The importance of the therapist and physician consultation before the actual simulation cannot be overemphasized. Radiation oncologists, even within the same institution, vary in their approach to simulation and treatment. For example,

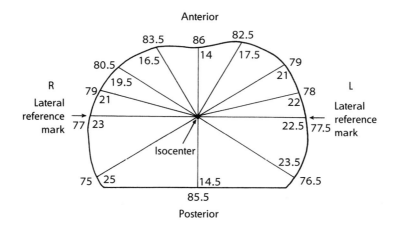

Fig. 9-8 Source-to-skin distance (SSD) varies with the patient's separation (IFD) when using an isocentric technique. Note that using a combination of SSD measurements, a patient's IFD can be calculated. In this example, the anterior SSD through the CA is 86 cm (depth of 14 cm) and the posterior SSD is 85.5 (depth of 14.5 cm). The IFD can be calculated by adding the two depths (14 + 14.5 = 28.5).

one physician may prefer to use a small amount of barium in the rectum for all endometrial cases, whereas another physician may use flexible beaded tubing to identify the rectum radiographically. In addition, the physician may be called away from the simulation area during the procedure and may not be immediately available to answer questions. So a plan should be established before beginning the simulation procedure if at all possible.

Additional attention in the presimulation planning process may involve the preparation of specialized immobilization devices. Certain accommodations for unique cases and an assessment of whether the simulation procedure is simple, intermediate, or complex should also be made. It is important to consider the patient's fears and anxieties, especially when doing simulations for small children and others with special needs. For all cases, if a clear treatment approach is known at the beginning of the simulation, the procedure will go more efficiently and accurately, enhancing the patient's confidence in the entire process and reducing the time needed to complete it.[8]

Preparing the room

Effective use of time on the simulator is essential. Proper room preparation can aid in the effective use of that time. A review of all the pertinent information needed for the simulation procedure allows the therapist to prepare the simulation room in advance. The time demands on the simulator can be pressing, bearing in mind that one simulator can serve two or three treatment units.[3] A typical simulation day involves simulating 3 to 10 cases, depending on the number of treatment units in the department, the total number of new patients seen at the institution each year, and other factors. To explain the specific needs concerning the simulator's room preparation, two examples are provided.

Head and neck. The room is first cleaned from the simulation previous to this patient. If a thermoplastic mask is used, the heating element in the water tank is turned on low. This is done so the water will be warm as the patient walks through the door. A clean sheet or piece of paper is placed on the simulator couch. The head rest (which can range from A to F and will be either transparent plastic or a solid foamlike material, see Fig. 7-2) selected for the simulation procedure is related to the patient's anatomy. For this simulation, a "C" or "D" headrest is selected. This should elevate the chin and isolate the treatment area (neck). The gantry head is positioned to the appropriate SSD for this patient's treatment machine. For example, some departments may have a 6 MV treatment unit with 100 SSD and an 80 SSD cobalt 60 unit.

If the patient requires a stent or special mouthpiece, this is made before the simulation begins. Wires help to visualize a surgical scar or any other pertinent anatomical areas. Pull straps or some kind of mechanism should be available (if needed) to pull the top of the shoulders down inferiorly and out of the treatment field. Tape is placed at the head of the couch. This is handy for drawing the marks on the thermoplastic mask (if used) or securing a wire on the patient's skin. A cloth or paper towels should be available to dry the excess water from the thermoplastic mask. The treatment volume may have already been decided during the presimulation session with the physician, making the simulation more accurate and time efficient.

Thorax. Because the patient will receive part of the treatment through the treatment couch from a direct posterior field or posterior oblique portal, a table pad is not recommended. The simulation must duplicate the treatment setup in all aspects. A cushion on the table may interfere with reproducibility. If the patient is in severe pain, accommodations required for a pad or cushion during treatment

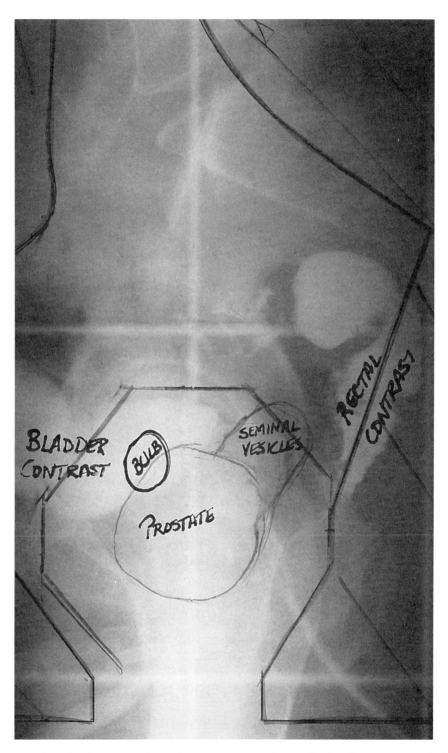

Fig. 9-9 A lateral radiograph of the pelvis with contrast medium used to localize the prostate. In this example, barium is used to visualize the rectum and an iodinated contrast medium helps to localize the bladder.

Procedure Outline for Simulation

1. Presimulation planning
2. Room preparation
3. Explanation of procedure
4. Patient positioning and immobilization
5. Operation of simulator controls
6. Setting field size parameters
7. Selecting exposure techniques
8. Radiographic exposure
9. Documenting pertinent data
10. Final procedures

and simulation can be calculated. The "B" head rest may be appropriate when the treatment portal will not cover the cervical lymph nodes. If the cervical lymph nodes must be encompassed in the treatment volume, a "C" headrest may be used to elevate the chin more, thus isolating the neck lymph nodes.

Depending on the patient's arm position, an Alpha Cradle can be constructed (see Chapter 7, Immobilization Devices) or the Vac-lok (a type of cushion constructed of thin plastic film with a fill material of tiny polystyrene spheres) used to provide patient immobilization. This increases the stability of the patient's arms (especially if they are positioned above the head) and increases reproducibility during treatment. An appropriate field size is set, positioning the collimator with no rotation.

If a CT scan is needed for treatment planning purposes, the therapist must arrange this ahead of time. This will involve additional time for the patient and therapist. To ensure the patient is in the same treatment position when scanned, the therapist must accompany the patient. Radiopaque markers may also be needed to obtain accurate CT data for treatment planning purposes. BBs, wires, arrows, or another type of radiopaque material is necessary to visualize specific points of interest on a radiograph and/or CT scan. This is done to help the dosimetrist transfer these anatomical points to the treatment planning computer. For example, a cross-table lateral film may be taken to provide data for a dose calculation to the spinal cord. A chain or wire is taped to the patient's posterior surface before the simulation begins.

Details concerning the preparation of the room become more important with a busy schedule. Establishing a definite treatment approach at the beginning of the simulation procedure allows the process to proceed more efficiently and accurately. The patient gains confidence in the radiation therapy staff if one of the first impressions of the department is a positive one. This can be enhanced if the simulation procedure is accurate, organized, and not rushed. It also provides an opportunity to educate the patient and answer questions concerning the treatment process, side effects, and skin care.

Explanation of simulation procedure

Assessment. Our entire health care system is based on effective communication. Miscommunication can have a major impact on the patient's care. The therapist must assess the patient's needs, recognize cultural differences, respond to nonverbal communication, and then attempt to communicate therapeutically and effectively with the patient.[24]

In the simulator, the therapist should assess the patient's physical condition and emotional state. The therapist should determine if the patient is nervous, fearful, or withdrawn. If a patient requires oxygen or medications or has difficulty standing, sitting, or walking, the therapist can try to make the patient more comfortable. If a patient has difficulty hearing or speaking, provisions can also be made. Good observation skills are essential to proper patient assessment.

Communication. The therapist should also establish an environment conducive to communication. If there are distractions in the area, such as unwanted noises or the usual distractions of a radiation oncology department, it may be preferable to retreat to a private area to communicate with the patient (the simulator room is much better for this than a busy waiting room). Therapists must establish an environment where they can facilitate the communication clearly, effectively, and therapeutically.[24]

A health care professional should make a conscious effort to speak clearly, confidently, and at a rate and tone conducive to listening. With practice a therapist can increase listening skills by not only listening to what the patient is saying, but also hearing what he or she is not saying.[20,24] For example, if during a conversation a patient cannot say the word "cancer," this could indicate this patient has not accepted the disease, which in turn can cause the therapist to communicate differently than with someone who talks freely about the disease diagnosed.

Observation is also an important skill in effective communication. The therapist should observe the patient at all times during a conversation, noting facial expressions, body gestures, space relations, and contradictions in the patient's communication. If a patient explains that he or she is in great pain but then is laughing and smiling, the therapist should pay close attention to the patient's nonverbal communication. Any barriers to communication may impact the patient's health care.

Nonverbal communication not only includes what the therapist and patient can observe, but also includes what the therapist and patient hear in the speech, what is felt as the person is touched, and what each person smells (for example, a lack of good personal hygiene or overuse of perfume/cologne) as they get closer to each other.[20,24] If a patient hears lack of interest and/or monotony in the therapist's voice, frequently because the same speech has already been made many times that day, the patient may feel that the therapist's disinterested in the situation. As the therapist touches the patient and the patient retreats back, the therapist should know the patient is anxious and refrain from touching him or her or ask before touching the patient again.

Cultural diversity. The therapist must be aware of cultural differences in both verbal and nonverbal communication to avoid being misunderstood, offending someone, or being offended by someone during communication.[20,24] This is especially important in culturally diverse areas and in teaching hospitals, where a larger percentage of patients may be foreign or from different parts of the country. Gestures displayed in the United States do not always have the same meaning in every culture. For example, in the United States, people tend to be more protective of their "personal space," whereas in other countries, it is considered rude to stand far away from a person while communicating. Language barriers can be overcome through an interpreter provided by the hospital or a local church group. This should be planned in advance if possible. A family member may also serve as an interpreter for a patient. In addition, the family member can be a source of support for the patient and may hear something the patient does not.

Therapeutic communication. Therapeutic communication enables the patient to feel part of the team or a partner in the situation. The care giver should not just repeat orders but rather establish a relationship with the patient. This takes some time and effort on the part of the care giver. For a radiation therapist, this realm of communication is the most valuable because once a relationship with a patient is established, he or she trusts the care giver and allows help to be given throughout the disease process (especially during the administration of the treatment). A therapist should first establish the basis for the communication by introducing the staff and explaining the simulation procedure in detail. Therapists should always face the patient and maintain eye contact whenever possible. A therapeutic communicator listens while the patient is speaking and never interrupts. It is inappropriate to be busy planning a response rather than listening while the patient is speaking.

During communication the therapist should also check for understanding; restating or repeating statements made by the patient is very useful. This lets the patient know you understand what he or she is saying verbally or nonverbally and also affirms to the patient that he or she is being heard. This can help a patient in making decisions because the same information is repeated back in another form, providing the opportunity to look at the problem from a different perspective and facilitating understanding. If at any time during communication the therapist does not understand the patient, clarification should be sought.

The main objective of therapeutic communication is to keep the conversation directed toward the patient. The therapist should avoid closed ended sentences, which are sentences answered with a "yes" or "no" response. The patient should be involved and the communication focused on him or her—not on the therapist. Therapeutic communication is kept short with open-ended questions, always directing the communication to the patient.

Educating the patient and family. Using therapeutic communication is also a vital process when educating the patient. Professionally the therapist is obligated to educate the patient not only about the physical aspects of radiation therapy the patient can see and feel, but also about the emotional aspects of radiation therapy. The simulation treatment procedure should be explained in detail. This explanation should be done slowly and clearly, using all therapeutic communication techniques. The equipment must be explained to the patient. It is helpful to mention that the simulation is not an actual treatment and that the simulator is an x-ray machine, not a therapeutic treatment machine. The patient should be shown where he or she will lie on the table, which way the head should be placed, whether the patient will be supine or prone, and whether he or she will be on a belly board or with the arms above the head. Basic patient positioning should be communicated along with an explanation of why that position is needed. This facilitates patient cooperation.

The patient should also be given an explanation of what procedures to follow after the simulation. The patient should receive instructions on how to take care of the skin marks as well as the skin itself before the treatments begin and while under treatment. When special orders are needed before the patient is to receive treatment, such as arriving for treatment with a full or empty bladder, this should be communicated at this time. When barium is used during the simulation, follow-up instructions are needed. An appointment time for the first treatment should be discussed, providing the therapist's name and department number in case communication is necessary before the next appointment.

Patient positioning and immobilization

One of the weakest links in treatment planning is patient positioning.[2,7] If the patient is not comfortable and does not remain still during treatment administration, then sophisticated treatment plans and elaborate immobilization devices are not as effective. If a stable position cannot be maintained and reproduced daily, the result is either a geometric miss of the target volume or irradiation of greater amounts of uninvolved normal tissue.[8,10]

For most simulation procedures the patient is positioned supine or prone. Occasionally other positions are used. On rare occasions, a sitting position may be necessary because of the patient's medical condition. For example, a patient may need to be positioned in an erect or semi-erect position (sitting on the end of the treatment table) because of an advanced lung mass that has compromised the patient's breathing and the return of blood through the superior vena cava. Helpful hints regarding patient positioning and immobilization are listed in the box on p. 176. These suggestions and recommendations can be considered in an effort to improve patient positioning and reproducibility.

Daily reproducibility is essential. The positioning of the patient for treatment is usually depicted by a patient alignment system (Fig. 9-10, *A* and *B*). Three-directional lasers

Helpful Hints in Patient Positioning During Simulation Procedures

1. If possible, one position should be established for all treatment fields, including boost fields. Internal structures can change dramatically if the patient's position is changed (for example, from supine for one field to a prone position for the other).[3,14] The supine position should be used whenever possible because it is more comfortable for the patient and easier to document reproducibility.

   Exceptions: May include mantle irradiation on a treatment unit where large fields are not possible, except at extended distances. This requires the patient to be treated in both supine and prone positions to adequately cover the treatment volume. It may not always be possible to treat breast and head and neck patients in the same position for their boost treatment, especially if electrons are used. Here, small fields are generally used for the boost, and electron cones do not offer the physical flexibility that photon fields offer.

2. Spending time before the simulation procedure educating, informing, and answering patient questions allows the patient to participate and cooperate more in maintaining a comfortable and reproducible treatment position.

   Exceptions: May include infants, small children, and severely handicapped individuals. In some situations premedication or anesthetics may be helpful in immobilizing the patient during the simulation procedure.

3. Consistent preparation of the treatment area should be carried out on a daily basis. Asking the patient to remove certain articles of clothing, dress in comfortable, loose-fitting clothing, or change into a specific type of hospital gown will add to consistent and reproducible positioning. Use of a bed sheet or suitable material prevents the shifting of skin marks when sliding a patient along the couch top.

   Exceptions: Include treatment areas that are not normally covered by clothing, such as the head and neck region and portions of the extremities. Patients requiring hospitalization may need special care and communication with the nursing staff regarding clothing or bandages that may interfere with visualizing external ink marks, tattoos, or anatomical landmarks.

4. Clinical considerations and medical conditions may restrict or inhibit patient positioning. Patient pain and discomfort or physical disabilities might result in very limited positioning.[3] For example, a breast cancer patient recovering from a lumpectomy or axillary node dissection may have limited arm movement. Special accommodations or a delay in initiating the simulation procedure may be considered.

   Exceptions: Include certain patients treated for palliation. Perez and Brady define the palliative aim of therapy as one in which there is no hope of the patient surviving for extended periods. However, symptoms that produce discomfort, impair the self-sufficiency of the patient, or cause severe pain require treatment. It must be remembered that in curative therapy, a certain probability of side effects, even though undesirable, may be acceptable. The same is not generally true in palliative treatment.[19] For example, a patient with metastatic breast cancer requiring treatment to the lumbar spine should not be denied a comfortable pad to lie on during treatment at the expense of a hard treatment couch and a small amount of skin sparing.

5. Accurate and complete setup instructions are necessary. The use of additional skin marks, reference to topographic anatomy, or special instructions for unusual patient positioning can be critical in the daily reproducibility of the treatment position. This requires accurate record keeping and careful documentation of the simulation procedure. A Polaroid picture of the setup, whenever possible, is helpful.

   Exceptions: None.

6. Sometimes it is necessary to move normal critical tissues out of the field or away from the edge of the beam. Examples include rotating the eye to spare the lens and moving the testicle(s) or ovaries to reduce the gonadal dose. A surgical procedure called an oophoropexy can relocate the ovaries to the midline of the body, where they may be more easily shielded.[3]

   Exceptions: Include critical structures that may be involved with tumor. In addition, many normal tissue structures can be shielded with custom blocking or special shielding devices. Radiographic documentation of the lens with the aid of a radiopaque BB or arrow provides the physician information regarding the construction of customized blocks. Special shielding devices are available to reduce the dose to the testes.

7. Simulation or CT scanning of patients on solid couch tops while treating them on flexible "tennis racquet" type windows can result in discrepancies between the planned volume and the irradiated volume.[3]

   Exceptions: Rare. Kahn recommends, for lateral portal exposure of the pelvis, that the Mylar section of the couch or "tennis racquet" be removed. The patient can be placed on a solid surface to avoid sag during positioning, reserving the "tennis racquet" for parallel opposed anteroposterior treatments where skin sparing is of concern.[16] Setup discrepancies in the pelvic area from the simulator to the treatment couch, especially with larger patients, can be as much as 1 to 1.5 cm. Part of this discrepancy may result from the inconsistent use of couch top surfaces between the simulator and treatment unit. For example, a solid couch top may be used during the simulation of a four-field pelvic procedure. Discrepancies may result if the patient is positioned on a "tennis racquet" couch top during treatment.

A

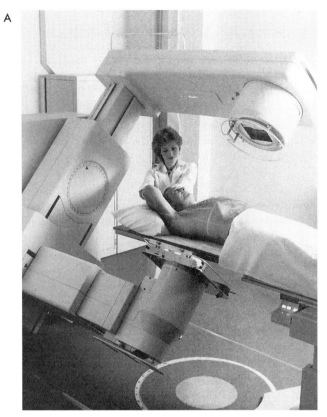

B

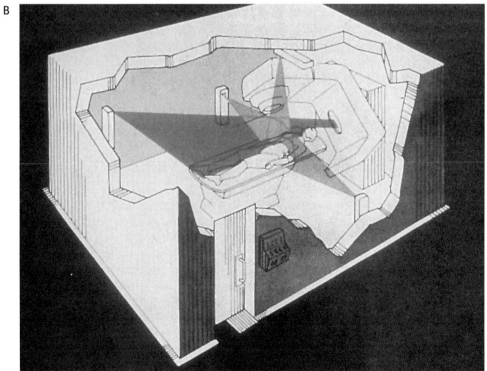

Fig. 9-10 Usually two side lasers and an overhead laser are used to accurately define the location of the isocenter during simulation (**A**), which demonstrates an oblique setup on a Philips SLS Simulator and (**B**) treatment delivery, which shows the THER-A-CROSS system. The directional lasers correspond to external reference marks on the patient. (**A**, courtesy of Philips Medical Systems, Shelton, CT; **B**, courtesy of Gammex RMI, Milwaukee, WI.)

accomplish this through the transverse and sagittal planes. A patient's age, weight, and general health as well as the anatomical area to be simulated can affect the patient's position. Usually India ink tattoos, visual skin marks, or references to topographic anatomy are used to delineate the treatment area. Immobilization devices improve the accuracy and reproducibility of a planned course of treatment. To achieve this, the integrity of a patient's position must be maintained throughout the course of treatment. As little as one or two patient positioning errors can increase the possibility of missing the treatment volume. This can reduce the dose to the tumor volume by 10% or greater as well as treat areas that do not need treatment.[10] Thus daily reproduction of the prescribed, planned, and simulated treatment is essential to its outcome. Also important is prohibiting patient movement during simulation, treatment setup, and treatment delivery.[15,23] Effective immobilization is essential to achieving this goal. There are many positioning aids and immobilization devices (see Chapter 7, Immobilization Devices) that are commercially available or easily created at the clinical site. The construction and use of immobilization devices should be discussed with the physician and/or physicist before the simulation procedure.

Operating simulator controls

Accurate patient positioning requires an understanding of how the mechanical, optical, and radiographic components of the simulator work. An understanding of their use is important. Mechanical components of the simulator include the motions of gantry rotation, collimator movements, and treatment couch. Optical components may include the laser system, optical distance indicator (ODI), and field light indicator.

Previous background in radiography is helpful, but not essential, in understanding the radiographic components of the simulator. State regulations may require the use of technique charts, which include guidelines for selecting kVp, mA, and time factors used in deciding radiographic exposure techniques. In some institutions, in an attempt to increase familiarity with simulation procedures, certain therapists will perform most of the simulation procedures. This means they rotate less frequently, if at all, through other (treatment) areas of the department.

It is also important to know the limits of the mechanical, optical, and radiographic components. For example, it is important to know the limits of gantry rotation with the use of specific immobilization devices or table angles. This is helpful in avoiding possible collisions on the treatment unit. In addition, it is important to know how to handle a burned out ODI light bulb partway through a simulation procedure. Can the simulation procedure be completed or should it be interrupted? This will depend on when during the simulation process the ODI fails you.

Radiographically, obtaining good quality lateral pelvic radiographs may require the use of a double exposure technique with some x-ray generators. This may be caused by heat limits on the x-ray tube. Two shorter exposures, instead of one longer one, may produce a better quality radiograph. A lateral view of the pelvis can be a most challenging radiograph to produce for the radiation therapist.

Setting field parameters

Familiarity with both the controls in the simulator room and those located on the control console is essential for a smooth, accurate, and efficient simulation procedure. Once the patient has been oriented to the simulation procedure and positioned on the simulator couch, the actual localization process can begin.

Establishing the field parameters may be done in one or more sessions, depending on the complexity of the case. It is the complex cases that often require more than one session. In these situations the target volume may not be visible on routine radiographs. It may be close to sensitive structures. Sometimes previous diagnostic studies identifying the location of the target volume were obtained with the patient in a different position than that of the simulation. In those cases the primary purpose of the first simulation is to establish a frame of reference between the data obtained during simulation and previously obtained diagnostic information.[8]

Field parameters such as width, length, gantry angle, collimator angle, and position of the isocenter should be established for both the SSD and SAD (isocentric) setup. Initially an estimate of the tumor volume may be established before fluoroscopy. This may be done by positioning the isocenter and setting a field width and length. The isocenter is positioned at the central axis (middle of the treatment field) on the patient's skin for an SSD approach and within the patient for an SAD technique. The locations of the central axis and field edges are then more accurately localized, usually with the aid of fluoroscopy.

Orthogonal films, which provide three-dimensional information, may be used with the isocentric technique. An example may help clarify the use of these radiographs in tumor localization. Small fields treated to high doses are often used to control prostate cancer. Here the patient's isocenter may be established using contrast medium and documented with an orthogonal pair of radiographs. At this point, two radiographs have been taken to document the position of the isocenter. The primary purpose of the first simulation is to establish a frame of reference. A CT scan is then performed with the patient in the treatment position (in the radiology department). A shift in the isocenter may be necessary based on information about the tumor volume obtained from the CT scan. Any shifts can be measured from the original isocenter (first simulation) on the first day of treatment or verified on the simulator during a second session.

There is no one universally accepted approach to establishing the field parameters. For simple parallel opposed treatment fields a short simulation session may be all that is necessary. More complex cases can be simulated using various approaches. A longer single simulation session can be used to document the isocenter, field width, and length along with other setup parameters in more complex cases. Multiple simulation sessions can also be used, incorporating orthogonal films and/or CT treatment planning. Even longer sessions may be required if using a virtual simulation technique.[17] Whatever approach is used, it is necessary to document the treatment fields with radiographs. Whenever possible, a radiograph should be taken for each treatment portal.

Producing quality radiographs

Radiographs taken at the time of simulation document the treatment portals. Not only do they serve as part of the patient's medical record, but also they are used as masters to compare with port films (taken on the treatment unit). Quality is important. Several aspects of producing good quality radiographs will be discussed in this section, including selecting exposure techniques, orienting the film, processing the film, and documenting the radiograph.

Selecting appropriate radiographic exposure techniques is a complex process. Several important details contribute to choosing the best technical factors. The use of critical thinking skills is the secret to producing good quality radiographs. This happens especially when those skills are applied to the four main technical factors (kVp, mA, time, and distance) in the right combination.

Categorizing patients into a specific **body habitus** (general physical appearance and body build; see Chapter 8, Surface and Sectional Anatomy) is helpful in selecting adequate exposure factors. Attenuation of the x-rays will vary, depending on the patient's thickness and, to a lesser degree, the body's composition. The composition of the patient's tissues can also change because of a specific disease process. For example, it is easier to penetrate the chest without the presence of pneumonia or congestive heart failure. Both pathologies result in increased radiation absorption. Knowing when to deviate from average exposure factors displays evidence of good critical thinking skills and is often necessary to producing useful images, especially in systems without phototiming.

Before the technical factors are selected, several elements concerning the type and orientation of the film must be considered. Will a grid be used? Some departments may have the option of using a grid or various cassettes with different screen/film combinations. The use of a fast screen/film combination may provide the extra edge in obtaining a good quality lateral radiograph of the pelvis. Other factors to consider before exposure include centering the film, reducing the size of the diaphragm opening, and setting an appropriate source-film distance. Some simulators will not allow an exposure unless the image intensifier is centered in relationship to the central axis. Evidence of collimation, by reducing the diaphragm opening on the radiograph, should appear as a clear 1 to 2 cm border on the processed film. This not only makes it easier to visualize the irradiated volume and some surrounding anatomy, but also reduces the amount of unwanted scatter radiation from reaching the film. Reducing scatter radiation generally improves radiographic contrast and the visibility of detail. Source-film distance should be recorded to document the magnification factor. This information may be needed for calculations or fabricating custom shielding blocks.

Phototiming is a form of automatic exposure control (AEC) where one or more ionization cells automatically stop the exposure. With phototiming, the operator can preselect the desired density. Anatomically programmed radiography is also available. These systems are simply computerized technique charts. For example, a button representing an anatomical site is selected and then correlated to a small, medium, or large patient. They provide more consistency in the production of radiographs with appropriate contrast and density.

Quality control experts agree that the radiographic film processor is the most sensitive variable factor in the production of a radiograph.[6] It may be the therapist's responsibility, especially in smaller satellite facilities and freestanding clinics, to monitor the quality control of the processor. This may be done through film sensitometry using a densitometer. The whole process adds a few minutes to the morning warm-up procedure on the simulator. For the sake of convenience, a darkroom should be located near the simulator. One processor should adequately serve two simulators and several treatment units.

All radiographs should be documented with pertinent patient information. Part of this process may occur in the darkroom, where information such as the patient's name, date, and identification number are permanently "stamped" on the film. Additional information, such as field size, gantry and collimator angle, SSD/SAD, SFD, treatment unit, and sometimes a reference to the radiation oncologist caring for the patient, is written on the radiograph after processing. Additional information included on the radiograph is helpful to someone comparing the port film (especially without the treatment chart or other details of the patient's history nearby) and includes the patient's diagnosis, incisions/palpable nodes, and other important reference points.[2] This can be done with a waxed pencil, felt-tipped marker, or other suitable means. Each film should be identified for further reference and as part of the patient's legal medical record.

Documenting pertinent data

Information gathered during the simulation procedure needs accurate documentation. This information is essential to accurately reproduce the geometry of the setup on the treatment unit (see box on p. 180). It is also used to maintain accurate medical records and to aid in the treatment planning and dose calculation processes. Documentation of pertinent information involves both marking the patient and documenting information in the patient's chart. Some institutions make use of a simulation worksheet designed to guide the therapist in documenting all of the patient's field parameters and measurements.

Machine parameters

Treatment SSD
Table top to isocenter distance
Collimator width
Collimator length
Gantry angle
Couch angle
Collimator angle
Multileaf collimator
Electron cone
Block tray

Patient's position

Supine/prone/other
Arm position
Leg position
Head support
Spirit level
Table pad/Egg crate
Immobilization devices
Other special devices
Shifts from isocenter

Diagram of the field arrangement

Schematic diagram for field arrangement
Blocked field diagram
Location of central axis
Location of field edges
Location of tattoos
Reference to bony anatomy
Wedge orientation

Other pertinent data

Bolus
Wedges
Tissue compensator
Special instructions
Setup photographs

One of the most important measurements obtained during the simulation process is the patient's intrafield distance (IFD) or separation. This measurement directly influences the dose to both the tumor and other, normal tissues. Therefore it is important to use a caliper correctly in determining the patient's IFD. A **caliper** consists of a graduated rule in centimeters with one stationary bar and a second one that slides up and down along the graduated rule. It is used to help determine the treatment volume by measuring the thickness of various body parts. If the treatment area is relatively flat, then one IFD measurement is generally taken at the central axis. If the treatment area is sloped, as is often the case in the thorax, then multiple IFD measurements are obtained (superior, center, and inferior field edge). Caution

must be used when obtaining an IFD value in an area where there may be an air gap, as is common in the cervical and lumbar regions. Here the lordotic curve is more pronounced. Accurate IFD measurements translate into accurate dose calculations.

There are two schools of thought in documenting and communicating the location of treatment fields. One method involves establishing marks on the patient's skin. The other method references bony landmarks in and around the treatment area.

Using bony landmarks the treatment field's CA and field edge(s) are referenced to specific anatomical landmarks. For example, in the treatment of head and neck cancer, the patient's CA might be referenced 2 cm inferior and 1.3 cm posterior to the external auditory meatus. Gerbi, in describing the location of the treatment field using bony landmarks, lists several advantages over the use of skin marks: (1) skin marks are highly mobile, especially for obese patients, whereas the location of the target volume remains essentially constant with respect to bony structures; (2) a resimulation is not required if the skin marks are lost; and (3) the treatment field can be easily reconstructed long after the current course of therapy.[8]

External skin marks or permanent tattoos can also be used to reference the patient's treatment position. Small tattoos on the patient's skin may be used to reference the position of the treatment field's CA or field edges. They are applied at the time of simulation using India ink with a small gauge needle. Semi-permanent marks, applied with felt-tipped markers or carfusion (a silver nitrate–based solution effective in "staining" the skin), also help to reference the treatment area on the patient's skin. A small tattoo less than 1 mm in size provides more accuracy than skin marks for laser alignment. However, tattoos must be used with caution in certain circumstances, especially in cases of obesity, weight loss, and change in tumor size, where the skin can shift in relation to the internal anatomy.[3] Some institutions employ a combination of both methods, depending on the individual case.

Information documented in the treatment chart to aid in the daily setup of the patient may be organized in several ways and is usually institutionally dependent. Fig. 9-11, *A* and *B,* illustrates treatment setup sheets where pertinent data gathered from the simulation procedure are documented at two different clinical sites. Pertinent information should include machine parameters such as SSD, table top to isocenter distance, collimator width and length (field size), and gantry, couch, and collimator angles. Any indicated shifts from the isocenter should also be documented. A description of the patient's position along with any immobilization and support devices used in reproducing the patient's position should be documented. Included in the setup instructions is a schematic diagram of the field arrangement. Also included is a blocked diagram. This is helpful in orienting the therapist to the position of shielding blocks, location of the central axis, and field edges. There should also be an area for setup

A

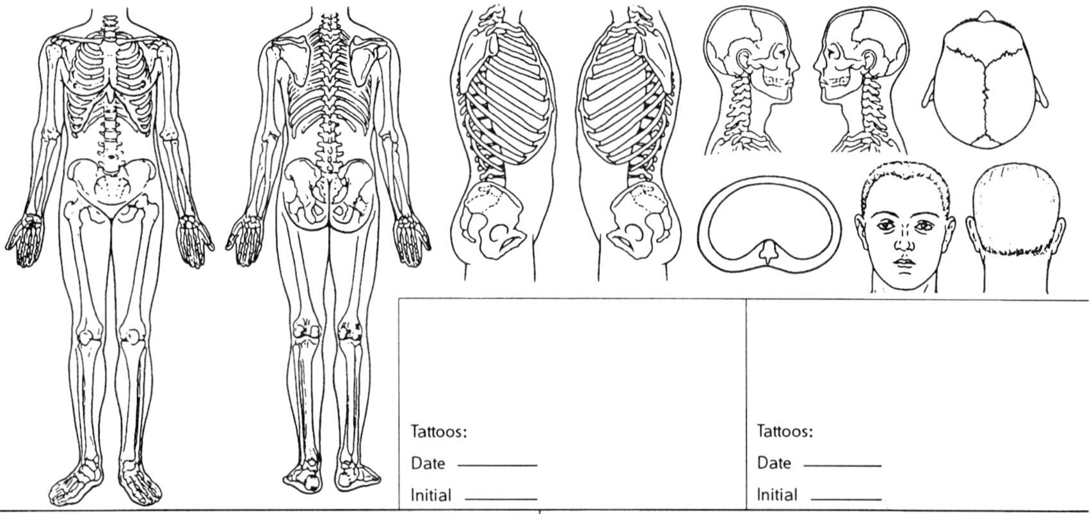

Tattoos:

Date ———————

Initial ———————

Tattoos:

Date ———————

Initial ———————

INSTRUCTIONS: Field Number(s):   Treatment Field Order

INSTRUCTIONS: Field Number(s):   Treatment Field Order

Patient position: ☐ Supine ☐ Prone ☐ Reverse on table ☐ Safety strap ☐ Full table pad
Head and neck support: _____Pillow ↓ Head ☐ Head immobilizer ___Neck rest ☐ Face rest ☐ Prone pillow ☐ Other_____
Leg support: ☐ Lg pillow ↓ knees ☐ Sm rd ↓ knees ☐ Lg pillow ↓ ankles ☐ No support ☐ Toe strap
Hand and arm position: ☐ Hands on chest ☐ Hands on abdomen ☐ Arms along side ☐ Arms above head ☐ Mantle position ___Armboard ☐ Breast board ___Arm ___Head
Accessory devices: ☐ Tongue cork or blade ☐ Dental rolls ☐ Carriers or prosthesis ☐ Jump rope ☐ Aquaplast _____Shims ☐ Alpha cradle ☐ Foot holder
Table position: ☐ Window ☐ Spline ☐ F.T.T. ☐ Decubitus board ☐ Lexan table extension ☐ CNS board

Special instructions

_____

_____

_____

_____

_____

_____

_____

_____

_____

_____

Patient position: ☐ Supine ☐ Prone ☐ Reverse on table ☐ Safety strap ☐ Full table pad
Head and neck support: _____Pillow ↓ Head ☐ Head immobilizer ___Neck rest ☐ Face rest ☐ Prone pillow ☐ Other_____
Leg support: ☐ Lg pillow ↓ knees ☐ Sm rd ↓ knees ☐ Lg pillow ↓ ankles ☐ No support ☐ Toe strap
Hand and arm position: ☐ Hands on chest ☐ Hands on abdomen ☐ Arms along side ☐ Arms above head ☐ Mantle position ___Armboard ☐ Breast board ___Arm ___Head
Accessory devices: ☐ Tongue cork or blade ☐ Dental rolls ☐ Carriers or prosthesis ☐ Jump rope ☐ Aquaplast _____Shims ☐ Alpha cradle ☐ Foot holder
Table position: ☐ Window ☐ Spline ☐ F.T.T. ☐ Decubitus board ☐ Lexan table extension ☐ CNS board

Special instructions

_____

_____

_____

_____

_____

_____

_____

_____

_____

_____

Fig. 9-11 The treatment portion of the patient's chart is used to document the patient's setup parameters. Note institutional differences between **A** (Mayo Clinic in Rochester, MN) and **B** (p. 182) (Central Maine Medical Center in Lewiston, ME). Both provide documentation of pertinent patient data.

Continued.

photographs (if used) and an area describing bolus, wedges, and tissue compensator.

Contour devices

The next step after a simulation is dose calculation. A dosimetrist or therapist cannot just calculate the necessary doses without considering the patient's anatomy and total treatment volume from multiple treatment portals. To complete the simulation process, it may be necessary to obtain a **contour** (an external representation of the patient's shape). This should be done in the central axis plane for three-dimensional treatment planning. There are many methods of obtaining a contour, and this may be done by the radiation therapist or physics personnel. They can range from a simple

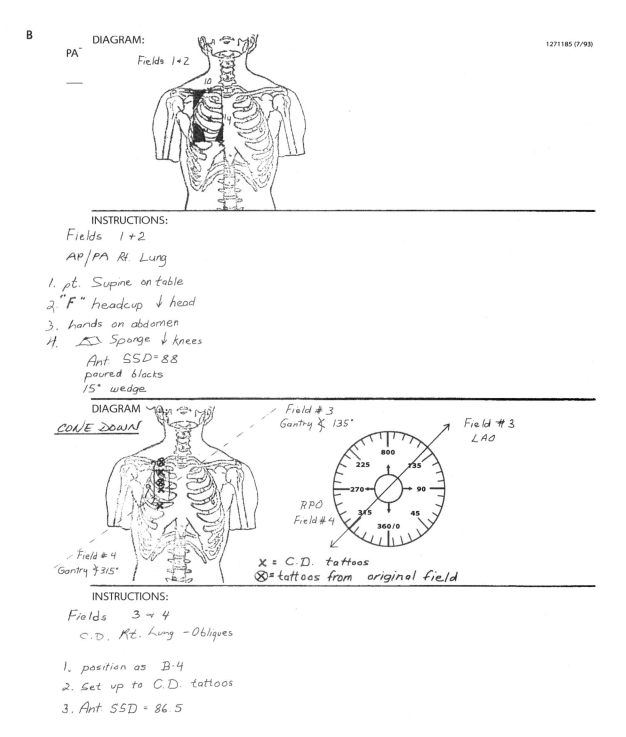

B

DIAGRAM:

PA⁻

Fields 1+2

1271185 (7/93)

10

14

x

INSTRUCTIONS:

Fields 1+2

AP/PA Rt. Lung

1. pt. Supine on table
2. "F" headcup ↓ head
3. hands on abdomen
4. ◁ Sponge ↓ knees
   Ant. SSD=88
   poured blocks
   15° wedge

DIAGRAM

CONE DOWN

Field #3
Gantry ∠ 135°

Field #3
LAO

800
225   135
270   90
315   45
360/0

RPO
Field #4

Field #4
Gantry ∠ 315°

X = C.D. tattoos
⊗ = tattoos from original field

INSTRUCTIONS:

Fields 3 & 4
C.D. Rt. Lung - Obliques

1. position as B·4
2. Set up to C.D. tattoos
3. Ant. SSD = 86.5

Fig. 9-11 The treatment portion of the patient's chart is used to document the patient's setup parameters. Note institutional differences between **A** (p. 181) (Mayo Clinic in Rochester, MN) and **B** (Central Maine Medical Center in Lewiston, ME). Both provide documentation of pertinent patient data.

lead wire, plaster of Paris, or aquatube to a complex imaging system such as ultrasound or CT scanning. Chapter 10 (Contours) provides a more detailed approach to the definition, purpose, and types of contours used in radiation therapy. In this section, two convenient methods of contouring are discussed: the lead solder and pantograph methods.

Lead solder. The method most widely used may be the lead wire positioned over the patient's skin along one or more transverse axes.[2] The outline of the external surface anatomy of the patient's shape will be documented with the help of the solder wire. Reference marks on the skin are transferred to the wire. This includes the central axis, field

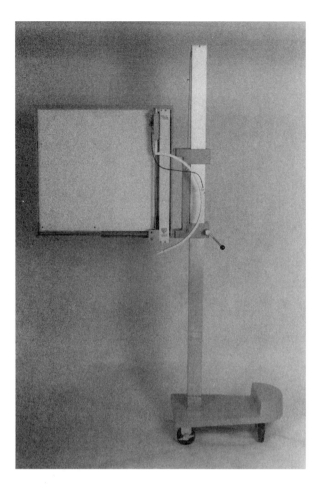

Fig. 9-12 Pantograph contour device. (Courtesy of Radiation Products Design, Inc., Albertsville, MN.)

edges, etc. The contour, along with the reference marks, is transferred to paper where the shape is outlined. Care must be used with this method because any distortion in the patient's shape results in inaccurate dose calculations.

Pantograph. A body pantograph is a more accurate contour technique. The **pantograph** allows a pointer to trace the patient's contour along the transverse plane of the body. It then draws the image on a piece of paper located in a device positioned near the simulator couch (Fig. 9-12). This method is very accurate when contouring smooth surfaces, especially in the abdomen and pelvis. However, some difficulties and inaccuracies may be encountered with this method when the slope changes rapidly, as is common in the head and neck region and the points being plotted are not in close intervals.

Whatever method is used, it cannot be overemphasized to take the time necessary to produce an accurate contour. Often the contour is the last step in the simulation procedure. Accuracy may be compromised by the pressure to hurry and finish because the patient is tired or the schedule is extremely busy.[22,23] Small errors that occur during the simulation and treatment planning process become magnified during the administration of a planned course of treatment.

TREATMENT VERIFICATION

As discussed earlier in the chapter, simulation can have more than one meaning. First, it is a general term describing the mockup process. This can include the selection of immobilization devices, radiographic documentation of treatment ports, measurement of the patient, construction of patient contours, and shaping of fields.[12] For a majority of cases in most institutions, the word "simulation" is applied to this type of procedure. However, it can also refer to a type of treatment verification. This may be a more specific term, where the simulator artificially duplicates the actual treatment conditions by confirming measurements, verifying treatment, and checking custom blocks.[7]

Verification simulation is a final check that each of the planned treatment beams covers the tumor or target volume and does not irradiate critical normal structures.[4] This is usually done as the second part of a two-step process on the simulator. It involves taking radiographs of each of the treatment beams using external marks and other immobilization devices intended for treatment reproducibility. An example might help further explain this idea.

A patient with cancer involving the head of the pancreas might benefit from external beam radiation therapy. Two simulation procedures might be necessary. The first simulation is done to establish a point of reference for the radiation oncologist and treatment planning staff. This is accomplished through orthogonal films. An isocenter is located in the patient and then documented by reference to external landmarks or tattoos. At the end of the first simulation, a target volume has not been established. A field size may not have been selected. Before the second simulation (in this case called treatment verification), additional treatment planning must be done.

Often the patient's tumor volume is drawn on the contour or planned with the aid of a CT or MRI scan with the patient in the treatment position. The information from the CT scan or contour is transferred to the treatment planning computer, where a new isocenter may be determined based on the extent of disease. Usually only a slight shift, if any, from the original isocenter is needed. The second simulation or verification is done as a final check. Does each of the treatment beams cover the target volume? Are any critical structures such as the spinal cord affected? Radiographs of each of the treatment beams using external marks and other immobilization devices are taken to complete the verification process.

Verification of custom blocks is also done on the simulator. This is done to correct block cutting and mounting errors before the patient is treated. Small adjustments to custom blocks are not uncommon. Several potential causes for error exist in the use and fabrication of custom blocks. For example, setting incorrect SFD and source-tray-distance (STD) marks before cutting the blocks or orienting the blocks incorrectly on the tray can result in a misadministration of the treatment. An error of approximately ± 3 mm in the size of the finished blocks can result if either too little or too much tension is applied to the hot cutting wire during the cutting procedure.[8] Johnson and Gerbi describe a three-step block-checking procedure designed to eliminate blocking errors and increase treatment precision. The steps involve (1) a static light check on the simulator using the custom blocks and the original simulation radiograph, (2) a parallel opposed film check to check for block misalignment, and (3) a final block check with the patient on the simulator.[13] Block verification can improve the precision, accuracy, and eventual outcome of the treatment.

Treatment verification, using radiographs (port films) produced in the radiation therapy treatment room, on the first day of treatment provides additional assurance that the correct area is irradiated. Ideally, port films of each treatment are compared with the simulation radiographs before treatment. This may identify mistakes in block fabrication and patient positioning. Greater differences between simulation radiographs and port films as compared to differences between one port film and the next have been documented.[19] Extra time should be scheduled the first day of treatment to evaluate the patient's position and verify the treatment plan. Errors and setup inaccuracies are more common during the transfer of information from the simulator to the treatment unit. This stresses the importance of verification on the first day of treatment.

EMERGENCY PROCEDURES

Any sudden, unexpected situation requiring immediate attention is an emergency. Fortunately the radiation oncology department generally does not experience this often. There are, of course, emergencies where a patient may need immediate treatment because of the sudden onset of symptoms. Examples of this include treatment for spinal cord compression, excessive bleeding, or a life-threatening obstruction caused by the unchecked growth of the tumor. Even in these situations there is some time for planning. The simulation procedure can be discussed and a plan developed for the patient's treatment. This plan may be as simple as several large fractions of radiation to a single field.

There are other situations arising during a simulation procedure that may require immediate attention. Certification in cardiopulmonary resuscitation equips the therapist to respond to specific medical conditions involving an obstructed airway or heart attack. In addition, a "crash cart" should be available. Usually the cart contains specific drugs and equipment needed to respond to certain emergencies, such as cardiac arrest or anaphylactic shock. The most common cause of anaphylactic shock during a simulation procedure is an allergic reaction to the contrast medium.

In any case there should be access to a nearby phone to initiate a response. Many hospitals have specific procedures to initiate a rapid response, such as "code 99" or "code blue." Knowing what to do before an emergency occurs can sometimes make the difference.

The mechanical operations of the simulator equipment can create a potential hazard to the patient and medical personnel. Knowing the location of "emergency off" switches is vital. These switches, which cut the power to the mechanical motions of the gantry and PSA, are generally incorporated into the room design and strategically located on the walls. It is also important to know the location of the main circuit breaker for the simulator. The circuit breaker generally controls power to both the mechanical components and the x-ray generator. Emergency switches are also incorporated into the simulator controls, both in the room and remotely in the shielded control area. An observation window allows the radiation therapist and others involved in the simulation process to view the patient and mechanical motions of the equipment. It is made of thick plate glass or leaded glass and installed in the control area along the wall facing the simulator. Anticollision devices, mounted on the collimator head and image intensifier, may prevent a potential collision by terminating the power and/or sounding an audio alarm. Some simulators are equipped with an integrated computer circuitry that prevents collisions by monitoring each component through a type of internal surveillance. In addition, some simulation rooms are equipped with cameras and monitors similar to those found in the treatment rooms.

The response to any sudden, unexpected situation requiring immediate attention during the simulation procedure should be well thought out in advance. Many potential emergency situations are minimized through careful planning of the procedure and observation of the equipment.

Summary of simulation procedures

Patients treated with radiation therapy, either for cure or for palliation, will be involved in various procedures, including simulation. It helps in figuring out the location and extent of the patient's disease. The simulation process may include presimulation planning, room preparation, patient positioning/immobilization, operation of controls, setting field parameters, radiographic exposure, documenting pertinent data, treatment verification, and emergency procedures.

The outcome of the simulation procedure should define the anatomical area so that it is reproducible for daily treatment. A complicated simulation is of little value unless it is reproducible. This means the ultimate success or failure of treatment may be directly related to the effectiveness of the simulation process.

Achieving ideal results in radiation therapy depends on delivering an appropriate dose to a well-defined region and at the same time reducing the dose to normal critical structures. Accomplishing this task demands a high degree of precision and accuracy in delivering the dose. In addition, a systematic and logical approach to the treatment of the particular disease is necessary. The use of the simulator is essential in achieving this goal.[8]

PRACTICAL APPLICATION/APPLIED TECHNOLOGY

Three areas are presented in the applied technology section.

1. Identification of topographical landmarks. This provides a knowledge base necessary in the clinical application of anatomical landmarks. These may be used to document and position the CA and field edges during a simulation procedure.
2. A case study designed to highlight and summarize some critical components involved in the simulation procedure.
3. A list of questions designed to generate discussion between your peers and to evaluate your knowledge of the subject matter.

Review of anatomical landmarks

A review of anatomical landmarks in the head and neck, thorax, abdomen, and pelvic regions is offered. Anatomical landmarks can be classified into two categories: bony and soft tissue landmarks, many of which are mobile. Anatomical landmarks are helpful when simulating any area.

Head and neck region. Bony landmarks of the head include the superior orbital margin (SOM), which is the roof of the orbit; the inferior orbital margin (IOM), which is a bony landmark that forms the lateral margin of the bony orbit; the external occipital protuberance (EOP), which is the prominence in the occipital bone; the mastoid process, which is the most lateral and inferior extension of the temporal bone; and the zygomatic arch, the bony prominence of the cheek. Table 9-3 identifies common anatomical landmarks of the head and neck region.

When simulating a brain, the inferior margin of the field may be set on the SOM so the entire frontal portion of the brain is included in the treatment portal. The SOM and mastoid process can be palpated to delineate the inferior field border of the treatment portal. When simulating a German helmet treatment portal (C2 whole brain) using bony landmarks, the SOM and zygomatic arch can be palpated to position the inferior border at C2 or the second cervical vertebra.

Bony landmarks of the neck include C1, which lies inferior to the mastoid process; C2, which is located at the level of the angle of the mandible; C3, which lies at the level of the hyoid bone; C4, which corresponds to the level of the thyroid cartilage; C6, which is at the level of the cricoid cartilage; and C7, the first prominent process of the cervical vertebrae.

Other landmarks of the head include the glabella, located between the orbits; the nasion, which is the depression at the base of the nose; the inner canthus (IC), located at the medial aspect of the eye where the upper and lower eyelids meet; the outer canthus (OC), located at the outer aspect of the eye where the upper and lower eyelids meet; the tragus, located near the external auditory meatus; and the commissure of the mouth, which is at the junction of the upper and lower lips. This area is often blocked out of the treatment area to reduce the side effects associated with irradiating this area. It may be marked with a radiopaque marker during simulation as a critical structure.

During a simulation involving the head and neck area, several other landmarks are of benefit. For example, the tragus is often used in the initial stages of simulation for brain or head and neck positioning. The tragus is a stable and symmetrical landmark that can be used with the side lasers to

Table 9-3	Anatomical landmarks of the head and neck region	
Landmark	**Description**
Superior orbital margin (SOM)	The roof of the of the orbit
Inferior orbital margin (IOM)	Forms the lateral margin of the bony orbit
External occipital protuberance (EOP)	The central prominence in the occipital bone
Mastoid process	The most lateral and inferior extension of the temporal bone
Zygomatic arch	The bony prominence of the cheek
Glabella	Located between the orbits
Nasion	The depression at the base of the nose
Inner canthus (IC)	Located at the medial aspect of the eye where the upper and lower eyelids meet
Outer canthus (OC)	Located at the outer aspect of the eye where the upper and lower eyelids meet
Tragus	Located near the external auditory meatus
Commissure of the mouth	Located at the junction of the upper and lower lip
C1	Lies inferior to the mastoid process
C2	Located at the level of the angle of the mandible
C3	Lies at the level of the hyoid bone
C4	Corresponds to the level of the thyroid cartilage
C6	Located at the level of the cricoid cartilage
C7	The first prominent process of the cervical vertebrae
Sternocleidomastoid muscle	A thick band of muscle in the neck, originating at the level of sternum and clavicle and inserting at the mastoid process of the temporal bone

check for rotation of the head. During a brain simulation the outer canthus and tragus can also delineate the inferior margin of the treatment portal.

The most notable landmark of the neck is the sternocleidomastoid muscle. This muscle is often palpated when simulating a supraclavicular portal during a breast simulation. This muscle is associated with many lymph nodes and can be palpated daily during radiation treatments to verify the position of the treatment field.

A therapist may benefit from relating soft tissue landmarks with bony landmarks during the planning process of the simulation procedure. For example, when simulating a true vocal cord lesion, the therapist may begin positioning the patient using soft tissue landmarks and check the final setup concerning bony landmarks. To reduce rotation and initially position the patient's head, each side laser and the tragus may be matched. Palpation of the thyroid cartilage (Adam's apple) will help position the superior field border. The therapist may then palpate the cricoid cartilage and place the inferior border just below this landmark. Once the field is established clinically, a check of the field placement using fluoroscopy can be performed. The superior field border should be at C4 and the inferior border at C6 to simulate this tumor of the larynx. Relating landmarks in reference to the patient's anatomy is very helpful in the simulation process, especially in the head and neck region.

Thoracic region. The principal bony landmarks used in simulating the thoracic region are the suprasternal notch, xiphoid, ribs, and clavicle. Aligning the suprasternal notch and tip of the xiphoid is useful in straightening the patient on the simulation table before the procedure begins. The thoracic vertebral column is itself a useful tool in straightening the patient. Bony landmarks in the thoracic region are sometimes used to delineate treatment borders when simulating a breast. A few examples may prove helpful.

When simulating a lung lesion, the hilar nodes often must be included in the treatment portal. The carina, located at T5, is a major anatomical landmark used in simulation. The hilar nodes are close to the carina. Therefore if the carina is in the treatment field, the hilar nodes are in the treatment field. This holds true for an A/P portal or an oblique off cord portal approach.

Pelvic region. Bony landmarks used in the pelvic region include the lumbar vertebrae, pelvic inlet, obturator foramen, ischial tuberosities, pubis symphysis, and ASIS. During a simulation involving the prostate the xiphoid and pubis are palpated along the overhead lasers to straighten the patient. The therapist will relate the topographical anatomy to the fluoroscopic images. Sometimes the lumbar spine and pubis symphysis are also used to ensure the patient is straight. Again the therapist will relate topographical and radiographic anatomy to patient positioning. Other landmarks of the pelvic region include the umbilicus, base of the penis, labia, and groin fold.

Case study–squamous cell carcinoma (superior sulcus tumor)

A 65-year-old white male came to his family physician with complaints of pain radiating from his shoulder region, including the neck and down his left forearm. He thought he was having a heart attack or had some medical problem concerning his cardiovascular system. After preliminary medical examinations, a chest radiograph revealed a tumor in the right apex of the lung. After bronchoscopy and sputum cytology a diagnosis of squamous cell carcinoma of the lung was made. A tumor located in the apex of the lung is considered a superior sulcus carcinoma, sometimes referred to as a Pancoast tumor. The patient was staged as T2 N1 M0. The tumor was confined to the chest with metastasis to the ipsilateral hilar lymph nodes. No distant metastases were documented.

It was recommended that the patient receive radiation therapy to a dose of 4500 cGy in 5 weeks, followed by a boost of 2000 cGy. The patient was scheduled for consultation with the radiation oncologist the following day and was told he would start his treatments within 3 days.

Through the application of the case study above, many of the major points in the chapter are reviewed. We will walk through the simulation process applied to this patient from room preparation to the documentation of pertinent data. If possible, the nurse or doctor should introduce you to the patient rather than have you just pop up in the examination or waiting room without prior notice. This can be overwhelming for some patients. Ask the patient if the nurse or doctor has spoken to him and if he or family members have any questions. Check for his understanding before you take the patient into the simulation room by asking open-ended questions, which require the patient to reply with something other than a "yes" or "no."

Room preparation. Before bringing the patient to the simulator, make sure you have properly prepared the room for the procedure. For a lung patient you will set the appropriate SAD on the simulator. The table should be lowered to its lowest point. A head rest (B or C) can be used, depending on the amount of chin elevation needed for the procedure and patient comfort. A clean linen sheet or clean sheet of paper should be on the simulation table. The gantry, floor, and collimator angles should all be preset to 0°. If a spinal cord calculation is required, decide beforehand which method the physician would like to use to calculate the amount of radiation the spinal cord will be receiving. For example, it might be possible to use a cross-table lateral radiograph, Clarkson point calculation, or CT information may be used. A Clarkson calculation will be used for this example.

Explanation of the procedure. If you can, bring the patient's friend or relative along with the patient into the simulator. Reiterate to both the procedure you are going to perform and how long it will take (usually a simulation takes 30 to 90 minutes, depending on the complexity). In this case, it should be about 1 hour (because additional time is necessary beyond the actual simulation procedure to gather the data for a Clarkson point calculation). Explain to the patient that he will be alone while in the simulator whenever a radiation exposure is made. This includes radiographs and fluoroscopy. Talk to the patient and try to put him at ease. Answer any questions he might have and explain to him that this is not a radiation treatment but part of the treatment planning process. Direct the friend or relative back to the waiting room.

Patient positioning and immobilization. Assist the patient to the table and offer any assistance while the patient is in the process of lying down. Cover the patient with a sheet over his abdomen, leaving the chest visible. Make sure the patient is secure and comfortable on the table. Place an angled sponge under his knees for comfort. Have him place his hands at his side if possible; sometimes the patient is too wide and the hands cannot fit on the table. The patient may also feel more comfortable with the hands clasped together resting on the abdomen and elbows resting on the table top for support. If not, the patient is more liable to move during the simulation. Also, you may consider using a medium-sized round rubber ring. The patient will hold onto the ring during the procedure. The ring can make a patient feel more comfortable because he is given a task to perform during simulation. After the patient has been positioned and straightened on the table, position the table height and direction slowly and smoothly.

Operation of simulator controls. Use the sagittal laser to ensure the patient is straight, aligning the midline facial structures, suprasternal notch, xiphoid, and pubic bone, and have the laser fall between the patient's feet. Even though the patient appears straight, you can double-check the patient's anatomy (vertebral bodies are a good starting point) using fluoroscopy. Fluoroscopy contributes a very small dose to the patient compared to that received from the treatment.

Turn the field light on and begin to set the field to a preliminary area (place the inferior border at the xiphoid). Tell the patient you are going to leave the simulation room, but you will be in the viewing area visible through the glass window (some come equipped with video monitors, much like those in the treatment room). Begin at the patient's head area and perform fluoroscopy as far inferior as possible, making sure the patient is straight. If the image is not very clear, try closing the diaphragms to within a few centimeters of the anatomy you are interested in observing. Reducing the image intensifier distance also helps improve image detail. As you do the fluoroscopy, make adjustments along the way, positioning the patient as straight as possible.

Setting field parameters. There are several methods of positioning the isocenter in or on the patient. A preliminary

field size is now established, and the treatment distance has been set by positioning the side lasers to fall on the chest surface, indicating 100 SSD. The patient's IFD or separation is measured using calipers. Explain to the patient you will be placing a measuring device under his back but ask him not to raise up and not to offer any assistance during the measurement. You have double-checked all of your measurements. Lock the table longitudinally, laterally, and up and down to ensure it is not moved inadvertently.

In attempting to establish the treatment volume, several landmarks are used, such as the carina, clavicles, hilar area, and vertebral column. As you do fluoroscopy, again check and make sure the patient is straight. You can see the carina (bifurcation of the trachea into the two main stem bronchi) as you follow the darker density from the trachea (air in the trachea is black), usually at T5. Count two vertebral bodies inferiorly from the carina (T7), and place the inferior border between vertebral bodies T7 and T8.

Next, both supraclavicular areas must be included in the treatment field. The acromion processes of the scapula can be palpated and the lateral borders placed near this area; the superior border can be placed between vertebral bodies C4 and C5. Now that the field parameters are established, double-check the isocenter depth again because the central axis may have shifted while you were setting the field parameters. This is important in the chest area, where there is a considerable slope in the inferior/superior direction. Fig. 9-13 illustrates the field borders and blocking used to treat this patient through both anterior and posterior fields.

Radiographic exposure. Prepare to make an exposure. First, document the field on the patient's skin. If a standard SFD measurement is not used during most simulation procedures, raise the intensifier as close as possible to the simulator table, which also decreases field magnification. Make sure the intensifier is turned in the correct direction to make an exposure. Some simulators require the intensifier to be in the longitudinal position before an exposure can be made. Place a positional marker ("ANT" and "RT" in this case, identifying the anteroposterior beam direction and the patient's right) on the patient or image intensifier. Determine the correct exposure from the patient's separation. Some simulators have an automatic photographic timing system that takes all the guessing out of setting the exposure time. After the exposure is taken, remove the cassette from the film holder and proceed to the developer. Stamp the film with the patient's identification card, listing the name, hospital number, physician, and date of the simulation. While the film is developing, record all of the patient's parameters on the simulation work sheet or retrieve the proper printout from the computer interfaced with the simulator. The pertinent information may include the SAD, SSD, SFD, field size, collimator angle, gantry angle, floor angle, table top measurement, table height, field orientation, AP/PA, RT/LT, separation, measurements at Clarkson points, and anatomical patient's position.

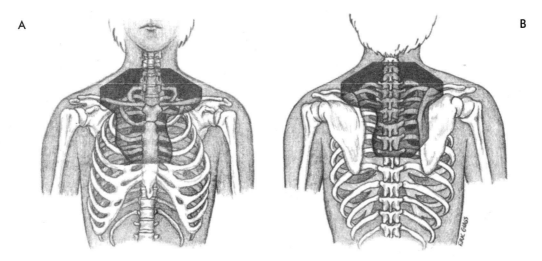

Fig. 9-13 Treatment fields (*shaded area*) used to treat a patient with a superior sulcus tumor include both anterior (**A**) and posterior (**B**) portals.

Documenting pertinent data. Once the simulation information and Clarkson measurements are recorded, evaluate the radiograph. Check the radiograph to make sure that the target volume is incorporated in the treatment field and an appropriate exposure technique was used (density/contrast). Verify the radiograph with the radiation oncologist.

Some institutions use tattoos to indicate the treatment volume and others reference anatomical landmarks. In this case, only the central axis and where the central axis intersects with the inferior border will be tattooed. Take photographs of the patient's position and the treatment area. Some institutions also take photographs of the simulation radiograph. Record the patient's position and any information pertinent to the setup (angled sponge under the knees, the distance from the suprasternal notch to the tip of the patient's chin). This measurement elevates the patient's chin in a consistent manner throughout the treatment. Before the simulation is completed, make sure the patient's name, hospital identification number, date, and physician's name are recorded on the simulation sheet, radiograph, and all of the photographs.

Final procedures. Explain the importance of skin care to the patient. Assist the patient while raising him to the sitting position. Usually the patient has been lying down from 30 to 60 minutes and may feel dizzy as he moves from the supine to the sitting position. Assist the patient to a wheelchair. Decide on an appointment time, and, if possible, introduce the patient to the therapists who will be treating him. If possible, show him the linear accelerator and explain what he should expect during his treatments. Again, ask the patient if he has any questions or if there is anything he needs before he goes back to his room. Pamphlets, brochures, and other important treatment-related information can also be given to the patient to read before his first treatment.

Make sure all appropriate documentation is finalized in the chart. Make any copies of previous radiographs or CT scans needed to complete the patient's records. Take the chart and radiographs to dosimetry. Log the chart, indicating whether Cerrobend blocks need to be constructed. In some institutions the therapist is responsible for constructing the Cerrobend blocks as well as filling out the chart and preparing all of the information required before the patient's first treatment.

Review Questions

True or False

1. Isocentric refers to placing the isocenter midline and mid-depth in the patient's anatomy.
   True _____ False _____
2. The geometric arrangement of the target and patient during the simulation must be identical to that of the treatment to ensure an accurate treatment delivery.
   True _____ False _____

Multiple Choice

3. A patient's separation = 25 cm. If the posterior SSD = 89 cm, what will the anterior SSD measure be?
   a. 87.5 cm
   b. 89 cm
   c. 88.25 cm
   d. 86 cm
4. Mr. Carson has metastatic cancer originating from the prostate. He has been coming to the radiation oncology department for months and is about to be simulated for the third time. Before you bring him into the room Mr. Carson says, "I don't know why I am here today. These treatments are not doing any good. This is my third time back to see you." Your best response would be:
   a. "Now, now, Mr. Carson. You know these treatments will make you feel better."
   b. "Once you start the treatments you will feel better—just wait and see."
   c. "It seems you feel discouraged because these treatments are not working, Mr. Carson."
   d. "Now, what do you expect, Mr. Carson? You do have metastatic disease."
5. The treatment volume will contain:
   a. Tumor
   b. Involved lymphatics
   c. Normal tissue
   d. All of the above

6. _____ is the initial phase of treatment planning where actual visualization of the treatment volume is documented before treatment.
   a. Initial consultation
   b. Simulation
   c. Brachytherapy
   d. Radiation treatment
7. The distance from a source of radiation to a radiograph is:
   a. SAD
   b. SFD
   c. SSD
   d. All of the above
8. The distance from a source of radiation to the patient's skin is:
   a. SAD
   b. SSD
   c. SDD
   d. SFD
9. Traits of a therapeutic listener are:
   a. Desire to listen, respond, and solve the patient's problems
   b. Partially listen so you can prepare your response ahead of time
   c. Listen while you work as quickly as possible, so you do not fall behind schedule
   d. All of the above
10. When simulating the chest, which major landmark(s) can be used to straighten the patient?
    a. Suprasternal notch
    b. Xiphoid
    c. Vertebrae
    d. All of the above

Questions to Ponder

1. Discuss the importance of the presimulation consultation between radiation team members.
2. Explain the differences between target, treatment, and irradiated volume.
3. While in the middle of a simulation the SAD is inadvertently changed from 100 cm to 110 cm. Will the size field change? If so, how can the simulation therapist detect this change?
4. Discuss several ways you can check a patient's separation and SSDs while simulating the patient.
5. Write out an appropriate explanation for a patient about to have a simulation for lung cancer.
6. Describe at least six treatment parameters documented during a simulation procedure and discuss their importance.

REFERENCES

1. American Registry of Radiologic Technologists: *Conventions specific to the radiation therapy technology examination.* St Paul, MN, 1995.
2. Bentel GC: *Radiation therapy planning.* New York, 1993, McGraw-Hill.
3. Bental GC, Nelson CE, Noell T: *Treatment planning and dose calculation in radiation oncology.* New York, 1989, Pergamon Press.
4. Bleehen NM, Glatstein E, Haybittle JL: *Radiation therapy planning.* New York, 1983, Marcel Dekker.
5. Bomford CK et al: Treatment simulators. *Br J Radiol*(Suppl 23) 17-22, 1989.
6. Carlton RR, McKenna-Adler A: *Principles of radiographic imaging.* Albany, NY, 1992, Delmar Publisher.
7. Dyk JV, Mah K: Simulators and CT scanners in radiotherapy physics in practice. In Williams JR, Thwaites, editors: *Radiotherapy physics in practice.* Oxford, 1993, Oxford University Press, pp 113-134.
8. Gerbi B: Use of the simulator in treatment planning and determination and definition of treatment volume. In Levitt SH, Khan FM, Potish, RA, editors: *Levitt and Tapley's technological basis of radiation therapy: Practical clinical application,* ed 2. Philadelphia, 1992, Lea & Febiger.
9. Goitein M: Applications of computed tomography in radiotherapy treatment planning. In Orton CG, editor: *Progress in medical radiation physics.* New York, 1982, Plenum.
10. Hendrickson FR: Precision in radiation oncology. *Int J Radiat Oncol Biol Phys* 8:311-312, 1982.
11. International Commission on Radiation Units and Measurements: Dose specification of reporting external beam therapy with photons and electrons (Report 29). Washington, DC, 1978, ICRU.
12. Inter-Society Council for Radiation Oncology: *Radiation oncology in integrated cancer management.* Philadelphia, 1991, American College of Radiology.
13. Johnson JM, Gerbi BJ: Quality control of custom block-making in radiation therapy. *Med Dosimetry* 14:199, 1989.
14. Karzmark CJ, Nunan CS, Tanabe E: *Medical linear accelerators.* New York, 1993, McGraw-Hill.
15. Keller R: Imobilization devices. In Washington CM, Leaver DT, editors: *Principles and practice of radiation therapy.* St Louis, 1996, Mosby.
16. Khan FM: *The physics of radiation therapy,* ed 2. Baltimore, 1994, Williams & Wilkins.
17. Manolis J: Personal communication. St Louis, 1994, The Mallinckrodt Institute of Radiology, Washington University School of Medicine.
18. Mizer S, Scheller RR, Deye JA: Radiation therapy simulation workbook. New York, 1986, Pergamon.
19. Perez CA, Brady LW: *Principles and practice of radiation oncology,* ed 2. Philadelphia, 1992, Lippincott.
20. Purtilo R: *Ethical dimensions in the health professions.* Philadelphia, 1981, WB Saunders.
21. Rabinowitz I et al: Accuracy of radiation field alignment in clinical practice. *Int J Radiat Bio Phys* 11:1857, 1985.
22. Rathe JC, Elliott P: *Radiographic tumor localization.* St Louis, 1982, Warren H Green.
23. Torres LS: *Basic medical techniques and patient care for radiologic technologists,* ed 4. Philadelphia, 1993, Lippincott.
24. Washington CM, Taylor F: Contours. In Washington CM, Leaver DT, editors: *Principles and practice of radiation therapy.* St Louis, 1996, Mosby.

Dosimetry and Treatment Planning

CHAPTER

10

Contours

Charles M. Washington
Frances Taylor

Outline

Contouring rationale
Types of contours
Identification of internal critical
  structures
Contouring materials
  Hand-molded materials
  Pantograph contouring device
  Image-related methods

Applied technology
  Mechanics of hand-molded
    contour production

Key terms

Air gap
Contour
Coronal contour
Critical structure
Demagnification
Exothermic reaction

Off-axis contour
Orthogonal radiographs
Plaster strips
Sagittal contour
Solder wire

 Treatment planning in radiation therapy requires accurate representation of the anatomy to be treated. The shape of the human form has a definite impact on this dimension of treatment planning. There are many different ways to gather this information for use in accurately localizing and treating a tumor volume. This chapter will specifically describe the process of taking physical contour measurements of the body for use with treatment planning procedures. Types of patient contouring devices and procedures will be presented to assist in understanding the importance of relating tumor location to anatomical structure and treatment geometry.

CONTOURING RATIONALE

A **contour** is a reproduction of an external body shape, usually taken through the transverse plane of the central axis of the treatment beam (or center of the treatment volume).[3,5,8] Contours may be taken through other planes of interest in the treatment volume to provide more information about the overall dose distribution. A contour is usually taken at the end of the simulation and treatment planning procedure when the treatment volume has been defined and verified with x-ray films and setup or alignment marks have been placed on the patient.

The purpose of a contour is to provide the therapist and dosimetrist with the most precise replica of the patient's body shape so that accurate information may be gathered concerning the dose distribution within the patient. The treatment volume and internal structures (tumor volume, critical organs) are transposed within the contour using data from the

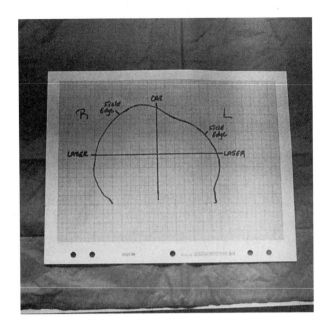

Fig. 10-1 Typical patient contour taken through mechanical means. Note the common points of interest that are labeled for accurate use.

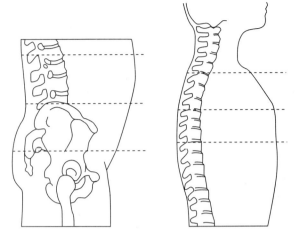

Fig. 10-2 Examples of sites where off-axis contours are typically taken. Contours at different levels through the body provide information that is essential in treatment planning.

simulation films and/or computed tomography (CT) or magnetic resonance imaging (MRI) films. Fig. 10-1 shows a typical patient contour taken with a conventional technique. The representation provides information essential to accurate treatment planning. At that point, isodose distributions from all treatment beams may be superimposed over the contour and summarized to produce the treatment plan.

Another purpose of a contour is to assist in repositioning the patient. A therapist or dosimetrist can check the location of field edges and treatment marks, the central axis location, and separations at a glance. It is important to realize, though, that the information will only be as accurate as the data recorded.[9]

Production of an accurate contour takes time. Often the contour is the last step in the simulation procedure, and accuracy may be compromised by the pressure to hurry and finish as a result of patient physical or department schedule concerns. If a contour is inaccurate, adequate treatment planning may be compromised. The setup distances may not correspond to the actual treatment distances encountered during patient positioning. This could translate into taking the patient back to simulation for a new contour, which in turn would require a new treatment plan and possibly a delay in the delivery of treatment.

TYPES OF CONTOURS

The most common type of contour is usually taken through one transverse plane of the body through the central axis of the beam, typically within the treatment volume.[3,8,9] This type of contour runs across the patient, from left to right, and sections the patient into the upper and lower halves. The planes of the body are shown in Fig. 9-5. In treating an area

with few variances in topography, it is reasonable to view the dose distribution through only one plane. However, when the patient's contour within the treatment volume varies more than a few centimeters, the dose distribution will not be the same as calculated through the central axis transverse contour. In this case, off-axis contours should be taken to verify the dose distribution in these areas. An **off-axis contour** is any contour parallel to the central axis transverse plane, in the inferior or superior directions. Fig. 10-2 demonstrates examples of sites where off-axis contours should be taken in the treatment of the chest (through anterior, posterior, or oblique fields) and in the treatment of the pelvis of an obese patient (through anterior and posterior fields).[3]

Another site where the patient contour varies considerably is in the head and neck area. This is true for both the transverse and the coronal planes. The lateral diameter of the patient's neck may differ significantly in the superior and inferior regions of the lateral treatment volume, as demonstrated in Fig. 10-3. When treating the head and neck with anterior/posterior (A/P) fields, the A/P diameter varies significantly from the superior to the inferior region of the treatment volume. Fig. 10-4 demonstrates this.

A **coronal contour** is one taken along the coronal plane of the body, cutting the patient in half from front to back. It is most likely to be used when parallel opposed beams enter the patient laterally or when a beam enters through the vertex of the head (Fig. 10-5). A coronal contour must include both the left and right sides of the body or it will not provide enough information to be useful.

A **sagittal contour** is taken along the median sagittal plane of the body, cutting the body into left and right halves, and is useful when there is a need to verify the dose distribution along the length of the body. Examples of sites where a sagittal contour may be useful are in A/P treatment of the

A

B

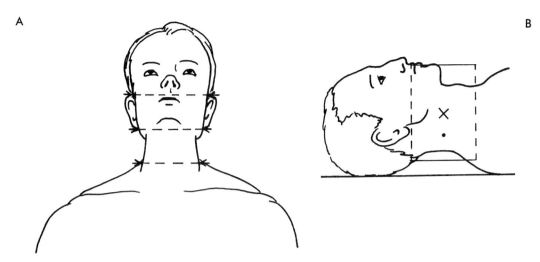

Fig. 10-3 A, Lateral diameter of patient's neck is significantly different in superior, central, and inferior regions of **B** the lateral treatment volume.

A

B

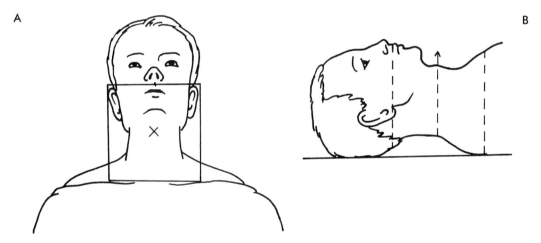

Fig. 10-4 A, Anterior/Posterior head and neck fields. **B,** Difference in anterior/posterior diameter within superior, central, and inferior regions of treatment volume.

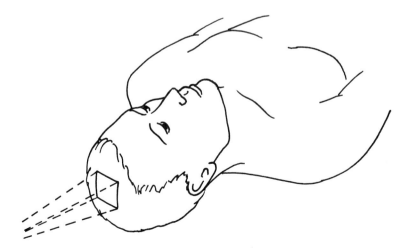

Fig. 10-5 Coronal contour taken along lateral aspect of the body and through vertex of the head.

A

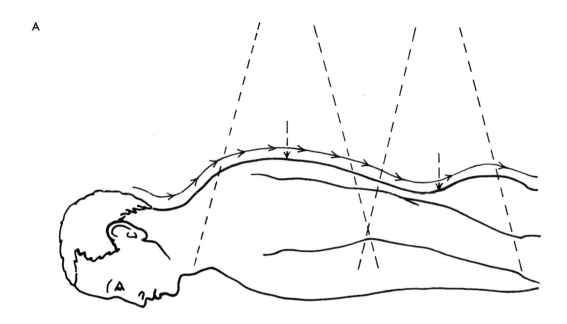

B

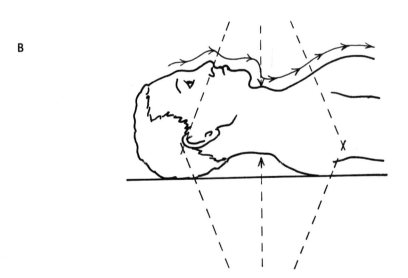

Fig. 10-6 A, Shows where a sagittal contour should be taken for posterior spinal axis fields. **B,** Identifies where a sagittal contour should be taken for anterior/posterior neck fields.

head and neck and in the posterior spinal axis, as shown in Fig. 10-6. Additional measurements are needed to complete the anterior to posterior part of the contour.

It is evident that various contours can provide much needed information to the radiation therapy practitioner. Body topography must be taken into account when planning a patient's treatment regimen.[5]

IDENTIFICATION OF INTERNAL CRITICAL STRUCTURES

A **critical structure** is any body structure that has a radiation tolerance limiting the total dose that can be administered to the treatment volume. Examples of critical structures that are commonly monitored in treatment planning are the eyes, kidneys, spinal cord, lungs, and rectum. These structures should be represented within the contour, along with the tumor volume, to assist in planning the optimum treatment for the patient.

To locate the internal structures and tumor volume, several different methods may be used. These methods include transverse tomography, CT, MRI, and ultrasound. The CT scan is the most accessible and accurate of the localization methods. Use of CT scans in treatment planning is an established procedure in most departments.[6]

The simulator is also an important therapy apparatus that can serve to identify internal anatomical structures. By introducing contrast material or radiopaque materials into the patient and taking **orthogonal radiographs** (two perpendicular radiographs) of the treatment volume, critical structures can be identified within and around the treatment volume.

To transfer critical internal structures within the contour, three-dimensional localization is necessary. Orthogonal radiographs can provide adequate information for "three-dimensional" localization through perpendicular images that are actually two-dimensional.[3] The typical arrangement of orthogonal films is an anterior and lateral film (90° apart) with a common isocentric point within the patient. Radiopaque markers are placed on the anterior and posterior skin surface to accurately delineate the patient's skin surfaces on the lateral film. **Demagnification**, the process of mathematically correcting for image size distortion resulting from divergence and distance, of the structure from the film is required before it can be outlined within the contour. The "width," or right-to-left dimensions of the structure, will be obtained from the anterior film. The "depth," or anterior-to-posterior dimensions of the structure, will be obtained from the lateral film. The "length," or cephalad-to-caudad dimension of the structure, is provided by both the anterior and lateral films but is not able to be visualized on the contour, since the contour represents only one plane (usually transverse) drawn in two dimensions.

A few examples of critical internal structures that can be identified from orthogonal simulator films and transferred to a contour are noted in Table 10-1.

| Table 10-1 | Critical structures commonly noted on contours |

Critical structure	Dose tolerance (cGy)
Kidney	2000
Lens of the eye	500
Spinal cord	4500

The kidney, with a minimum tolerance dose (TD 5/5) of 2000 cGy, is a critical internal structure in the abdomen that should be localized using an intravenous pyelogram (IVP) during the simulation procedure.[3] The radiation oncologist will be able to accurately shape the field to block out as much of the kidney as possible, using the orthogonal films. The lens of the eye is another critical internal structure, with a TD 5/5 of 500 cGy, that should be located so the radiation oncologist and dosimetrist can monitor the dose it receives.[3] A radiopaque marker can be placed on the surface of the eyelid to assist in identifying the most anterior aspect of the eye on the lateral film. As a general rule of thumb, by looking at the lateral orthogonal film, the anterior portion of the lens is located 3.0 mm posterior to the lid surface, and the posterior portion of the lens is 9.0 mm posterior to the lid surface. From the midpoint of the bony orbit on the anterior film, the width is approximately 1 cm, 0.5 cm on either side of the midpoint. The lens drawn within the contour will measure approximately 0.6 cm deep and 1 cm wide in an oval shape. The spinal cord, another important critical internal structure with a TD 5/5 of 4500 cGy, lies just posterior to the midpoint of the vertebral bodies and is about 1 cm in diameter. By locating the vertebral body from the orthogonal films the spinal cord can be placed within the contour. Fig. 10-8 demonstrates a lateral orthogonal film with the spinal cord sketched in.

It is sometimes helpful to transfer the position of structures within the contour that do not lie exactly within the plane of the contour. It is usually reasonable to view the dose distribution through only one plane because of minor variances between other transverse planes parallel to the central axis plane. However, this does not hold true if the contour is very irregular. It is extremely important to remember that the contour is representing only one thin "slice" of the patient's body.[3] Therefore, when transferring structure positions onto the contour that are located above or below the plane of the contour, it must be stated where the structure is located in relationship to the plane of the contour (e.g., the vertebral body is located 2 cm cephalad to the central axis plane).

CONTOURING MATERIALS

Many different devices and materials can be used to produce a patient contour. While most are commercially available, an institutional machine shop can fabricate tailor-made devices. Contouring materials and devices can be grouped into hand molded, mechanical, and image related. The use of the simulator machine will also be discussed as a means of obtaining a contour. Most radiation therapy departments have preferences regarding the one or two contouring methods that fit their needs and will adhere to those methods for consistency.

Hand-molded materials

Solder wire is probably the most commonly used type of contouring material and is suitable for all body sites. It is inexpensive and readily available. Solder comes in various thicknesses; the thinner variety is more useful in the head and neck regions, while the thicker wire works well in areas that have large separations.

The advantages of using solder wire in contouring include the ability to cut it to any size needed, its pliability, and its reuse capacity. The major disadvantage is its pliability, which means the shape can be easily distorted. Extreme care must be taken when removing the molded solder wire from the patient so as to retain the exact shape. Sometimes it is difficult to mold the thicker solder wire around structures like the nose, lips, eyes, and ears. A slight amount of pressure must be applied when molding the solder wire, which can cause some patient discomfort and distortion. The box below notes points of interest that may be useful to the practitioner using this medium.

A **plaster strip** is another common contouring material that can be used in any body site. These are the same type of strips used to make plaster immobilization devices. When determining the length of plaster strip to use, enough material should be used to span from the table top on one side of the patient to that on the other. Plaster strips work best when folded to approximately 2.5 cm wide and 6 to 8 layers thick. Although this thickness makes molding more difficult, the contour's shape will be easily retained. Use of

hot water reduces the plaster drying time. Caution should be exercised so that the water temperature does not cause undue patient discomfort. As the plaster dries, it will give off some heat of its own. This is called an **exothermic reaction**, and patients should be made aware of this before contouring. Also, if the strip is to be made over any body hair, a layer of plastic wrap should cover the hair to avoid epilation on removal.[1] Fig. 10-7 demonstrates a contour being taken using a plaster strip.

Plaster is fairly inexpensive and is very easy to apply; very little pressure is needed to form an accurate shape. It is good for areas where there is a lot of detail, and it retains its shape very well. If the points on the patient have been marked with a dark ink, the marks will usually transpose right onto the plaster with very little distortion. This eliminates one step in the general process, that of having to

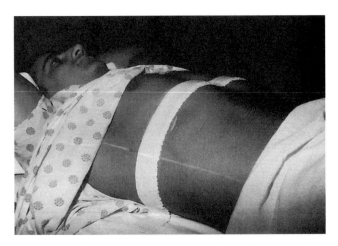

Fig. 10-7 Contour being taken using a plaster strip.

Contouring with Solder Wire: Points to Remember

- The solder wire end may be rounded by holding a match under it for a few seconds after being measured out and before patient use. This lowers the opportunity to accidentally stick the patient.

- An "R" and an "L" can be formed onto the ends of the wire to aid in remembering the corresponding side of the patient.

- The solder wire should be cleaned with alcohol between uses. This eliminates confusion with old marks and achieves asepsis.

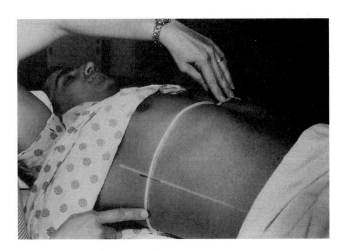

Fig. 10-8 Contour being taken using a thermoplastic tube.

remember to transpose the points onto the contour material. There are a few disadvantages when using plaster strip contouring. It can be messy. It also requires substantial drying time before it can be removed from the patient. While there are fast-setting plaster strips with a drying time of 2 to 4 minutes, because of the thickness required of the strip it usually takes at least 5 to 6 minutes to dry adequately. If a patient is very uncomfortable or tired, this might not be the best method to use. It is also difficult to get an accurate contour around an area with a lot of hair.[1]

W.R. Aquaplast makes inexpensive 4.8 mm diameter Contour Tubes in 3-foot lengths that can be used in most sites of the body. The tubes are hollow and made of a low-temperature thermoplastic that molds very easily. The shape of the contour is maintained very well, and the material can be used several times by reheating. Fig. 10-8 demonstrates a contour being taken with a thermoplastic tube. There are some disadvantages when using this product. It requires proper facilities for heating the water to the proper temperature (160°) to make the tube pliable. The drying time of 2 to 5 minutes is similar to that for the plaster strip method. While it is pliable, it is not quite pliable enough for very detailed areas, such as the ears, nose, lips, and eyes. There is also some shrinkage as the material hardens, which may produce contour inaccuracies.

Mechanical contouring device

While there are many different types of mechanical devices used for contouring, two types are commonly used.

The most widely used and most accurate mechanical contouring device is the pantograph contour plotter. The physical contour of the patient is traced with a stylus, and the device transfers the body's transverse contour to an overhead drawing board by way of a pen attached to the arm of the stylus. There are several types of pantographs available; some can be mounted to a wall, and some are mounted on a rolling stand as shown in Fig. 10-9. These devices save a lot of time in that the contour is immediately transferred to the paper and only one person is required to use the device to obtain an accurate contour. Pantographs can be very good for tracing detailed areas of the body, such as the ears, nose, lips, and eyes (as long as the plotted points are close together). A major disadvantage is the cost of these devices. Also, they tend to be bulky and require adequate room for storage when not in use. Occasionally the lines may not be accurate if the patient is ticklish and moves while the therapist is tracing the stylus over the body.[3]

The second type of mechanical device consists of an array of low-friction nylon or aluminum rods, the tips of which are pulled down to touch the patient's skin surface in a 180 degree cross-section, as shown in Fig. 10-10. The rods are locked into place, removed and placed on a sheet of paper where the shape of the patient is traced. It is fairly easy to use devices of this type for any transverse contour site, and requires only one person to operate. One disadvantage is that the size of the area to be contoured is limited by the size of the device. Also, these devices tend to be large and bulky, which could cause concern if used with an uncooperative patient. Translation of the information is also time consuming.

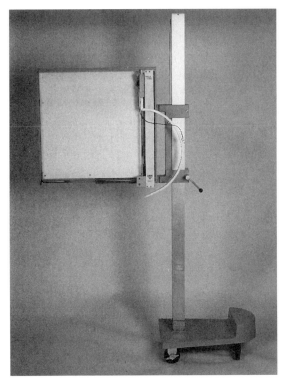

Fig. 10-9 Pantograph contouring device on a rolling stand. (Courtesy of Radiation Products Design, Inc., Albertville, MN.)

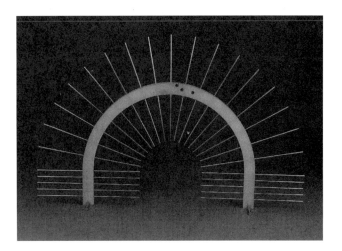

Fig. 10-10 An example of a mechanical contour maker. The tips of the rods touch the skin surface and are locked in place to give a rendering of the patient's contour. (Courtesy of Radiation Products Design, Inc., Albertville, MN.)

Table 10-2	Advantages and disadvantages of contouring materials/methods		
Material/Method	**Advantage**	**Disadvantage**	
Solder wire	Reusability, pliability	Pliability (distortions)	
Plaster strips	Inexpensive, transferability of surface ink markings	Drying time, messy, not reusable	
Aquaplast contour tubes	Inexpensive, reusable, shapes well	Drying time, not well-suited for intricate areas	
Pantograph contouring device	Time-saving operation, reproduces detail well	Cost, size, storage space required	
CT	Accurate transverse views	Cost of interface	
MRI	Accurate transverse, coronal, and sagittal contours	Cost of interface	
Ultrasound	Discernible transverse correlation of internal structures	Poor quality of imaged deep structures	

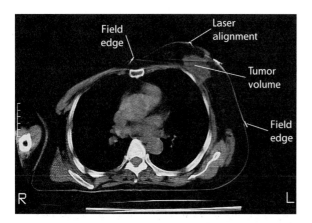

Fig. 10-11 CT slice used for treatment planning. Note how the radiopaque markers on this breast patient show up. This provides useful information for the treatment planning team (tumor volume is marked).

Image-related methods

The first application of computers in medicine was in radiation therapy rotational treatment. Since then a wide variety of computer programs have been developed, taking advantage of the computer technology and applying it to all aspects of radiation therapy.[2,9] The ability to visualize the internal organs of the body in relation to surface anatomy affords the radiation therapy practitioner the knowledge necessary to maximize doses to the tumor volume while sparing normal tissues. The image-related methods of contouring include the use of CT, MRI, and ultrasound.

With CT, patient contour and other anatomy are reduced to numerical coordinates using electromechanical devices for converting pen position to electrical signals recognized by the computer.[9] Thus CT accurately provides transverse anatomical contours. The advantage of the CT scan for generating contours is that the contour is immediately available in suitable form for input to the treatment planning computer. A separate digitizing procedure for the outline is not necessary. CT-generated contours are probably the most accurate of all transverse contouring methods,

since there is no hand molding or manipulation to introduce significant error. An important point to note is that the patient must be in the exact treatment position on the scanner with a flat table top comparable to the simulator and treatment tables. Since most scanners have concave table tops, a flat surface insert must be used.[9] Also, a large-diameter CT aperture should be used to allow patient positioning in the CT scanner that exactly matches simulation and treatment. Patient immobilization devices should be used that will not cause image artifacts.[6] Sometimes the total contour of the patient is missing from the field of view, especially on large patients, which would cause errors in the accuracy of the information. The external alignment marks on the patient should be marked with plastic, radiopaque catheters so they can be delineated on the CT scan for reference (Fig. 10-11). A disadvantage may be the cost of the interfacing computer software necessary for linking CT images to computer hardware.

MRI has versatility in producing contours in transverse, sagittal, and coronal planes. The same considerations for contouring should be followed as outlined for CT scanning.

Ultrasound imaging for delineating patient contours has been widely used in radiation therapy, although the image quality is not as good as CT. Deeply seated anatomical structures are not as easily defined as in CT and MRI. This being the case, the advantage of visualizing intricate anatomical detail is lost in the process.

Many different materials and devices are used in the production of contours, each having both advantages and disadvantages. Each department must assess its own needs in deciding which means are to be employed. While CT is becoming the mainstay of patient contouring, any of the materials and methods described can be used effectively. Table 10-2 summarizes the advantages and disadvantages of each method.

APPLIED TECHNOLOGY
Mechanics of hand-molded contour production

A contour may be taken with the patient lying in any position; the most common positions for contours are supine and prone. For the sake of explanation, we will assume the patient is lying supine in the anatomical position. If the therapist is at the foot of the simulator table looking at the patient, the patient's left is on the therapist's right and the patient's right is on the therapist's left. CT/MRI scans are also typically viewed in this fashion. This general explanation of the method of contouring in the transverse plane is intended for the most commonly used types of hand-molded contour materials: solder wire, plaster, and Aquaplast.

Before taking the patient's contour, all necessary materials should be readily available to the therapist and dosimetrist. If transposing the contour to a paper medium, labeling the appropriate position and anatomical orientation with respect to reference points will save time. In this way, if the allotted time for the procedure is short, correct contour labeling is assured.[8] The box above lists commonly used reference points noted on contours. Graph paper is often preferred because it has accurately drawn horizontal and vertical lines that can be used to correctly place the contour in relationship to the isocenter.[3] When using graph paper, it is helpful to mark a point representing the isocenter where horizontal and vertical lines intersect. This can be used as a point of reference for all measurements. Most measurements are collected with the aid of calipers. When using calipers for patient measurements, they should just lightly touch the skin surface. In this way the surface is not "squeezed," distorting the measurements.

A contour should always be taken with the patient in the correct treatment position. No matter what material is being used for the contour, if the patient is not in the correct treatment position, less inaccurate information for treatment planning results.[1,6,8,9] Therefore it is extremely important to check the A/P and lateral setup points on the patient by using the optical alignment lasers before contouring. All must be in alignment. These points, as well as a table top measurement, will be used to align the contour and accurately represent depths. The depth of the volume, or isocenter, must be rechecked to make sure it has not changed; patients often get very tired by the end of the simulation procedure and have a harder time holding still. It is paramount to double-check the position and to work quickly and accurately in taking the contour.

With the patient in the correct position, the depth to isocenter (the distance measured from the skin surface to the isocenter within the patient) must be determined. This is accomplished by using the three setup points, anterior and lateral central axes/laser points, to help align the contour on the paper.[4] Since the distance to the isocenter (the SAD) is known for each therapy unit, the depth of the isocenter for those points can be determined by subtracting each lateral source-to-skin distance (SSD) from the SAD. This technique is demonstrated in the following series of examples.

The SAD = 100 cm. The left lateral SSD = 88 cm.
The depth to isocenter from the left is 100 − 88 = 12 cm.

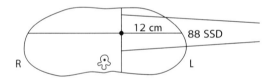

The SAD is 100 cm. The right lateral SSD is 78 cm.
The depth to isocenter from the right is 100 − 78 = 22 cm.

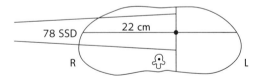

By adding the two depth measurements together, the patient's lateral **interfield distance** (IFD) or patient thickness is derived. This measurement should be verified with a set of calipers to ensure that the two measurements correspond (see example on p. 202).

The depth to isocenter from the left is 12 cm.
The depth to isocenter from the right is 22 cm.
The patient's lateral IFD is 12 + 22 = 34 cm.

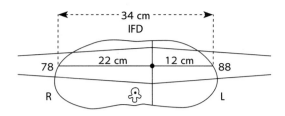

If the patient's lateral IFD is 34 cm, a mark should be made on the horizontal line of the graph paper 12 cm to the left of isocenter and 22 cm to the right of isocenter on the paper (refer back to Fig. 10-9).

To determine the depth of the isocenter from this point, the anterior central axis SSD should be subtracted from the SAD (see example below).

The SAD is 100 cm. The anterior setup SSD is 90 cm.
The anterior depth to isocenter is 100 − 90 = 10 cm.

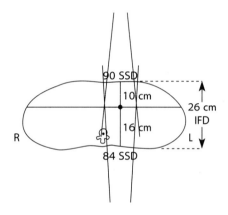

At that point, a mark is drawn on the paper along the vertical line 10 cm anterior to the isocenter. An A/P IFD measurement is taken to complete the posterior aspect of the contour.

The A/P IFD measured with calipers is 26 cm.
The anterior depth is 10 cm.
The posterior depth to isocenter is 26 − 10 = 16 cm.

A mark is drawn on the paper along the vertical line 16 cm posterior to the isocenter.

Although the posterior center is not drawn on the patient (since the patient is lying supine), a posterior SSD reading can be taken if the table is equipped with a racquet. This will allow for cross referencing of the work.

Rotate the gantry 180°. The SAD is 100 cm. The posterior depth to isocenter is 16 cm. The SSD on the posterior aspect of the patient's skin surface is 100 − 16 = 84 cm.

Another measurement that can be helpful in aligning the contour is a midline A/P IFD. Fluoroscopy should be used to verify the patient's midline position, using the vertebral bodies as a reference. A midsagittal alignment mark is important in that it helps to determine the location of a critical midline structure, the spinal cord. Therefore, along with the three points commonly used for alignment, a midline point can be added along the transverse plane and used in dosimetry planning. A midline-point IFD measurement can also be used to help complete the posterior aspect of the contour, especially if midline is more than a few centimeters away from the isocenter.

Having defined the setup points on the paper, the contouring material can be molded around the patient so that it lightly touches the skin surface without excessively pressing the skin inward. It should follow all of the contours of the patient's body surface without leaving any air gaps between the molding material and the skin surface.[4] An **air gap** is an area or void that occurs when the surface to be measured is not flush with the initial point of measurement. A common site for this to occur is in the lumbar region of the back or in the head and neck region.

The contour material should reach from the table top on one side of the patient to the table top on the other side, or as close to it as possible. The therapist and dosimetrist need as much accurate information about the patient's body contour as possible. If the contour abruptly stops just beyond the lateral reference points, the dosimetrist will have to "guess" concerning the rest of the shape. The more guessing required, the less accurate the contour.[4,5]

While the material is molded around the patient, the three or four points (two lateral points, an A/P center, optional midline) should be marked onto the molded material corresponding to their location on the patient's skin surface. Depending on the type of contour material used, the marks on the skin may be transposed automatically when they come in contact with the material, as when plaster strips are used. Otherwise marking pens that will not run should be used.

The contour material should then be removed from the patient and aligned with the marks on the paper, making sure that the correct left and right orientation is noted and that the inside of the contour is matched. If the outside of the contour is used, the contour will have to be squeezed to make it match, thus distorting it. The contour material should be held securely to the paper for tracing. The *inside* of the contour should be traced with a pen or pencil onto the paper.[4,5] This can be a difficult task for one person, which can increase the potential for inaccuracy. If possible, the therapist should enlist the assistance of another to hold the contouring material down while tracing the contour onto the paper. The lateral, anterior, and optional midline points must be marked onto the graph paper from the marks on the contour material.

The last component in accurate contour production is to make sure that important labeling information has been transposed onto the paper. Patient name, identification number, and date of the contour must be noted. The date becomes important when boost fields are planned as well as helping to avoid confusion between multiple contours.[5] Field sizes and gantry angles should also be noted when possible. The more information the treatment planning team has, the fewer are the possibilities for errors. Reference points and information commonly noted on contours are listed in the box on p. 201.

Errors in contouring are frequently made because it is often the last step in a long simulation procedure. The patient may get tired of holding still in an uncomfortable position, and a busy schedule may be forcing the therapist to hurry. Errors are especially seen in the use of hand-molded methods of contouring. Some errors to avoid are (1) leaving air gaps between the contour material and the patient's skin surface, (2) not double-checking the patient's position before beginning the contour, (3) inaccurately tracing the contour to the graph or other paper, and (4) not double-checking the measurements on the drawn contour to see that they correspond to the actual patient measurements. Changes do occur during the course of treatment because of weight fluctuation, swelling, or tumor growth or regression, and the measurements should be checked weekly. Common sources of error in contour production are listed in box at top right.

SUMMARY

Contouring is an essential part of modern radiation therapy treatment planning. It is an important step in the process of planning the best individualized treatment for the patient. It provides the treatment planning team with the most accurate information possible by exercising precision in patient positioning, taking proper measurements, and including all of the detailed information necessary to interpret the contour. Relationships to surface and internal structure are paramount in the delivery of ionizing radiation. While accuracy has been enhanced with the use of image-related methods, it is important for the radiation therapy practitioner to be well versed in contouring techniques (see box at bottom right and box on p. 204).

Common Sources of Error Experienced in Contour Production

- Air gaps between the contour material and the patient's skin surface

- Not double-checking the patient's position before beginning the contour

- Inaccurately tracing the contour onto the graph paper or other paper

- Not double-checking the measurements on the drawn contour to see that they correspond to the actual patient measurements

- Changes that occur during the course of the treatment (weight loss or gain, swelling, tumor growth, etc.)

Step-by-Step Contour Procedure

1. Prepare all necessary materials (graph/transfer paper, calipers, contour material).
2. Make sure patient is in correct position.
3. Secure accurate measurements to use as references.
4. Mold the material around the patient, following all the contours, from table top to table top.
5. Mark the three or four points onto the contouring material.
6. Remove the contour material, and align contour marks with graph paper/cardboard marks in the correct orientation.
7. Hold the contour securely and trace the inside of the contour onto the graph paper/cardboard.
8. Mark the points onto the graph paper from the contour.
9. Double-check that the measurements drawn on the contour correspond to the actual measurements of the patient (IFDs, depths).
10. Double-check material labeled on the contour.

True Versus Surface–to–Table Top Separations

The use of calipers is typically straightforward when measuring diameters during contouring procedures. During these measurements, it must be noted whether the measurement is a true diameter or a surface–to–table top diameter. A true diameter is a measurement of the inside surface of the calipers used (see Fig. below). This is usually the case when measuring lateral points or the separation when there is an air gap.

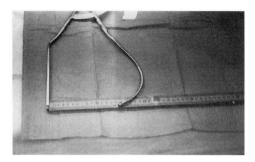

For surface–to–table top measurements, commonly done when the patient's anatomy is flat on the table top, the measurement is taken from the inside surface of the calipers on the patient surface side to the outside caliper surface on the table side (see Fig. below). When measuring a diameter where there is no air gap, the calipers are slid under the patient, but the displaced tissue must be accounted for.

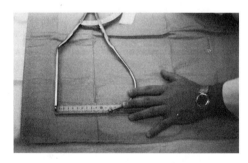

Notation of these differences can mean the difference between an accurate and an erroneous contour. Just a little attention to detail can mean a lot.

Review Questions

Multiple Choice

1. When measuring a patient's diameter including an air gap, the caliper measurement must be read from:
   a. Table top to anterior skin point
   b. Table top to posterior skin point
   c. Anterior skin point to posterior skin point
   d. Anterior skin point to midline
2. When taking a patient contour on a parallel opposed field arrangement, which of the following items must be labeled on the drawing?
   I. Tabletop
   II. Central axis diameter
   III. Treatment field edge
   a. I and II
   b. I and III
   c. II and III
   d. I, II, and III
3. When simulating a SAD mantle set up to be treated to the midplane point, the central axis measures 15 cm with an air gap and 14 cm without an air gap. What should the SSD read on the anterior surface of the patient?
   a. 92
   b. 92.5
   c. 93
   d. 94
4. When taking a contour, which of the following are important points of information that must be known before beginning the procedure?
   I. Patient anterior separation
   II. Patient lateral separation
   III. Measurement from table top to the posterior surface at the central axis
   a. I and II
   b. I and III
   c. II and III
   d. I, II, and III

5. Which of the following would warrant additional contours being taken during the course of treatment?
   I. Change in treatment delivery portals
   II. Change in patient weight or topography
   III. Moving the patient from one linear accelerator to another of the same design
   a. I and II
   b. I and III
   c. II and III
   d. I, II, and III
6. Orthogonal radiographs provide valuable contour information by locating structures in the following perspectives:
   I. Length
   II. Width
   III. Depth
   a. I and II
   b. I and III
   c. II and III
   d. I, II, and III
7. Plastic strips are commonly used in contouring. During the plaster's drying, the strips radiate heat. This occurrence is known as a(n) _____ reaction.
   a. Endothermic
   b. Exothermic
   c. Hyperthermic
   d. Hypothermic

True or False

8. Ideally, all treatment fields should be contoured while the patient remains in one position.
   True _____ False _____
9. Graph paper used in contouring assists the therapist in measuring and locating areas by providing accurately drawn vertical and horizontal lines for reference.
   True _____ False _____

Questions to Ponder

1. Contrast the advantages and disadvantages between hand-molded contours and image-related contours.
2. Describe the impact that patient shape and contour have on overall treatment planning procedures in radiation therapy.
3. Describe methods that may minimize errors in taking hand-molded contours.
4. Measuring patient diameters with calipers is at times confusing for novice radiation therapy practitioners. Outline the procedure for measuring patient separations with these tools.
5. Analyze the considerations a department must review in deciding the type of contour methods that will be used. What considerations must be taken into account if the department handles a substantial number of breast management cases.

REFERENCES

1. Barish RJ: An improvement in the use of plaster bandage for patient contouring. *Med Phys* 20(1):Jan/Feb 1993.
2. Bentel GC: *Radiation therapy planning,* New York, 1992, Macmillan.
3. Bentel GC, Nelson CE, Noell KT: *Treatment planning and dose calculation in radiation oncology,* ed 4. New York, 1989, Pergamon.
4. Gastorf R: Conversation on contouring techniques, July 1995.
5. Kempa A: Conversation on contouring techniques, July 1995.
6. Khan FM: *The physics of radiation therapy,* ed 2. Baltimore, 1994, Williams & Wilkins.
7. Levitt SH, Tapley duVT: *Technological basis of radiation therapy: practical clinical applications.* Philadelphia, 1984, Lea & Febiger.
8. Stanton NR, Stinson D: *An introduction to radiation oncology physics.* Madison, WI, 1992, Medical Physics Publishing.
9. Walter J: *A short textbook of radiotherapy.* New York, 1979, Churchill Livingstone.

Dose Calculations

Julius Armstrong
Charles M. Washington

Outline

Key terms

INTRODUCTION AND PERSPECTIVE

 The administration of ionizing radiation for therapeutic purposes requires detailed knowledge of anatomy, physics, and biological responses. The success or failure of a course of radiation therapy depends on accurate delivery of specific amounts of radiation to a localized site outlined by a radiation oncologist. To that end, the treatment planning team must be able to quantify the overall prescribed dose of radiation and determine how much dose will be delivered over the time frame outlined. Since there are many parameters of dose calculation that must be addressed, the radiation therapist and dosimetrist must be proficient in determining treatment machine settings to deliver the prescribed dose with both computers and manual efforts.

This chapter will incorporate clinical experiences in its presentation. Monitor unit and time settings will be reviewed as well as point dose (i.e., dose to D_{max} and spinal cord) calculations. It is not possible to cover every established method of performing dose calculation; most clinical settings have established site-specific methods for dose calculation, normally determined by a medical radiation physicist. This chapter will give monitor unit and time dose calculation models with examples that encompass the essential components used in treatment planning. Thus practitioners will be able to use the principles presented in this chapter with the calculation methods employed in any radiation therapy center.

It is important to mention that this chapter was written with the beginning practitioner in mind. A brief review of basic terminology and concepts will provide a conceptual overview. The majority of this chapter will be dedicated to the practical application of monitor unit and dose calculations. Very basic calculations will be presented initially, then we will move toward the more advanced calculations.

RADIATION THERAPY PRESCRIPTION

When a patient requires medicine to address an ailment, the physician writes a medical prescription. The *prescription* is a communication tool between the physician and the pharmacist. The medical prescription provides the pharmacist the name of the medication as well as its dosage, route, and quantity and must also state how often and how long the patient should take the medicine. The pharmacist must also be familiar with the effects of the drug or combination of drugs prescribed.

The **radiation therapy prescription** is a communication tool between the radiation oncologist and the radiation therapist. The prescription provides the therapist with the information required to deliver the appropriate radiation treatment. This legal document defines the treatment volume, intended tumor dose, number of treatments, dose per treatment, and frequency of treatment.[2] The prescription also states the type and energy of radiation, beam-shaping devices such as wedges and compensators, and any other appropriate factors. The radiation therapist must be able to discuss with the patient the treatment procedure, function of the devices, and treatment side effects. In practice, there is no standard radiation therapy prescription. The organization and detail of prescriptions vary from one radiation therapy center to another. It is very important that the radiation prescription be clear, precise, and complete. For example, if a thorax is to be treated using anterior and posterior opposed fields, the prescription commonly sets a spinal cord limit not to exceed 4500 cGy. This instruction should be clear and exact; there should be no instruction that is open to interpretation. Every parameter and phase of the treatment must be clearly defined in the radiation therapy prescription.

Often the radiation prescription is not on a single prescription sheet. The radiation oncologist will commonly define the region to be treated, technique, treatment machine, energy, fractionation, and daily and total doses on a "radiation prescription form." The field sizes and gantry, collimator, and couch angles may be written in the patient setup instructions.

Often a computerized isodose or three-dimensional treatment plan may be part of the patient's record. The isodose plan may show field sizes, machine angles, doses, beam weighting, wedges, compensators, or blocks. The isodose plan is considered part of the radiation therapy prescription and should always be signed by the radiation oncologist.

The radiation therapist must make sure that all parts of the prescription match before treatment. For example, the doses, treatment machines, etc. should be the same on the prescription form and the isodose plan.

NOMENCLATURE AND CONCEPTS USED IN DOSE CALCULATIONS

When ionizing radiation is administered to a patient, many factors must be taken into account. As identified earlier, beam energy, distance from the source of radiation, and field size are just a few of the variables that must be addressed to accurately calculate a treatment time or monitor unit setting. The radiation physicist uses mathematics, computers, and specialized equipment to develop dose calculation data used by the dosimetrist and radiation therapist. Many of the data are organized in tables to provide quick reference for these calculations. Before there is any attempt at performing a dose calculation, a number of terms used in the process must be defined. It is important to be consistent in the use and understanding of these terms. The nomenclature used outlines the parameters necessary for accurate administration of radiation. It is important to remember that there are different approaches, methods, and terms used for dose and monitor unit calculations. The therapy practitioner must be meticulous in assuring that the appropriate information for each individual application is used.

Dose

The radiation therapy practitioner must have a clear idea of what is meant by dose. The *dose*, or **absorbed dose**, is measured at a specific point in a medium (typically a patient) and refers to the energy deposited at that point. Dose is typically measured in Gray (Gy), which is defined so that 1 Gy equals 1 J/kg.[1,2]

Depth

Depth is the distance beneath the skin surface where the prescribed dose is to be delivered. Sometimes the radiation oncologist will specify the depth of calculation. For example, when an area is being treated by a single treatment field, the radiation oncologist will state the exact point, or depth, for the calculation. Using a posterior field for treatment of vertebral body metastasis, the radiation therapy prescription may state that 3 Gy are to be delivered per fraction to a depth of 5.0 cm. For opposed fields the patient's midplane is often used for the depth of calculation. Most multiple field arrangements use the isocenter, or intersection of the beams, for the calculation depth. Plain radiographs and CT scans are useful in determining the point of calculation. It is necessary to take measurements of the patient's thickness or separation.

Separation

Separation is a measurement of the patient's thickness from the point of beam entry to the point of beam exit. When calculating a treatment time or monitor unit setting, the separation is normally measured along the beam's central axis. The separation can be measured directly using calipers or indirectly using the readings supplied by optical distance indicators (ODI) located on the treatment units. It is important to know the patient's separation when performing dose calculations. Often, for parallel opposed treatment fields (two fields focused at a point of specification directed 180° apart), the calculation is done to deliver the prescribed dose at the patient's midplane or mid-separation. To find the mid-separation, the total separation is divided by two. For example, if the treatment prescription requires delivery of 2 Gy per fraction at mid-separation using opposed fields, the patient's separation at the central axis would be measured. If the separation was measured as 20 cm, the mid-separation would be 10 cm. In that case, a depth of 10 cm would be used for the monitor unit calculation.

Source-to-skin distance

Source-to-skin distance (SSD) is the distance from the source or target of the treatment machine to the surface of the patient or phantom (a volume of tissue equivalent material). The SSD is normally measured using an ODI. This device projects a distance scale onto the patient's skin (Fig. 11-1, *A*). The number read is the distance from the source of gamma rays or x-rays to the patient's skin surface.

Isocenter

The **isocenter** is the intersection of the axis of rotation of the gantry and the axis of rotation of the collimator for the treatment unit. This is usually a point in space at a specified distance from the source or target that the gantry rotates around. Cobalt 60 treatment machines typically have a source to axis distance of 80 cm, while the source to axis distance for most modern linear accelerators is 100 cm.

Source-to-axis distance

The **source-to-axis distance** (SAD) is the distance from the source of gamma rays or x-rays to the isocenter of the treatment machine (Fig. 11-1, *B*). Each isocentric machine has its own SAD. When the gantry rotates around the patient, the SSD will continually change; however, the SAD and isocenter are at a fixed distance and therefore do not change. In an isocentric setup the isocenter is established inside the patient. The treatment machines are designed so that the gantry will rotate around this reference point.

Field size

Field size refers to the physical size set on the collimators of the therapy unit that delineates size of the treatment field at a reference distance. The field size is defined at the machine's isocenter. For example, when a field size of 10 cm × 10 cm

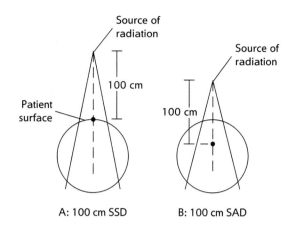

Fig. 11-1 These diagrams graphically define SSD and SAD. **A**, SSD is the distance from the source of radiation to the surface of the patient or phantom for a linear accelerator (100 cm to surface). **B**, SAD is the distance from the source of radiation to the isocenter of the treatment unit. The isocenter is typically placed within the patient.

is set on the treatment unit collimator, the square treatment field measures 10 cm × 10 cm at that particular machine's isocentric distance. On a cobalt 60 machine, it would be at 80 cm; on most linear accelerators, it would be at 100 cm.

Field size changes with distance from the source of radiation because of divergence. The 10 cm × 10 cm field size would measure smaller at distances shorter than the isocentric distance and larger at distances greater than the isocentric distance. In the isocentric or SAD patient setup, the field size set would be inside the patient at the isocenter. The physical size measured on the patient's surface at that point would be smaller, since it would be at a distance shorter than the isocenter. In the nonisocentric (SSD) patient setup, the field size set on the collimator would be the same as measured on the skin surface, since the isocentric distance is set at the skin surface in this instance.

Scatter

Therapeutic radiation is composed of primary and scatter radiation. Any interaction of the primary radiation may result in scatter. When the primary beam interacts with matter, the result is scatter radiation made up of photons or electrons. Usually there is a change of direction associated with scatter radiation. When an electron interacts with the target in the linear accelerator, photons are produced. These photons are the primary beam. As the primary photons travel to the patient, some of them will interact with the collimator. When the primary photon interacts with the collimator, an electron from the collimator may be ejected and travel toward the patient. The primary photon beam may also be deflected back toward the patient. Both the electron and the deflected photon are considered scatter radiation. Radiation that is scattered back toward the surface of the patient is called *backscatter*. The absorbed dose received by the patient results from secondary radiation caused by interactions where the photon imparts energy to an electron. Then the electron undergoes tens of thousands of collisions while giving up some energy at each collision. Most of the absorbed dose received by the patient results from the collisions of the scattered electrons.

D_{max}

D_{max}, also known as the depth of maximum equilibrium, is the depth at which electronic equilibrium occurs for photon beams. D_{max} is the point where the maximum absorbed dose occurs for single field photon beams and chiefly depends on the energy of the beam. Normally the depth of maximum ionization increases as the energy of the photon beam increases. D_{max} occurs at the surface for low energy photon beams and beneath the surface for megavoltage photon beams. Other factors such as field size and distance may influence the depth at which maximum ionization occurs. Table 11-1 below lists the approximate depth of D_{max} for various photon beam energies.

There are times when it is important to know what the dose is at D_{max}. When a patient is treated using a single field, the dose at D_{max} should be calculated and recorded because the dose at D_{max} will be higher than the prescribed dose. The dose at D_{max} is also greater than the prescribed dose when opposed treatment fields are used to treat the patient and will be greater than the dose delivered to the patient's mid-plane. The dose at D_{max} will be slightly greater than the mid-plane dose for high energy treatment beams and for patients with a small separation. When low energy treatment beams (cobalt 60, 4 MV and 6 MV) are used, the dose at D_{max} can be significantly higher than the mid-plane dose. This is especially true for large patient separations. When using megavoltage photon beams, it may not be necessary to calculate the dose at D_{max} when using multiple field arrangements to treat the patient. By using many fields, the dose at D_{max} will normally be less than the prescribed dose.

Output

The **output** can be referred to as the dose rate of the machine and is measured in the absence of a scattering phantom and

Table 11-1	Approximate depths of D_{max}
Beam energy	**Depth of D_{max} (cm)**
200 kV	0.0
1.25 MV	0.5
4 MV	1.0
6 MV	1.5
10 MV	2.5
18 MV	3.5
24 MV	4.0

in tissue equivalent material.[1] It is the amount of radiation exposure produced by a treatment machine or source as specified at a reference field size and at a specified reference distance. The reference field size and distance are used so that we may relate standardized measurements to those that vary from the standards. Changing the field size, distance, or medium will change the dose rate. Dose rate increases with increased field size. A therapeutic beam of radiation is made up of primary and scatter and measured at a point of reference. If the field size is increased on a treatment machine, the primary component would remain the same. However, the increased area would cause increased scatter, which would add to the output (all other parameters remaining constant). If the distance from the source of radiation to the point of measurement increases, the dose rate would decrease because of the inverse square law (as discussed in earlier chapters). An example of output on a cobalt 60 unit may be 150 cGy/min, while a linear accelerator output may be 1 cGy/mu at reference field size and distance.

Output factor

The **output factor** is the ratio of the dose rate of a given field size to the dose rate of the reference field size. The output factor allows for the change in scatter as the collimator setting changes. The output factor is usually normalized or referenced to a 10 cm × 10 cm field size. This means that the output factor for a 10 cm × 10 cm field size is 1.00 for the linear accelerator or cobalt 60 unit. The output factor will be greater than 1.00 for field sizes larger than 10 cm × 10 cm because of an increase in scatter as the collimator setting is increased. The output factor will be less than 1.00 for field sizes smaller than 10 cm × 10 cm because of a decrease in scatter as the collimator setting is decreased.

The term *output factor* may be a generic term. Many institutions use other terminology, such as relative output factor, collimator scatter factor, field size correction factor, and phantom scatter factor. Khan defines a collimator scatter factor (Sc), a phantom scatter factor (Sp), and a total scatter factor (Sc, p).[6] Sc and Sc,p are measured data; Sp is a derived value.

Output factors relate the dose rate of a given collimator setting to the dose rate of the reference field size. Output factors are very useful and practical for calculations involving cobalt 60 treatment machines. The reference dose rate for the cobalt 60 treatment machine is constantly changing. Usually the reference dose rate is updated monthly. Even though the reference dose rate is changed every month, the output factors do not change. Therefore, by using output factors, only the reference dose rate must be changed. Normally the reference dose rate is 1.0 cGy per monitor unit for linear accelerators. The reference dose rate does not normally change for linear accelerators. This means that in some centers the output factor is the dose rate for that field size (any number multiplied by one does not change). For example, let us say that the reference dose rate is 1.0 cGy per monitor unit for a 10 cm × 10 cm field size measured at 100 cm from the target in free space. Let us also say that the output factor for the 15 cm × 15 cm collimator setting is 1.02 (larger than 1.00 because the field size is greater than the reference). The dose rate for the 15 × 15 cm collimator setting can be calculated as follows:

Dose rate $_{(Given\ field\ size)}$ =
Dose rate $_{(Reference\ field\ size)}$ × Output factor$_{(Given\ field\ size)}$

Dose rate $_{(Given\ field\ size)}$ = 1.0 cGy/MU × 1.02

Dose rate $_{(Given\ field\ size)}$ = 1.02 cGy/my

Today some treatment centers use more than one output factor. For example, some calculation models require the use of a collimator output factor (COF) and a phantom scatter factor (PSF). The COF is used to determine the scatter, usually measured in air, from the collimators. The PSF is used to determine the scatter from the patient.

Inverse square law

The inverse square law is a mathematical relationship that describes the change in beam intensity caused by the divergence of the beam. As the beam of radiation diverges or spreads out, there is a decrease in the intensity. Therefore, as the distance from the source of radiation increases, the intensity will decrease. For example, a photon beam that is made up of 400 photons is administered in a field size of 10 cm × 10 cm at a distance of 100 cm. The area of the beam is 100 cm^2 (given by the formula width × length). If the photon coverage is uniform, there is an intensity of 4 photons/cm^2. At a distance of 200 cm, the field size will double to dimensions of 20 cm × 20 cm. The area of this field would then be 400 cm^2. There are still only 400 photons to cover this larger area. Now if the photon coverage is uniform, there will be 1 photon/cm^2. By doubling the distance, the intensity or number of photons per square centimeter has decreased by one fourth.

One practical application of the inverse square law is its effect on the output or dose rate of the treatment machine. The dose rate is commonly measured at the isocenter of the treatment machine. For linear accelerators, the dose rate at the isocenter for a 10 cm × 10 cm field is often 1.0 cGy/MU. When the monitor units are calculated for setup at distances greater than the standard, the inverse square law is used to account for the decrease in dose rate at distances beyond the isocenter. The dose rate of the beam is inversely proportional to the square of the distance. This means that even a small change in distance can have a large effect on the dose rate. For example, if the dose rate is 1.0 cGy/MU at 100 cm, then the dose rate is 0.64 cGy/MU at 125 cm. The equation commonly used for the inverse square law is as follows:

$$\frac{I_1}{I_2} = \frac{(d_2)^2}{(d_1)^2}$$

This equation may be used to find the change in dose rate with a change in distance:

$$\frac{Dose\ rate\ at\ distance_1}{Dose\ rate\ at\ distance_2} = \frac{(Distance_2)^2}{(Distance_1)^2}$$

Distance$_1$ is defined as 125 cm for this example. Rearranging the above equation, we get the following:

$$Dose\ rate\ at\ distance_1 = Dose\ rate\ at\ distance_2 \times \frac{(Distance_2)^2}{(Distance_1)^2}$$

Substituting the values in our example we have:

$$Dose\ rate\ at\ 125\ cm = Dose\ rate\ at\ 100\ cm \times \frac{(100\ cm)^2}{(125\ cm)^2}$$

$$Dose\ rate\ at\ 125\ cm = 1.0\ cGy/MU \times \frac{(100\ cm)^2}{(125\ cm)^2}$$

$$Dose\ rate\ at\ 125\ cm = 0.64\ cGy/MU$$

Equivalent squares of rectangular fields (ESRF)

A square field is a field that has equal dimensions for the field width and length, such as a 10 cm × 10 cm field. A rectangular field has a field width and length that are different, as is the case with a 10 cm × 15 cm field. In a clinical setting, most patients are treated with rectangular fields; square fields are not as commonly used. Treatment calculation tables employ field size as a qualifying parameter. Using different rectangular fields would require extensive tables with thousands of number combinations. Because of this, a method was needed to make the amount of data and number of tables manageable. The method devised was to take different rectangular field sizes and compare them to square fields that demonstrate the same measurable scatter characteristics, known as an **equivalent square**.

A formula may be used to calculate the equivalent square of a rectangular field. One formula is commonly called the 4 × Area ÷ Perimeter method. Using this formula the area and perimeter of the rectangular field are calculated. The area is divided by the perimeter, and this quotient is multiplied by four. The number derived would be one side of the square field that has approximately the same measurable scatter characteristics as the original rectangular field. This essentially takes field shape into account. This formula is an approximation and should be used when an ESRF table is not available. In general, if the ratio of width or length exceeds 2, standardized tables of equivalent squares are recommended. Table 11-2 on p. 211 demonstrates an example of a chart showing equivalent squares of rectangular fields.

Equivalent squares of rectangular fields are used to find the output, output factor, and tissue absorption factors. Most radiation beam data tables are constructed so that the equivalent square of the rectangular field must be known to use the table. For example, to look up the output factor for a collimator setting of 7 cm × 19 cm, converting the rectangular field to a square one is required. Its equivalent square is found to be 10 cm × 10 cm.[5,9] The output factor for a 10 × 10 cm field would be used, since it is effectively the same as that of a 7 cm × 19 cm field, all other parameters remaining

Table 11-2	Sample equivalent squares of rectangular fields chart												
Long axis (cm)	0.5	1.0	2.0	3.0	4.0	5.0	6.0	7.0	8.0	9.0	10.0	11.0	12.0
0.5	**0.5**												
1	0.7	**1.0**											
2	0.9	1.4	**2.0**										
3	1.0	1.6	2.4	**3.0**									
4	1.1	1.7	2.7	3.4	**4.0**								
5	1.2	1.8	2.9	3.8	4.5	**5.0**							
6	1.2	1.9	3.1	4.1	4.8	5.5	**6.0**						
7	1.2	2.0	3.3	4.3	5.1	5.8	6.5	**7.0**					
8	1.2	2.1	3.4	4.5	5.4	6.2	6.9	7.5	**8.0**				
9	1.2	2.1	3.5	4.6	5.6	6.5	7.2	7.9	8.5	**9.0**			
10	1.3	2.2	3.6	4.8	5.8	6.7	7.5	8.2	8.9	9.5	**10.0**		
11	1.3	2.2	3.7	4.9	6.0	6.9	7.8	8.5	9.3	9.9	10.5	**11.0**	
12	1.3	2.2	3.7	5.0	6.1	7.1	8.0	8.8	9.6	10.3	10.9	11.5	**12.0**
13	1.3	2.2	3.8	5.1	6.2	7.2	8.2	9.1	9.9	10.6	11.3	11.9	12.5
14	1.3	2.3	3.8	5.1	6.3	7.4	8.4	9.3	10.1	10.9	11.6	12.3	12.9
15	1.3	2.3	3.9	5.2	6.4	7.5	8.5	9.5	10.3	11.2	11.9	12.6	13.3
16	1.3	2.3	3.9	5.3	6.5	7.6	8.6	9.6	10.5	11.4	12.2	12.9	13.7
17	1.3	2.3	3.9	5.3	6.5	7.7	8.8	9.8	10.7	11.6	12.4	13.2	14.0
18	1.3	2.3	3.9	5.3	6.6	7.8	8.9	9.9	10.9	11.8	12.6	13.5	14.3
19	1.4	2.3	4.0	5.4	6.6	7.8	8.9	10.0	11.0	11.9	12.8	13.7	14.5
20	1.4	2.3	4.0	5.4	6.7	7.9	9.0	10.1	11.1	12.1	13.0	13.9	14.7

unchanged. The output factor for a 10 cm × 10 cm field is 1.000. Therefore the output factor for a 7 cm × 19 cm field is 1.000.

When blocks are used to customize the shape of the treatment area, two portions of the field are created. The first is the area being shielded, and the second is the area being treated. When examining the area being treated, its dimensions must be determined. This derived field size is called the blocked field size (BFS) or **effective field size (EFS)**, which is the equivalent rectangular field dimension of the open or treated area within the collimator field dimensions. Usually some method of approximation is used to determine the EFS (a square or rectangular field that approximates the same physical volume as the blocked shape). The EFS is normally smaller than the collimator field size, although it may be larger for some extended distance setups. The unblocked equivalent square may be used to determine the output factor. The EFS equivalent square is normally used to determine the tissue absorption factors, such as the percentage depth dose (PDD), tissue-air ratio (TAR), tissue phantom ratio (TPR), or tissue maximum ratio (TMR), which are discussed in the following section.

TISSUE ABSORPTION FACTORS

As the beam of radiation travels through the body, it gives up energy. The more tissue the beam traverses, the more it is attenuated. There are a number of different methods for measuring the attenuation of the beam as it travels through tissue. These are **percentage depth dose** (PDD), **tissue-air ratio**

(TAR), tissue phantom ratio (TPR), and **tissue maximum ratio (TMR)**. The first of these methods used in a treatment setting was PDD. It may be helpful to remember that in the early days of radiation therapy the patients were treated using an SSD technique. PDD was developed for SSD setups. Using appropriate corrections, any of the four methods (PDD, TAR, TPR, and TMR) may be used for SSD or SAD setups. However, PDD works best with SSD (nonisocentric) treatments, whereas TAR, TPR, and TMR work very well with SAD (isocentric) treatments.

PDD

PDD is the ratio, expressed as a percentage, of the absorbed dose at a given depth to the absorbed dose at a fixed reference depth usually D_{max}[7,8] (Fig. 11-2), as follows:

$$PDD = \frac{\text{Absorbed dose at depth}}{\text{Absorbed dose at } D_{max}} \times 100\%$$

Normally the depth of D_{max} is used for the fixed reference depth. PDD is dependent on four factors: energy, depth, field size, and SSD. PDD increases as the energy, field size, and SSD increase. This is a direct relationship. Higher energies are more penetrating, so a greater percentage is available at a specific depth when compared to a lower energy. As field size increases, more scatter is added to the deposited beam, thus increasing PDD. PDD decreases as the depth increases (inverse relationship), because since dose is deposited in tissue as it traverses it, a smaller percentage is available at greater depths.

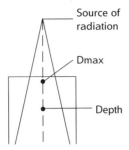

Fig. 11-2 Diagram of percentage depth dose (PDD). PDD measures the dose along the central ray at depth as it compares to the dose at maximum equilibrium (D_{max}).

TAR

TAR is the ratio of the absorbed dose at a given depth in phantom to the absorbed dose at the same point in free space (Fig. 11-3):

$$TAR = \frac{\text{Dose in tissue}}{\text{Dose in air}}$$

Free space (in air) is a term used for measurements using a build-up cap or miniphantom. It may not be possible to do a true air measurement. A build-up cap is a device made of acrylic or other phantom material that is placed over an ionization chamber to produce conditions of electronic equilibrium. The miniphantom is a sphere of tissue-equivalent material surrounding a point of interest. There is just enough material to produce build-up at the center (depth of D_{max}).[5] The ionization chamber then measures the flow of electrons and eventually the dose rate of the treatment machine (Fig. 11-4).

When determining the TAR, the dose is measured at a reference distance from the target, but under two sets of conditions. The first measurement is in air or free space, and the second measurement is in phantom (the point of measurement does not change between the two measurements). The amount of phantom material used for the second measurement corresponds to the depth of interest.

TAR depends on energy, field size, and depth.[4] TAR increases as the energy and field size increase and decreases as the depth increases. These characteristics are consistent with PDD. However, TAR is independent of SSD (distance). TAR is normally used to perform calculations for SAD treatments involving low energy treatment units such as a cobalt 60 or 4 MV linear accelerators. Some treatment centers use TAR for energies greater than 4 MV.

Backscatter factor

The **backscatter factor** (BSF) is the ratio of the dose rate with a scattering medium (water or phantom) to the dose rate at the same point without a scattering medium (air) at the level of maximum equilibrium.[1-4,7,8] Backscatter is then a TAR at the level of D_{max}. The BSF is measured at the surface for orthovoltage and other low energy x-ray treatment machines (energies less than 400 kV) (Fig. 11-5). The BSF is measured at the depth of D_{max} for megavoltage photon beams. Therefore the BSF is often called the **peak scatter factor** (PSF) for megavoltage radiation. The PSF is sometimes normalized to a reference field size, usually 10 cm $\times$ 10 cm, for energies of 4 MV and above.[1] In the applications section of this chapter, the term *PSF* is used in a number of the calculations. However, many tables still use BSF for both low energy and megavoltage photon beams.

Tissue phantom ratio and tissue maximum ratio

Tissue phantom ratio (TPR) is the ratio of the absorbed dose at a given depth in phantom to the absorbed dose at the same point at a reference depth in phantom, as follows:

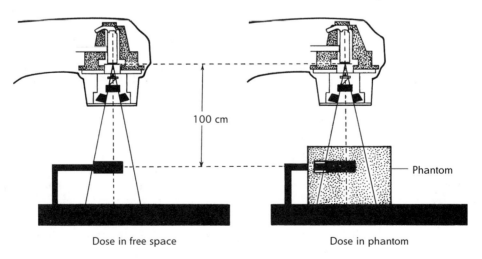

Dose in free space   Dose in phantom

Fig. 11-3 Diagram of tissue-air ratio (TAR). TAR compares the dose in tissue at a specific depth to the dose in air at the same distance from the source (at the isocenter). When the depth in tissue corresponds to the level of D_{max}, the TAR is known as the backscatter or peak scatter factor.

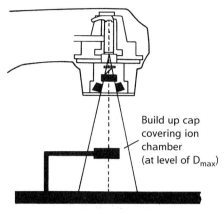

Dose rate measured in free space (air)

Fig. 11-4 Dose rate measured in air. There is a build-up cap over the ionization measuring chamber to allow for maximum scatter component to be accounted for.

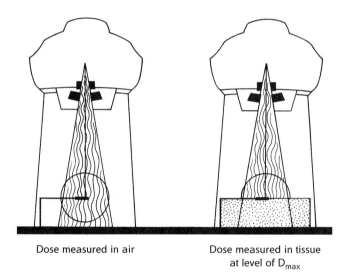

Dose measured in air — Dose measured in tissue at level of D$_{max}$

Fig. 11-5 Backscatter or peak scatter factor relates dose in tissue to dose in air at the level of maximum equilibrium.

$$\text{TPR} = \frac{\text{Dose in tissue}}{\text{Dose in phantom}}$$

The reference depth may be any depth but 5.0 cm is commonly chosen. If the reference depth is chosen to be the depth of D$_{max}$, then the TPR is referred to as the **tissue maximum ratio** (TMR), as seen in Fig. 11-6.

$$\text{TMR} = \frac{\text{Dose in tissue}}{\text{Dose in phantom (D}_{max}\text{)}}$$

The TMR is related to the TAR by the formula: TAR = TMR × BSF for low energy beam, or TAR = TMR × PSF for high energy beams.

TMR and TPR were developed because of difficulties in measuring the TAR for high energy beams. TAR is measured using some form of a build-up cap. With high energy beams

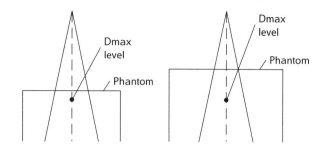

Fig. 11-6 Tissue maximum ratio compares dose at the depth of D$_{max}$ to dose at depth where the distance from the source to each point is the same. If another point of reference is used instead of D$_{max}$, the relationship is known as tissue phantom ratio.

a large build-up cap would be required to accurately measure it. As the build-up cap becomes increasingly larger, phantom scatter is introduced into the "in-air measurement" of the TAR. A build-up cap is not needed for measuring TMR, since both measurements are done in phantom. Thus TMR overcame the problem of getting a true "in-air" measurement.

Since the depth of D$_{max}$ depends on field size, the reference depths for TMR change accordingly. One advantage of a TPR over a TMR is that the reference depth will not change with field size. By using a reference depth of D$_{max}$ for the 10 × 10 cm field size, the dependence of the depth of D$_{max}$ with field size has been eliminated with TPR.

When determining the TMR and TPR, the dose is measured at one distance from the target, but at two different depths under phantom-specific conditions. The first measurement is at the depth of D$_{max}$ or another established standard, and the second measurement is at the desired depth. The point of measurement does not change between the two measurements. The amount of phantom material used for the second measurement is determined by the depth of interest. The value of TMR is never greater than 1.00, and the value of TPR has no upper limit. The deeper the reference depth, the greater the TPR.[8]

Dose rate modification factors

Any device placed in the path of the radiation beam will attenuate some of it. The transmission factor is the ratio of the radiation dose with the device to the radiation dose without the device and accounts for the material in the beam's path. Examples of such factors would include tray transmission, wedge, and compensating filter factors.

Tray transmission factor

The *tray transmission factor (tray factor)* defines how much of the radiation is transmitted through a block tray. Most block trays are made of plastic. When the beam of radiation hits the tray, some of the radiation will be attenuated by the tray. The radiation not attenuated by the tray will pass through and continue to the patient. To correctly calculate a monitor unit or time setting, the amount of radiation transmitted through the tray must be measured. The physicist takes two measurements: the first measurement is with the tray in the path of the beam, while the second measurement is without the tray in the path of the beam. The ratio of these two measurements is known as the tray transmission factor. For example, if a dose with the tray in place is measured as 97 cGy and the dose without the tray is 100 cGy, the ratio of the two doses (97/100) will yield a tray transmission factor of 0.97. This means that 97% of the radiation is transmitted through the tray, while 3% of the radiation is attenuated. Tray factors vary with beam energy. As energy increases, the effect of the material in the beam's path is lessened because of the increased penetrating power of the higher energy. Thus departments may use the same trays on different treatment units (Fig. 11-7). They simply use an appropriate tray factor for the energy with which it is used.

To deliver the correct dose to the patient, the radiation attenuated by the tray must be taken into consideration. This is normally done by having the tray transmission factor as a dose rate modifier. When the tray transmission factor is handled in this manner, it should always be represented by a number less than 1.00. While this will be the method used in this chapter, some therapy departments opt to multiply the monitor unit or time setting by a tray factor that is greater than 1.00. For example, if the calculated monitor unit setting before taking the tray into account is 100 MU and the tray factor is 1.03 (denoting a 3% attenuation), by multiplying the 100 MU by 1.03, a corrected MU setting of 103 would be obtained. When the tray factor is greater than 1.00, it is not a tray transmission factor and cannot be multiplied by the dose rate to account for the

attenuation. In these cases, the machine setting needs to be increased by this factor.

Wedge and compensator filter transmission factors

The wedge transmission factor (wedge factor) depicts the amount of the radiation transmitted through a wedge. A wedge is made of a dense material, usually lead or steel, which attenuates the radiation beam progressively across a field. The thinner side of the wedge attenuates less of the beam than the thicker side, resulting in an alteration of the beam isodose patterns.[1,2] The physicist takes several measurements and defines the wedge transmission factor, which is specific for each beam energy with which it is used. For example, if a wedge has a wedge transmission factor of 0.67, this means that 67% of the radiation is transmitted through the wedge and 33% of the radiation is attenuated. To deliver the correct dose to the patient, a correction must be made for this amount of beam attenuation.

The compensator filter transmission factor is measured in the same manner as the wedge transmission factor. A compensator filter alters the isodose patterns just as in the wedge (Fig. 11-8). However, the compensator filter is individually produced for each patient and alters the patterns so that they are at maximum efficiency for that patient. Both factors are normally multiplied into the dose rate when doing a treatment unit calculation. Examples of treatment unit calculations involving wedges and compensators can be found in the section on applications.

PRACTICAL APPLICATIONS OF EXTERNAL BEAM DOSE CALCULATIONS

Having a clear understanding of the factors that affect the administration of ionizing radiation is extremely important to the radiation oncology team. Small changes in parameters can change the dose administered to the patient. A field size set incorrectly will change the machine output in reference to the patient. A sagging table top that inaccurately sets the patient at a wrong distance can have the same effect. With all this in mind and keeping the concepts presented as the focus, this section will present practical applications of treatment unit calculations.

Calculating the given dose for an SSD setup using PDD

Often it is important to know the dose to points other than the prescription point. Dose-limiting structures, also known as critical structures, are anatomical sites that cannot withstand the same amount of exposure as neighboring tissues without damage. The spinal cord, bowel, and lens of the eye are examples of dose-limiting structures that are commonly monitored. The points monitored will be determined chiefly by the region of the body being irradiated.

Often SSD calculations are done at D_{max}. When a single field is used to treat a patient, such as a posterior spine field, the dose at D_{max} is known as the given dose. Other names for the given dose are applied dose, entrance dose, peak absorbed dose, or D_{max} dose. This is the point where the

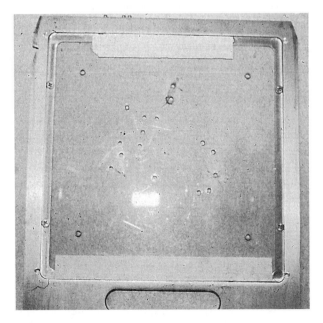

Fig. 11-7 Typical blocking tray used to support standardized or custom shielding blocks.

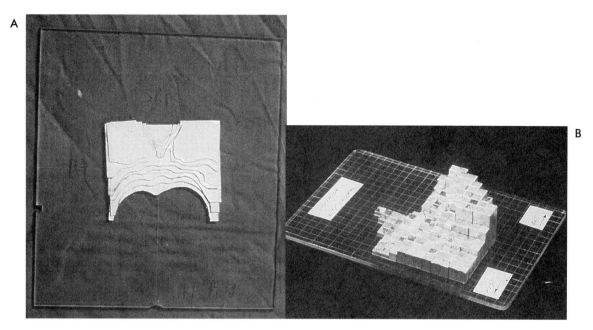

Fig. 11-8 Compensating filters. **A,** Lead sheet comp filter. **B,** Aluminum cube comp filter. These filters attenuate the beam so that topographic variances are accounted for. Through this process, the distribution of dose at depths below the surface is even.

PDD is equal to 100%. As the depth increases from that point, the PDD will decrease. If a prescription calls for the administration of 300 cGy to a certain depth below D_{max} through a single field, the given dose will have to be more than the 300 cGy based on these concepts The dose at depth is also called the *tumor dose* (TD). This is done for cobalt 60 as well as linear accelerators. Each treatment field has its own given dose. Calculating the given dose can be accomplished by using the ratio of the prescribed dose for the field and the PDD at the depth of the prescribed dose, as follows:

$$\text{Given dose} = \frac{\text{TD}}{\text{PDD}} \times 100$$

When writing the PDD, the following convention will be used: PDD (d,s,SSD), indicating that this refers to the PDD at depth (d), for equivalent square (s), at the setup distance (SSD). If the PDD at a depth of 5 cm for 10 cm × 10 cm field setup is 80 cm, the PDD is 78.3%; the convention for writing this information is PDD (5,10,80) = 78.3%.

There is a direct relationship between the dose and the PDD at a point. Thus a ratio or direct proportion can be established, as follows:

$$\frac{\text{Dose at point A}}{\text{PDD at point A}} = \frac{\text{Dose at point B}}{\text{PDD at point B}}$$

The following example calculates the given dose.

Example 1: A patient is treated on the cobalt 60 treatment machine at 80 cm SSD. The collimator setting is 10 cm × 10 cm. There is no blocking used for this treatment. The prescription states that a dose of 3000 cGy is to be delivered to a depth of 5 cm in 10 fractions (the dose per fraction is 300

cGy). Calculate the given or applied dose.

$$\text{Given dose} = \frac{\text{TD}}{\text{PDD}} \times 100$$

$$\text{Given dose} = \frac{300 \text{ cGy}}{78.3} \times 100$$

$$\text{Given dose} = 383.1 \text{ cGy}$$

Again it should be noted that in this case to deliver 300 cGy to a depth of 5 cm with a 10 cm × 10 cm field at 80 cm SSD, a dose of 383.1 cGy is delivered to D_{max}. This calculation would be done exactly the same for any linear accelerator.

The given dose formula can be rearranged to solve for the TD if the given dose is known. The following example will demonstrate this. Before any calculations, it should be noted that the TD should be less than the given dose in a single field calculation because the TD will be located at a depth greater than the level of D_{max}.

Example 2: A patient is treated on the 6 MV linear accelerator at 100 cm SSD. The collimator setting is 15 cm × 15 cm. There is no blocking used for this treatment. The prescription states that a dose of 300 cGy per fraction is to be delivered at D_{max}. What is the dose delivered at a depth of 5 cm²?

$$\text{TD} = \text{Given dose} \times \frac{\text{PDD (5,15,100)}}{100}$$

$$\text{TD} = 300 \text{ cGy} \times \frac{87.9}{100}$$

$$\text{TD} = 263.7 \text{ cGy}$$

As expected, the TD is lower than the given dose.

Any other point along the central axis can be found if the depth and PDD are known. If a dose at a depth of 3 cm was sought in the preceding example, it would be somewhere between the dose at D_{max} and the dose at 5 cm. By looking up the PDD at the desired depth, the information can be derived.

In earlier years of radiation therapy the higher given doses presented problems. To treat tumors at depth, it was necessary to give the superficial tissues higher doses. Coupled with the use of lower energy therapy machines that had a shallower D_{max}, brisk skin reactions were common and sometimes limited the administration of radiation therapy.

There are times when nonisocentric treatments are done for parallel opposed fields. At those times, it may be beneficial to the radiation oncology team to note the total dose at D_{max}. In this case, the given dose is added to the exit dose. The *exit dose* is the dose absorbed by a point that is located at the depth of D_{max} at the exit of the beam. For example, the depth of D_{max} for a 6 MV photon beam is approximately 1.5 cm. If a patient is treated using parallel opposed anterior and posterior photon beams and the patient's central axis separation is 20 cm, the total D_{max} dose can be calculated. The given dose would be calculated at a depth of 1.5 cm and the exit dose at a depth of 18.5 cm (20 cm − 1.5 cm). The following example calculates the total D_{max} dose and cord dose using a linear accelerator. Each field contributes to the total dose of each. Remember that the calculation using a cobalt unit would be done the same way.

Example 3: A patient is treated on the 6 MV linear accelerator at 100 cm SSD. The collimator setting is 15 cm × 15 cm. The field is blocked to an 8 × 8 blocked equivalent square. A 5 mm solid plastic tray is used to hold the blocks. The prescription states that a dose of 4000 cGy is to be delivered to a depth of 10 cm in 20 fractions using an anterior and posterior (AP:PA) treatment field arrangement. The patient's central axis separation is 20 cm. The cord lies 3.0 cm beneath the posterior skin surface. Calculate the total D_{max} dose and the cord dose.

We see that in this arrangement, the calculation point lies 3.0 cm from the posterior surface and 17.0 cm from the anterior surface. It is important to note here that all points of calculation are along the central axis. To obtain the anterior depth of the cord, the posterior depth of the cord should be subtracted from the patient's total separation (20.0 − 3.0 = 17.0). The depth of D_{max} for the 6 MV linear accelerator is 1.5 cm. Therefore the depth of the posterior field exit point is 18.5 cm (20.0 − 1.5).

The factors required for this calculation are as follows:

PDD (1.5,8,100) = 100.0 (Table 11-7 on p. 233)

PDD (3,8,100) = 95.0 (Table 11-7)

PDD (10,8,100) = 66.7 (Table 11-7)

PDD (17,8,100) = 45.2 (Table 11-7)

PDD (18.5,8,100) = 41.6 (Table 11-7)

PSF (15 × 15) = 1.039 (Table 11-7)

PSF (8 × 8) = 1.016 (Table 11-7)

Determining total D_{max} dose
A. Calculate the anterior dose contribution to D_{max} (given dose)
In this problem, the direct proportion formula will be used, as follows:

$$\frac{\text{Dose at point A}}{\text{PDD at point A}} = \frac{\text{Dose at point B}}{\text{PDD at point B}}$$

$$\frac{\text{Dose}_{1.5\,cm}}{\text{PDD}_{1.5\,cm}} = \frac{\text{Dose}_{10\,cm}}{\text{PDD}_{10\,cm}}$$

$$\frac{\text{Dose}_{1.5\,cm}}{100} = \frac{100\ cGy}{66.7}$$

$$\text{Dose}_{1.5\,cm} = 149.9\ cGy$$

B. Calculate the posterior dose contribution to D_{max} (exit dose)
Using the exit point (A) and D_{max} point (B), we have depths of 18.5 cm and 1.5 cm, respectively.

$$\frac{\text{Dose}_{1.5\,cm}}{\text{PDD}_{1.5\,cm}} = \frac{\text{Dose}_{18.5\,cm}}{\text{PDD}_{18.5\,cm}}$$

$$\frac{149.9\ cGy}{100} = \frac{\text{Dose}_{18.5}}{41.6}$$

$$\text{Dose}_{18.5} = 62.4\ cGy$$

C. Add the anterior and posterior dose contributions to obtain total D_{max} dose

$$D_{max}\text{ dose (total)} = D_{max}\text{ dose (anterior)} + D_{max}\text{ dose (posterior)}$$

$$D_{max}\text{ dose (total)} = 149.9\ cGy + 62.4\ cGy$$

$$D_{max}\text{ dose (total)} = 212.3\ cGy$$

Determining cord dose (contribution from both fields)
A. Calculate the anterior dose contribution to the cord
Using the cord point (A) and D_{max} (B), we have depths of 17.0 cm and 1.5 cm, respectively.

$$\frac{\text{Dose}_{1.5\,cm}}{\text{PDD}_{1.5\,cm}} = \frac{\text{Dose}_{17\,cm}}{\text{PDD}_{17\,cm}}$$

$$\frac{\text{Dose}_{17\,cm}}{45.9} = \frac{149.9\ cGy}{100}$$

$$\text{Dose}_{17\,cm} = 68.8\ cGy$$

B. Calculate the posterior dose contribution to the cord
Using the cord point (A) and D_{max} point (B), we have depths of 3.0 cm and 1.5 cm, respectively.

$$\frac{\text{Dose}_{1.5\,cm}}{\text{PDD}_{1.5\,cm}} = \frac{\text{Dose}_{3\,cm}}{\text{PDD}_{3\,cm}}$$

$$\frac{\text{Dose}_{3\,cm}}{95.0} = \frac{149.9\ cGy}{100}$$

$$\text{Dose}_{3\,cm} = 142.4\ cGy$$

C. Add the anterior and posterior dose contributions to obtain the total cord dose

Cord dose (total) = Cord dose (anterior) + Cord dose (posterior)

Cord dose (total) = 68.8 cGy + 142.4 cGy

Cord dose (total) = 211.2 cGy

If this calculation were done on a cobalt 60 treatment machine (1.25 MeV) and compared to the preceding calculation, the following chart could be built:

Point of calculation	Cobalt 60	6 MV	% Difference
Total dose at D_{max}	232.5	212.3	9.5%
Total cord dose	218.9	211.2	3.7%
Total dose to mid-plane	200.0	200.0	0.0%

While the mid-plane dose is constant in both cases, the total doses to D_{max} and the cord are different for the two energies. The data demonstrate that the total dose at D_{max} and the cord dose are less for higher treatment energies. One of the advantages of using higher energy beams, especially for parallel opposed treatment field arrangements, is that the total dose at D_{max} will be significantly less. In this case the patient will receive approximately 3.7% less dose to the cord if a 6 MV beam is used instead of the cobalt 60 beam.

Treatment unit calculations general equation

When attempting to perform treatment unit calculations, we have seen that a number of variables must be considered. Field size variations, energy changes, and modifiers in the beam's path can alter the amount of radiation administered to a patient, as either an underdose or an overdose. While the complexity of each calculation varies within these parameters, there is one basic equation that addresses virtually every scenario. The general equation for performing monitor unit or treatment time calculation can be represented as follows:

$$\text{Monitor unit/Time setting} = \frac{\text{Dose at a point}}{\text{Dose rate at that point}}$$

The monitor unit setting represents the setting to be used on a linear accelerator, while the time setting represents the minutes for a cobalt 60 treatment unit. The dose at a point represents the prescribed dose as determined by the radiation oncologist. The dose rate at that point represents the dose rate of the treatment unit at the point of calculation. There are three general points necessary when performing a treatment calculation: (1) know the dose at a point, (2) know the dose rate at that point, and (3) the dose and dose rate must be in the same medium.

Normally the dose and dose rate will be expressed in air or tissue. If the dose is expressed in tissue and the dose rate in air, then we have an "apple and orange" situation. As a rule for simplifying these calculations, it is desirable to have the dose rate expressed in air when using TAR for the megavolt-

age setting calculation. It is also desirable to have the dose rate expressed in tissue when using PDD, TPR, or TMR for the mu setting calculation.

SOURCE TO SKIN DISTANCE (SSD) CALCULATIONS

An SSD setup occurs when the patient's skin surface is set up at the reference distance or isocenter distance. Therefore in an SSD setup the field size is defined on the patient's skin. The reference distance convention used in this chapter will be 80 cm SSD for cobalt 60 treatment machines and 100 cm for linear accelerators. Some older linear accelerators are designed for use at 80 cm target to skin distance. The output or dose rate of the machine for SSD setups should be expressed at the depth of D_{max}; the field size will be defined at the skin surface, and the dose rate will be measured in tissue at the depth of D_{max}.

To perform nonisocentric SSD calculations with either a cobalt 60 or a linear accelerator unit, a five-step process can be employed:

Step 1. Find the equivalent square of the collimator setting (used for output factor).
Step 2. Find the equivalent square of the blocked field size (used for PDD) if applicable.
Step 3. Using the appropriate tables, determine the PDD.
Step 4. Determine the prescribed dose.
Step 5. Use the appropriate equation for determining the treatment unit setting.

Cobalt 60 treatment machine nonisocentric calculations

Example 4: A patient is treated on the cobalt 60 treatment machine at 80 cm SSD to his thoracic spine. The patient is prone and will be treated through a single treatment field. The collimator setting is 10 cm × 10 cm. There is no blocking used for this treatment. The prescription states that a dose of 3000 cGy is to be delivered to a depth of 5 cm in 10 fractions. Calculate the treatment time.

This is the most basic calculation and involves only the reference dose rate, output factor, and PDD. Since there is no blocking used, the equivalent square for the collimator setting or actual field size is used to look up the output factor and PDD.

Step 1. Find the equivalent square of the collimator setting

The equivalent square of a 10 cm × 10 cm field is 10 cm × 10 cm.

Step 2. Find the equivalent square of the blocked field size

There is no blocking in this field. Therefore the blocked field size in equivalent square is the same as the collimator equivalent square.

Step 3. Using the appropriate tables, look up the dose rate factors

The factors for the dose rate at a point are reference dose rate, output factor, and tissue absorption factor, in this case, PDD. The following information can be obtained in the example data table located at the end of the chapter (Tables 11-3 through 11-17 on pages 230 to 243).

Reference dose rate = 51.7 cGy/min (Table 11-3 on p. 230)

Output factor (10 cm × 10 cm) = 1.000 (Table 11-4 on p. 231)

PDD (5,10,80) = 78.3 (Table 11-6 on p. 232)

Step 4. Determine the prescribed dose

From the prescription, the total prescribed dose to a depth of 5 cm is 3000 cGy. This dose is to be delivered in 10 fractions. Therefore the dose per fraction is 300 cGy. To obtain the dose per fraction, you divide the total dose by the number of fractions, as follows:

$$\text{Dose per fraction} = \frac{\text{Total prescribed dose}}{\text{Number of fractions}}$$

$$\text{Dose per fraction} = \frac{3000 \text{ cGy}}{10 \text{ fractions}}$$

$$\text{Dose per fraction} = 300 \text{ cGy}$$

$$\text{Dose per treatment field} = \frac{\text{Dose per fraction}}{\text{Number of fields}}$$

$$\text{Dose per treatment field} = \frac{300 \text{ cGy}}{1}$$

$$\text{Dose per treatment field} = 300 \text{ cGy}$$

Step 5. Use the appropriate equation for determining the treatment setting

$$\text{Time setting} = \frac{\text{Dose at a point}}{\text{Dose rate at that point}}, \text{ so}$$

$$\text{Time setting} = \frac{\text{Prescribed dose}}{\text{Output} \times \text{Output factor} \times \frac{\text{PDD}}{100}}$$

$$\text{Time setting} = \frac{300 \text{ cGy}}{51.7 \text{ cGy/min} \times 1.00 \times \frac{78.3}{100}}$$

$$\text{Time setting} = \frac{300 \text{ cGy}}{40.4811 \text{ cGy/min}}$$

$$\text{Time setting} = 7.41 \text{ min}$$

The treatment unit would have to be set for 7.41 min to treat a 10 cm × 10 cm field size at 80 cm SSD to deliver 300 cGy to a depth of 5 cm.

Example 5: A patient is treated on the cobalt 60 treatment machine at 80 cm SSD to his thoracic spine. The patient is prone and will be treated through a single treatment field. The collimator setting is 15 cm × 15 cm. There is no blocking used for this treatment. The prescription states that a dose of 3000 cGy is to be delivered to a depth of 5 cm in 10 fractions.

Example 5 is essentially the same setup as Example 4. The only difference is that the collimator setting has changed. In this setting, the output factor and PDD will change.

Step 1. Find the equivalent square of the collimator setting

The equivalent square of a 15 cm × 15 cm field is 15 cm × 15 cm.

Step 2. Find the equivalent square of the blocked field size

There is no blocking in this field. Therefore the blocked field size in equivalent square is the same as the collimator equivalent square, that is, 15 cm × 15 cm.

Step 3. Using the appropriate tables, look up the dose rate factors

The factors for the dose rate at a point are reference dose rate, output factor, and PDD, as follows:

Reference dose rate = 51.7 cGy/min (Table 11-3 on p. 230)

Output factor (15 × 15) = 1.046 (Table 11-4 on p. 231)

PDD (5,15,80) = 80.7 (Table 11-6 on p. 232)

Note that the reference dose rate is the same in both examples. This is because the reference dose rate is always the dose rate for the 10 cm × 10 cm collimator setting. The reference dose rate is multiplied by the output factor of the actual collimator setting to correct for the variance from the standard. This takes the different amount of scatter into account. Also note that both the output factor and the PDD have increased in Example 5 because of increased scatter from the larger collimator surface and larger volume of tissue treated.

Step 4. Determine the prescribed dose

The dose per fraction is 300 cGy.

Step 5. Use the appropriate equation for determining the treatment setting

$$\text{Time setting} = \frac{\text{Prescribed dose}}{\text{Output} \times \text{Output factor} \times \frac{\text{PDD}}{100}}$$

$$\text{Time setting} = \frac{300 \text{ cGy}}{51.7 \text{ cGy/min} \times 1.046 \times \frac{80.7}{100}}$$

$$\text{Time setting} = \frac{300 \text{ cGy}}{40.6411 \text{ cGy/min}}$$

$$\text{Time setting} = 6.87 \text{ min}$$

The time setting has decreased from Example 4 to Example 5 because of the increased scatter increasing the dose rate at the point of calculation. Since the dose rate has increased, the time necessary to deliver the dose will decrease. This is similar to driving a car. If a person needs to travel 300 miles and drives at 50 miles per hour, the trip will take 6 hours. However, if the driving speed is increased to 60 miles/hr, the driving time will be reduced to 5 hours.

Example 6: A patient is treated on the cobalt 60 treatment machine at 80 cm SSD to his thoracic spine. The patient is prone and will be treated through a single treatment field.

The collimator setting is 15 cm × 15 cm. The field is blocked to an 8 cm × 8 cm blocked equivalent square. A 5 mm solid plastic tray is used to hold the blocks. The prescription states that a dose of 3000 cGy is to be delivered to a depth of 5 cm in 10 fractions. Calculate the treatment time.

In example 6, blocks are added to the treatment field. This makes the calculation slightly more complex. The reference dose rate will remain unchanged. The output factor is a combination of the scatter from the collimator and the scatter from the phantom or patient. While the blocking has little effect on the collimator scatter, it does affect the phantom scatter. One approach for correcting the measured output factors is to take out the phantom scatter for the collimator setting and then put back in the phantom scatter for the blocked field size. To accomplish this, the output factor is multiplied by the ratio of the BSF. The output factor for the equivalent square of the collimator setting (15 cm × 15 cm) is multiplied by the BSF (or PSF) of the blocked equivalent square and divided by the BSF of the collimator setting equivalent square. There are other solutions to this problem of handling the effect of blocking on the output factor. There is also a change in the PDD because the blocks have affected the area or amount of tissue being treated. In this case the area of tissue treated has been reduced to less than the 15 cm × 15 cm collimator setting. If less tissue is irradiated, then there will be a decrease in scatter. Therefore the PDD will be decreased. The equivalent square of the blocked field size is used to look up the PDD.

Step 1. Find the equivalent square of the collimator setting

The equivalent square of a 15 cm × 15 cm field is 15 cm × 15 cm

Step 2. Find the equivalent square of the blocked field size

There is blocking in this field. Therefore the blocked field size equivalent square is 8 cm × 8 cm.

Step 3. Using the appropriate tables, look up the dose rate factors

The factors for the dose rate at a point are reference dose rate, output factor, PDD, and tray factor. Since there is blocking, a PSF is needed.

Reference dose rate = 51.7 cGy/min (Table 11-3 on p. 230)

Output factor (15 × 15) = 1.046 (Table 11-4 on p. 231)

PDD (5,8,80) = 76.9 (Table 11-6 on p. 232)

PSF (8 × 8) = 1.028 (Table 11-6 on p. 232)

PSF (15 × 15) = 1.051 (Table 11-6 on p. 232)

Tray factor = 0.96 (Table 11-17 on p. 243)

Step 4. Determine the prescribed dose

The dose per fraction is 300 cGy.

Step 5. Use the appropriate equation for determining the treatment setting

Note that the basic equation has been modified to account for tray factor and PSF, since both are needed to accurately calculate the time setting in the following example:

Time setting =

$$\frac{\text{Prescribed dose}}{\text{Output} \times \text{Output factor} \times \frac{\text{PSF}_{(EFS)}}{\text{PSF}_{(CS)}} \times \frac{\text{PDD}}{100} \times \text{Tray factor}}$$

$$\text{Time setting} = \frac{300 \text{ cGy}}{51.7 \text{ cGy/min} \times 1.046 \times \frac{1.028}{1.051} \times \frac{76.9}{100} \times 0.96}$$

$$\text{Time setting} = \frac{300 \text{ cGy}}{39.049 \text{ cGy/min}}$$

Time setting = 7.68 min

The treatment time has increased because the dose rate is decreasing. The decrease in dose rate was caused by two factors. First, the PDD was decreased because of the blocked field size and therefore less scatter radiation. Second, the blocking tray attenuated some of the radiation. To compensate for the attenuation by the blocking tray, the time setting had to increase. A tray factor of 0.96 means that there is approximately 4% attenuation by the tray. Another way to look at this tray factor is that the time setting will need to be increased by approximately 4% to compensate for the radiation attenuated by the tray.

Example 7: A patient is treated on the cobalt 60 treatment machine at 80 cm SSD. The collimator setting is 15 cm × 15 cm. The field is blocked to an 8 cm × 8 cm blocked equivalent square. A 5 mm solid plastic tray is used to hold the blocks. The prescription states that a dose of 4000 cGy is to be delivered to a depth of 10 cm in 20 fractions using an anterior and posterior (AP:PA) treatment field arrangement.

Example 7 is similar to Example 6; however, in Example 7 the patient is going to be treated using more than one treatment field. The fields are equally weighted, meaning that the same dosage is administered through each portal. The treatment setting for each treatment field should be done individually.

Step 1. Find the equivalent square of the collimator setting

The equivalent square of a 15 cm × 15 cm field is 15 cm × 15 cm.

Step 2. Find the equivalent square of the blocked field size

There is blocking in this field. Therefore the blocked field size equivalent square is 8 cm × 8 cm.

Step 3. Using the appropriate tables, look up the dose rate factors

The factors for the dose rate at a point are reference dose rate, output factor, PDD, and tray factor.

Reference dose rate = 51.7 cGy/min (Table 11-3 on p. 230)

Output factor (15 × 15) = 1.046 (Table 11-4 on p. 231)

PDD (10,8,80) = 54.5 (Table 11-6 on p. 232)

PSF (8 × 8) = 1.028 (Table 11-6 on p. 232)

PSF (15 × 15) = 1.051 (Table 11-6 on p. 232)

Tray factor (TF) = 0.96 (Table 11-17 on p. 243)

Step 4. Determine the prescribed dose

From the prescription, the total prescribed dose to a depth of 10 cm is 4000 cGy. This dose is to be delivered in 20 fractions. Therefore the dose per fraction is 200 cGy. Since there are two treatment fields that will get the same dose, the dose per treatment field is 100 cGy.

Step 5. Use the appropriate equation for determining the treatment setting

Time setting =

$$\frac{\text{Prescribed dose}}{\text{Output} \times \text{Output factor} \times \frac{\text{PSF}_{(EFS)}}{\text{PSF}_{(CS)}} \times \frac{\text{PDD}}{100} \times \text{Tray factor}}$$

$$\text{Time setting} = \frac{100 \text{ cGy}}{51.7 \text{ cGy/min} \times 1.046 \times \frac{1.028}{1.051} \times \frac{54.5}{100} \times 0.96}$$

$$\text{Time setting} = \frac{100 \text{ cGy}}{27.6745 \text{ cGy/min}}$$

Time setting = 3.61 min

The time setting will be 3.61 minutes for the anterior field and 3.61 minutes for the posterior field.

The treatment time for the cobalt 60 machine is given in real time (that is, minutes). The dose rate for the cobalt 60 machine is defined in centigrays per minute. Real time is used with the cobalt 60 machine because the dose rate is caused by the radioactive decay of the cobalt 60 isotope. The half-life of cobalt 60 is approximately 5.3 years. This means that after 5.3 years, the dose rate of the cobalt 60 machine will be half of its original dose rate. For example, if the dose rate of the cobalt 60 machine is 50 cGy/min today, then the dose rate will be 25 cGy/min 5.3 years from today. As the dose rate decreases, the time it takes to deliver the prescribed dose increases.

Since the rate of decay for the cobalt 60 machine is relatively slow, it can be assumed that the dose rate is constant over a short period of time. The time frame for this constant dose rate is 1 month. This means that every month the minute settings used to treat the patient with the cobalt 60 machine must be adjusted. The rate of adjustment is approximately 1.1% each month. The following equation can be used to make the monthly adjustment in the minute setting for patients who are already on treatment:

New minute setting = Old minute setting × 1.01

If it takes 2.00 minutes to deliver 100 cGy on January 1, then it will take 2.02 minutes to deliver 100 cGy on February 1. Also, because of the slow decay or long half-life, the dose rate of the cobalt 60 machine is constant for a given treatment.

LINEAR ACCELERATOR NONISOCENTRIC MONITOR UNIT (MU) SETTING CALCULATIONS

The major difference in the time setting calculation for the cobalt 60 machine and the monitor unit setting calculation for the linear accelerator is in the measurement of the reference dose rate. The reference dose rate for the cobalt 60 treatment machine is measured in centigrays per minute while the reference dose rate for the linear accelerator is measured in centigrays per monitor unit.

In looking at the dose rate for the linear accelerator, it might be helpful to look at a simple time, distance, and speed calculation. The following formula can be used to calculate the time it takes to drive a given distance:

$$\text{Time} = \frac{\text{Distance}}{\text{Speed}}$$

If a driver makes a 450-mile trip, driving the entire distance at exactly 50 miles per hour, it will take exactly 9 hours to complete the trip.

$$\text{Time} = \frac{450 \text{ miles}}{50 \text{ miles/hr}}$$

Time = 9 hours

No matter how many times this trip is made, it will take us 9 hours as long as a constant speed of 50 miles/hr is maintained. This type of constant speed (dose rate) happens in the cobalt 60 machine and is the principle behind the cobalt 60 time setting calculation. In the linear accelerator, the dose rate varies slightly from one moment to the next. If the dose from the linear accelerator were measured using real time, the dose could be different each time. Therefore real time cannot be used to deliver the prescribed dose with a linear accelerator. Instead, a different system of time called the monitor unit (MU) is used. Normally the dose rate for the linear accelerator is 1.0 cGy/MU for a 10 cm × 10 cm field size defined at the isocenter.

Linear accelerator nonisocentric calculations

The parameters for examples of cobalt 60 will be repeated for the linear accelerator. The same trends seen between the cobalt 60 calculations will be noted in the linear accelerator calculations.

Example 8: A patient is treated on the 6 MV linear accelerator at 100 cm SSD. The collimator setting is 10 cm × 10 cm. There is no blocking used for this treatment. The prescription states that a dose of 3000 cGy is to be delivered to a depth of 5 cm in 10 fractions. Calculate the MU setting.

The factors for the dose rate at a point are reference dose rate, output factor, and PDD.

Reference dose rate = 0.993 cGy/MU (Table 11-3 on p. 230)

Output factor (10 × 10) = 1.000 (Table 11-4 on p. 231)

PDD (5,10,100) = 87.1 (Table 11-7 on p. 233)

$$\text{MU setting} = \frac{\text{Prescribed dose}}{\text{Output} \times \text{Output factor} \times \dfrac{\text{PDD}}{100}}$$

$$\text{MU setting} = \frac{300 \text{ cGy}}{0.993 \text{ cGy/MU} \times 1.00 \times \dfrac{87.1}{100}}$$

$$\text{MU setting} = \frac{300 \text{ cGy}}{0.8649 \text{ cGy/MU}}$$

MU setting = 347 MU

Example 9: A patient is treated on the 6 MV linear accelerator at 100 cm SSD. The collimator setting is 15 cm × 15 cm. There is no blocking used for this treatment. The prescription states that a dose of 3000 cGy is to be delivered to a depth of 5 cm in 10 fractions. Calculate the MU setting.

The factors for the dose rate at a point are reference dose rate, output factor, and PDD.

Reference dose rate = 0.993 cGy/MU (Table 11-4 on p. 231)

Output factor (15 × 15) = 1.035 (Table 11-4 on p. 231)

PDD (5,15,100) = 87.9 (Table 11-7 on p. 233)

$$\text{MU setting} = \frac{\text{Prescribed dose}}{\text{Output} \times \text{Output factors} \times \dfrac{\text{PDD}}{100}}$$

$$\text{MU setting} = \frac{300 \text{ cGy}}{0.993 \text{ cGy/MU} \times 1.035 \times \dfrac{87.9}{100}}$$

$$\text{MU setting} = \frac{300 \text{ cGy}}{0.9034 \text{ cGy/MU}}$$

MU setting = 332 MU

Note that the MU setting is lower in Example 11-9 when compared to Example 8. This change is caused by the increase in field size and scatter component.

Example 10: A patient is treated on the 6 MV linear accelerator at 100 cm SSD. The collimator setting is 15 cm × 15 cm. The field is blocked to an 8 cm × 8 cm blocked equivalent square. A 5 mm solid plastic tray is used to hold the blocks. The prescription states that a dose of 3000 cGy is to be delivered to a depth of 5 cm in 10 fractions.

The factors for the dose rate at a point are reference dose rate, output factor, PSF, and PDD.

Reference dose rate = 0.993 cGy/MU (Table 11-3 on p. 230)

Output factor (15 × 15) = 1.035 (Table 11-4 on p. 231)

PDD (5,8,100) = 86.8 (Table 11-7 on p. 233)

PSF (15 × 15) = 1.039 (Table 11-7)

PSF (8 × 8) = 1.016 (Table 11-7)

Tray factor = 0.97 (Table 11-17)

MU setting =

$$\frac{\text{Prescribed dose}}{\text{Output} \times \text{Output factor} \times \dfrac{\text{PSF}_{(EFS)}}{\text{PSF}_{(CS)}} \times \dfrac{\text{PDD}}{100} \times \text{Tray factor}}$$

$$\text{MU setting} = \frac{300 \text{ cGy}}{0.993 \text{ cGy/MU} \times 1.035 \times \dfrac{1.016}{1.039} \times \dfrac{86.8}{100} \times 0.97}$$

$$\text{MU setting} = \frac{300 \text{ cGy}}{0.8462 \text{ cGy/MU}}$$

MU setting = 355 MU

Example 11: A patient is treated on the 6 MV linear accelerator at 100 cm SSD. The collimator setting is 15 cm × 15 cm. The field is blocked to an 8 cm × 8 cm blocked equivalent square. A 5 mm solid plastic tray is used to hold the blocks. The prescription states that a dose of 4000 cGy is to be delivered to a depth of 10 cm in 20 fractions using an anterior and posterior (AP:PA) treatment field arrangement.

The factors for the dose rate at a point are reference dose rate, output factor, PSF, PDD, and tray factor.

Reference dose rate = 0.993 cGy per MU (Table 11-3 on p. 230)

Output factor (15 × 15) = 1.035 (Table 11-4 on p. 231)

PDD (10,8,100) = 66.7 (Table 11-7 on p. 233)

PSF (15 × 15) = 1.039 (Table 11-7)

PSF (8 × 8) = 1.016 (Table 11-7)

Tray factor = 0.97 (Table 11-17 on p. 243)

MU setting =

$$\frac{\text{Prescribed dose}}{\text{Output} \times \text{Output factor} \times \dfrac{\text{PSF}_{(EFS)}}{\text{PSF}_{(CS)}} \times \dfrac{\text{PDD}}{100} \times \text{Tray factor}}$$

$$\text{MU setting} = \frac{100 \text{ cGy}}{0.993 \text{ cGy/MU} \times 1.035 \times \dfrac{1.016}{1.039} \times \dfrac{66.7}{100} \times 0.97}$$

$$\text{MU setting} = \frac{100 \text{ cGy}}{0.6502 \text{ cGy/MU}}$$

MU setting = 154 MU for each port

EXTENDED DISTANCE CALCULATIONS USING PDD AND SSD SETUP

There are occasions when large areas of a patient's body must be treated that are larger than the collimator areas achievable by conventional radiation therapy treatment units.

This is the case in total body irradiation, total skin fields, and some mantle field arrangements. In these cases, larger field areas are possible by extending the distance of the treatment area. Because of divergence, as the distance from the source increases, the field size increases. In this manner, very large areas can be treated in a single field. The alternative would be to split the treatment fields up into areas that could be accommodated at conventional distances. When arrangements like these are done, we are treating at *extended distances*. For example, the isocenter on a cobalt 60 treatment unit is 80 cm. In a standard SSD setup the patient is treated at 80 cm SSD. However, to set up a larger field, the patient may be set up at 100 cm SSD. An extended distance setup is one where the patient is set up at a distance beyond the isocenter or reference distance.[8]

In performing this type of calculation, several points must be considered. PDD is used for the calculation because its arrangement is nonisocentric. PDD depends on four factors: energy, field size, depth, and SSD. If any of these factors change, the PDD changes. If the energy is increased from cobalt 60 (1.25 MeV) to 6 MV, the PDD increases because of increased penetrating power. If the field size, at a given energy, changes from 10 cm × 10 cm to 15 cm × 15 cm, the PDD increases because of an increase in scatter. If the depth is increased from 6 cm to 10 cm, the PDD will decrease, since more attenuation and beam absorption occur. As the SSD is increased the PDD will increase due to a change in the inverse square law with a change in distance and because of an increase in scatter. As a result of these changes, special considerations must be employed to calculate treatment times and monitor units at extended distances.

Mayneord's factor

Mayneord's factor is an application of the inverse square law. There are many forms of Mayneord's factor used by different authors. This chapter will present a method where formula memorization is not necessary. If it is understood where the numbers for Mayneord's factor are derived from, they will always be able to correctly apply the numbers.

Reference or standard distance PDD values are determined from direct measurement. When patients are treated at an extended distance, the distance from the source of radiation to the depth of D_{max} and the depth of the calculation point changes. Note that the distances change and not the depths. If a patient is treated on a cobalt 60 unit with a 10 cm × 10 cm field size at 80 SSD to a depth of 10 cm and the distance is extended to 100 SSD, the level of D_{max} and the point of calculation remain the same; the depths are 0.5 cm and 10 cm, respectively. However, the distance to these points for a 100 cm SSD setup will be 100.5 cm and 110 cm, respectively.

There are other factors to consider. The energy of the treatment machine is the same in the standard and extended distance setup. Cobalt 60 has the same energy at 100 cm as

it does at 80 cm. If the field size was 10 cm × 10 cm in both cases and the depth of calculation is 10 cm for both setups, these factors should have little or no effect on the calculation. Since the 10 cm × 10 cm field was defined on the skin in both setups, the field size at the calculation point will be slightly different because of divergence. This would slightly change the amount of scatter. The major change will result from the change in distance. The original distances from source to D_{max} and depth were 80.5 and 90 cm, respectively. These distances should be removed from the measured PDD by multiplying by the inverse, as follows:

$$\frac{(90)^2}{(80.5)^2}$$

Then the correct distance is used in the calculation by multiplying by the square of the ratio of the new distances:

$$\frac{(100.5)^2}{(110)^2}$$

This allows for the correct attenuation of the beam for the new distances. These derived correction factors are then multiplied by the PDD referenced from the table, the result being the new PDD for the extended distances.

This PDD correction holds true for higher energy linear accelerators as well. A 6 MV linear accelerator has D_{max} of 1.5 cm and the standard setup distance is 100 cm. An extended distance of 125 cm is to be used to treat a patient. The depth of calculation is 8 cm. Mayneord's factor can be calculated using these distances. Note that the depth of D_{max} is 1.5 cm for a 6 MV linear accelerator and is reflected in the numbers. The PDD (8,10,100) is 75.1%.

The original distances were 101.5 cm and 108 cm.
The new distances are 126.5 cm and 133 cm.

$$\text{New PDD}_{(8,10,125)} = 75.1\% \times \frac{(108)^2}{(101.5)^2} \times \frac{(126.5)^2}{(133)^2}$$

$$\text{New PDD} = 76.9\%$$

Again, Mayneord's factor is an inverse square correction of the PDD. It can also be used in shortened treatment distances. It should be noted that Mayneord's factor does not account for changes in scatter because of a change in beam divergence. Therefore Mayneord's factor gives us the approximate value for the new PDD. To obtain the exact value for the new PDD, actual beam measurements using an ionization chamber or other appropriate devices would be necessary.

The following example uses the Mayneord's factor in the calculation of a treatment time for a cobalt 60 unit. The same principles would be used in finding monitor units for a linear accelerator operated at an extended distance.

Example 11: A patient is treated on the cobalt 60 treatment machine at an extended distance of 100 cm. The collimator setting is 20 cm × 20 cm, and the field size on the patient's skin is 25 cm × 25 cm. The prescription states that a dose of 3000 cGy is to be delivered to a depth of 5 cm in 10 fractions using a single posterior treatment field arrangement. Calculate the time setting.

We can use a similar process for extended distance calculations. We will use the same five steps discussed earlier and add a sixth step for Mayneord's factor.

Step 1. Find the equivalent square of the collimator setting (used for output factor)

The collimator setting is 20 cm × 20 cm, which is conveniently the equivalent square.

Step 2. Find the equivalent square of the blocked field size (used for PDD)

The field size at the setup SSD of 100 cm is 25 cm × 25 cm. The equivalent square of a 25 × 25 cm field is 25 cm × 25 cm.

Step 3. Using the appropriate tables, look up the dose rate factors

Reference dose rate = 51.7 cGy/min (Table 11-3 on p. 230)

Output factor (20 × 20) = 1.081 (Table 11-4 on p. 231)

PDD (5,25,80) = 82.15 (Table 11-6 on p. 232)

PSF (20 × 20) = 1.063 (Table 11-6)

PSF (25 × 25) = 1.0715 (Table 11-6)

Step 4. Determine the prescribed dose

The prescribed dose is 3000 cGy in 10 fractions. Therefore the daily prescribed dose is 300 cGy/fraction.

Step 5. Calculate the new PDDs using Mayneord's factor

Determine the PDD at a depth of 5 cm:

$$\text{New PDD}_{(5,25,100)} = 82.15\% \times \frac{(85)^2}{(80.5)^2} \times \frac{(100.5)^2}{(105)^2}$$

$$\text{New PDD} = 83.91\%$$

Step 6. Use the appropriate equation for determining the time setting

The equation to be used is again a variation of dose divided by dose rate. The dose rate is affected by the factors mentioned in the problem. Since the treatment is at an extended distance, the intensity of the beam is affected by the inverse square law, just as the PDD was. While the PDD increased because of increased scatter, the intensity of the beam would decrease because of the increased distance. The correction relates the distance from the source to the point of treatment unit calibration (where referenced data were measured) and the treatment SSD plus D_{max}. The inverse square correction would then be included as a dose rate correction in the denominator of the equation. It may be written as follows:

$$\text{Inverse square correction} = \frac{(\text{Reference source calibration distance})^2}{(\text{Treatment SSD} + D_{max})^2}$$

The treatment time can now be calculated, as follows:

$$\text{Time setting} = \frac{\text{Prescribed dose}}{\text{Output} \times \text{Output factor} \times \text{Inverse square correction} \times \frac{\text{PSF}_{(EFS)}}{\text{PSF}_{(CS)}} \times \frac{\text{PDD}}{100}}$$

$$\text{Time setting} = \frac{300 \text{ cGy}}{51.7 \text{ cGy/min} \times 1.081 \times \frac{(80.5)^2}{(100.5)^2} \times \frac{1.0715}{1.063} \times \frac{83.91}{100}}$$

$$\text{Time setting} = \frac{300 \text{ cGy}}{30.3283 \text{ cGy/min}}$$

$$\text{Time setting} = 9.89 \text{ min}$$

SOURCE-TO-AXIS DISTANCE (SAD) CALCULATIONS

An SAD treatment occurs when the treatment machine's isocenter is established at some reference point inside the patient. When this is established, it can also be referred to as an isocentric technique. Since the field size is defined at the isocenter, the collimated field matches the field size setting inside the patient and not on the skin surface as seen in the nonisocentric, SSD treatment setup.

One advantage that SAD treatment techniques have over SSD techniques is that when the patient has been properly positioned and the isocenter for the treatment has been established, there is usually no movement of the patient relative to the treatment isocenter for each of the subsequent treatment field. For example, a patient treated using an anterior and posterior treatment field arrangement on a 6 MV, 100 cm isocentric linear accelerator. The patient's central axis separation is 20 cm, and the dose is calculated at the patient's mid-plane (equal distance established from both anterior and posterior skin surfaces). If we were to treat this arrangement with an SSD technique, the anterior field would be established at 100 cm to the anterior skin surface. After treating the anterior field, the gantry would be rotated 180° to treat the posterior field. However, the treatment table would have to be raised until the optical distance indicator reads 100 cm on the patient's posterior skin surface.

In treating the same patient with an SAD (isocentric) technique, the anterior SSD would be established at 90 cm. The isocenter is positioned 10 cm beneath the anterior skin surface and 10 cm beneath the posterior skin surface, making it mid-plane as prescribed. (Note that the 10 cm anterior depth and 10 cm posterior depth add up to the 20 cm central axis separation.) The SAD is 100 cm (90 cm SSD plus 10 cm depth). After treating the anterior field the gantry would be rotated 180° to treat the posterior field. However, in an isocentric technique, the gantry is rotating about the isocenter, which has been established inside the patient. Therefore the patient is at the correct posterior SSD of 90 cm without raising or lowering the treatment table. Less movement between treatment fields lowers the chance of having treatment errors because of positioning variations that occur during patient movement.

TAR, TMR, and TPR work very well with isocentric techniques. PDD can also be used for isocentric treatment techniques. There are two main differences from PDD that will affect calculations using TAR, both caused by the way PDD and TAR are calculated. PDD is calculated from two measurements at two different points in space. TAR is calculated using two measurements at the same point in space. This affects the beam geometry, field divergence, and application of the inverse square law.

First, when using TAR for calculations, the field size at the point of calculation must be used. Under some conditions the field size at the point of interest must be determined. One example would be when trying to determine a dose delivered to points other than the isocenter along the central axis. In this case the treatment field size at the alternate point would change because of beam divergence and would need to be calculated. Another effect on the calculation involves the application of the inverse square law. There will be an inverse square correction needed when calculating the dose to a point other than the isocenter. These points will be covered in greater detail in the example problems.

ISOCENTRIC CALCULATION PROCESS

The same basic five-step process described earlier in the section on nonisocentric calculations involving PDD is used in the isocentric technique:

Step 1. Find the equivalent square of the collimator setting (used for output factor).

Step 2. Find the equivalent square of the blocked field size (used for TAR, TMR, or TPR).

Step 3. Using the appropriate tables, look up the dose rate factors.

Step 4. Determine the prescribed dose.

Step 5. Use the appropriate equation for determining the time setting.

Several examples will be performed using both cobalt 60 and linear accelerator treatment units.

Cobalt 60 isocentric calculations

Example 13: A patient is treated on the cobalt 60 treatment machine at 80 cm SAD. A single field is used with the collimator setting of 15 cm × 15 cm. There is no blocking used for this treatment. The prescription states that a dose of 3000 cGy is to be delivered to a depth of 5 cm in 10 fractions. Calculate the treatment time.

Step 1. Find the equivalent square of the collimator setting

The equivalent square of a 15 cm × 15 cm field is 15 cm × 15 cm.

Step 2. Find the equivalent square of the blocked field size

There is no blocking in this field. Therefore the blocked field size equivalent square is the same as the collimator equivalent square.

Step 3. Using the appropriate tables, look up the dose rate factors

The factors for the dose rate at a point are reference dose rate, output factor, and TAR (TAR is commonly used in lower therapeutic isocentric calculations)

Reference dose rate = 50.6 cGy/min (Table 11-3 on p. 230)

Output factor (15 × 15) = 1.030 (Table 11-4 on p. 231)

TAR (5,15) = 0.941 (Table 11-10 on p. 236)

(The reference dose rate is modified by multiplying it by the output factor of the actual collimator setting.)

Step 4. Determine the prescribed dose

From the prescription the total prescribed dose to a depth of 5 cm is 3000 cGy. This dose is to be delivered in 10 fractions. Therefore the dose per fraction is 300 cGy.

Step 5. Use the appropriate equation for determining the time setting

$$\text{Time setting} = \frac{\text{Dose at a point}}{\text{Dose rate at that point}}, \text{ so}$$

$$\text{Time setting} = \frac{\text{Prescribed dose}}{\text{Output} \times \text{Output factor}_{(CS)} \times \text{TAR}_{(EFS)}}$$

$$\text{Time setting} = \frac{300 \text{ cGy}}{50.6 \text{ cGy/min} \times 1.03 \times 0.941}$$

$$\text{Time setting} = \frac{300 \text{ cGy}}{49.043 \text{ cGy/min}}$$

$$\text{Time setting} = 6.12 \text{ min}$$

Example 14: A patient is treated on the cobalt 60 treatment machine at 80 cm SAD. The setup SSD is 75 cm. A single treatment field is used with a collimator setting of 15 cm × 15 cm. The field is blocked to an 8 cm × 8 cm blocked equivalent square. A 5 mm solid plastic tray is used to hold the blocks. The prescription states that a dose of 3000 cGy is to be delivered to a depth of 5 cm in 10 fractions. Calculate the treatment time.

In Example 14, shielding blocks are added to the treatment field, making the time setting calculation slightly more complex. The reference dose and output factor rate will not change in this example from Example 13. However, there is a change in the TAR. The area of tissue treated has been reduced to less than the 15 cm × 15 cm collimator setting, decreasing the scatter. The factors for the dose rate at a point are reference dose rate, output factor, TAR, and tray factor.

Reference dose rate = 50.6 cGy per minute

Output factor (15 × 15) = 1.030

TAR (5,8) = 0.876

Tray factor = 0.96

$$\text{Time setting} = \frac{\text{Prescribed dose}}{\text{Output} \times \text{Output factor}_{(CS) \text{ collimator setting}} \times \text{TAR}_{(EFS)} \times \text{TF}}$$

$$\text{Time setting} = \frac{300 \text{ cGy}}{50.6 \text{ cGy/min} \times 1.03 \times 0.876 \times 0.96}$$

$$\text{Time setting} = \frac{300 \text{ cGy}}{43.8292 \text{ cGy/min}}$$

Time setting = 6.84 min

Example 15: A patient is treated on the cobalt 60 treatment machine at 80 cm SAD. The collimator setting is 15 cm × 15 cm. The field is blocked to an 8 cm × 8 cm blocked equivalent square. A 5 mm solid plastic tray is used to hold the blocks. The prescription states that a dose of 4000 cGy is to be delivered to a depth of 10 cm in 20 fractions using an anterior and posterior (AP:PA) equally weighted treatment field arrangement. Calculate the time setting.

The factors for the dose rate at a point are reference dose rate, output factor, TAR, and tray factor.

Reference dose rate = 50.6 cGy/min

Output factor (15 × 15) = 1.030

TAR (10,8) = 0.687

Tray factor = 0.96

$$\text{Time setting} = \frac{\text{Prescribed dose}}{\text{Output} \times \text{Output factor}_{(CS)} \times \text{TAR}_{(EFS)} \times \text{TF}}$$

$$\text{Time setting} = \frac{100 \text{ cGy}}{50.6 \text{ cGy/min} \times 1.03 \times 0.687 \times 0.96}$$

$$\text{Time setting} = \frac{100 \text{ cGy}}{34.373 \text{ cGy/min}}$$

Time setting = 2.91 min/port

Linear accelerator isocentric calculations

Example 16: A patient is treated on the 6 MV linear accelerator treatment machine at 100 cm SAD. The setup SSD is 95 cm. The collimator setting is 15 cm × 15 cm. The field is blocked to an 8 cm × 8 cm blocked equivalent square. A 5 mm solid plastic tray is used to hold the blocks. The prescription states that a dose of 3000 cGy is to be delivered to a depth of 5 cm in 10 fractions through a single field. Calculate the MU setting using TAR.

The factors for the dose rate at a point are reference dose rate, output factor, TAR, and tray factor.

Reference dose rate = 1.0 cGy/MU

Output factor (15 × 15) = 1.021

TAR (5,8) = 0.941

Tray factor = 0.97

$$\text{MU setting} = \frac{\text{Prescribed dose}}{\text{Output} \times \text{Output factor}_{(CS)} \times \text{TAR}_{(EFS)} \times \text{TF}}$$

$$\text{MU setting} = \frac{300 \text{ cGy}}{1.0 \text{ cGy/MU} \times 1.021 \times 0.941 \times 0.97}$$

$$\text{MU setting} = \frac{300 \text{ cGy}}{0.9319 \text{ cGy/MU}}$$

MU setting = 322 MU

Example 17: A patient is treated on the 6 MV linear accelerator treatment machine at 100 cm SAD. The setup SSD is 90 cm. The collimator setting is 15 cm × 15 cm. The field is blocked to an 8 cm × 8 cm blocked equivalent square. A 5 mm solid plastic tray is used to hold the blocks. The prescription states that a dose of 4000 cGy is to be delivered to a depth of 10 cm in 20 fractions using an anterior and posterior (AP:PA) treatment field arrangement. Calculate the MU setting using TAR.

The factors for the dose rate at a point are reference dose rate, output factor, TAR, and tray factor.

Reference dose rate = 1.0 cGy/MU

Output factor (15 × 15) = 1.021

TAR (10,8) = 0.787

Tray factor = 0.97

Prescribed dose = 100 cGy/field

$$\text{MU setting} = \frac{\text{Prescribed dose}}{\text{Output} \times \text{Output factor}_{(CS)} \times \text{TAR}_{(EFS)} \times \text{TF}}$$

$$\text{MU setting} = \frac{100 \text{ cGy}}{1.0 \text{ cGy/MU} \times 1.021 \times 0.787 \times 0.97}$$

$$\text{MU setting} = \frac{100 \text{ cGy}}{0.7794 \text{ cGy/MU}}$$

MU setting = 128 MU/field

When high energy linear accelerators are used (energies above 10 MV), tissue maximum ratio and tissue phantom ratio are commonly used in the isocentric MU calculations as opposed to tissue air ratio.

When TMR or TPR is used for dose calculation, the output for the 10 cm × 10 cm field size is normally 1.0 cGy/MU. In the TMR calculations presented in this chapter, two output factors will be used. One of the output factors corrects for collimator scatter and is commonly referred to as the collimator output factor (COF). The other output factor corrects for patient scatter and is often called the phantom scatter factor (PSF). The total output factor is obtained by multiplying the COF by the PSF.

Example 18: A patient is treated on the 6 MV linear accelerator treatment machine at 100 cm SAD. The setup SSD is 95 cm. The collimator setting is 15 cm × 15 cm. There is no blocking used for this treatment. The prescription states that a dose of 3000 cGy is to be delivered to a depth of

5 cm in 10 fractions through a single field. Calculate the MU setting using TMR.

The factors for the dose rate at a point are reference dose rate, output factor, and TMR.

Reference dose rate = 1.0 cGy/MU (Table 11-3 on p. 230)

COF (15 × 15) = 1.021 (Table 11-4 on p. 231)

PSF (15 × 15) = 1.014 (Table 11-5 on p. 231)

TMR (5,15) = 0.937 (Table 11-14 on p. 240)

Prescribed dose = 300 cGy

$$\text{MU setting} = \frac{\text{Prescribed dose}}{\text{Output} \times \text{COF}_{(CS)} \times \text{PSF}_{(EFS)} \times \text{TMR}_{(EFS)}}$$

$$\text{MU setting} = \frac{300\ \text{cGy}}{1.0\ \text{cGy/MU} \times 1.021 \times 1.014 \times 0.937}$$

$$\text{MU setting} = \frac{100\ \text{cGy}}{0.9701\ \text{cGy/MU}}$$

MU setting = 309 MU

Example 19: A patient is treated on the 6 MV linear accelerator treatment machine at 100 cm SAD. The setup SSD is 90 cm. The collimator setting is 15 cm × 15 cm. The field is blocked to an 8 cm × 8 cm blocked equivalent square. A 5 mm solid plastic tray is used to hold the blocks. The prescription states that a dose of 4000 cGy is to be delivered to a depth of 10 cm in 20 fractions using an anterior and posterior (AP:PA) treatment field arrangement. Calculate the MU setting using TMR.

The factors for the dose rate at a point are reference dose rate, output factor, and tissue absorption factor.

Reference dose rate = 1.0 cGy/MU (Table 11-3 on p. 230)

COF (15 × 15) = 1.021 (Table 11-4 on p. 231)

PSF (8 × 8) = 0.992 (Table 11-5 on p. 231)

TMR (10,8) = 0.775 (Table 11-14 on p. 240)

Tray factor = 0.97 (Table 11-17 on p. 243)

Prescribed dose = 100 cGy/port

$$\text{MU setting} = \frac{\text{Prescribed dose}}{\text{Output} \times \text{COF}_{(CS)} \times \text{PSF}_{(EFS)} \times \text{TMR}_{(EFS)} \times \text{TF}}$$

$$\text{MU setting} = \frac{100\ \text{cGy}}{1.0\ \text{cGy/MU} \times 1.021 \times 0.992 \times 0.775 \times 0.97}$$

$$\text{MU setting} = \frac{100\ \text{cGy}}{0.76141\ \text{cGy/MU}}$$

MU setting = 131 MU

The next example is similar to the previous one except that TPR will be used.

Example 20: A patient is treated on the 10 MV linear accelerator treatment machine at 100 cm SAD. The setup SSD is 90 cm. The collimator setting is 15 cm × 15 cm. The field is blocked to an 8 cm × 8 cm blocked equivalent square. A 5 mm solid plastic tray is used to hold the blocks. The prescription states that a dose of 4000 cGy is to be delivered to a depth of 10 cm in 20 fractions using an anterior and posterior (AP:PA) treatment field arrangement. Calculate the MU setting, the total dose to the depth of D_{max}, and the total dose to the cord. For this example, the cord lies at a depth of 5 cm beneath the patient's posterior skin surface.

MU setting using TPR

The factors for the dose rate at a point are reference dose rate, output factor, and TPR.

Reference dose rate = 1.0 cGy/MU (Table 11-3 on p. 230)

OF (15 × 15) = 1.021 (Table 11-4 on p. 231)

PSF (8 × 8) = 0.992 (Table 11-5 on p. 231)

TPR (10,8) = 0.8740 (Table 11-16 on p. 242)

Tray factor = 0.97 (Table 11-17 on p. 243)

Prescribed dose = 100 cGy/port

$$\text{MU setting} = \frac{\text{Prescribed dose}}{\text{Output} \times \text{COF}_{(CS)} \times \text{PSF}_{(EFS)} \times \text{TPR}_{(EFS)} \times \text{TF}}$$

$$\text{MU setting} = \frac{100\ \text{cGy}}{1.0\ \text{cGy/MU} \times 1.021 \times 0.992 \times 0.874 \times 0.97}$$

$$\text{MU setting} = \frac{100\ \text{cGy}}{0.8587\ \text{cGy/MU}}$$

MU setting = 116 MU

In the next part of the problem, the total dose delivered to two points, at D_{max} and at the level of the spinal cord, must be calculated. There is a dose contributed to each point from both the anterior and posterior treatment fields (obtained by adding the dose delivered by the anterior field to the dose delivered by the posterior field). Deriving this information will be explained in the next series of steps. It should be noted that deriving this information can be done with TPR, TMR, and TAR.

Deriving given dose in isocentric problems

The given dose is the dose delivered at the depth of D_{max} for a single treatment field. In this example problem, each treatment field has its own given dose. Calculating the given dose using TAR, TMR, or TPR is more complex than when using PDD. To calculate the given dose using TPR for this example, the prescribed dose for the field, the source to calculation point distance, and the TPR at the depth of the prescribed dose must be known.

As discussed earlier, both measurements for the TPR are made at the same distance from the source. The field size increases because of divergence as the distance from the source increases. Therefore when using TPR (or either TAR or TMR) the field size at the point of calculation must be known. To find the field size at any distance, the following relationship can be used:

$$\frac{\text{Field size at distance}_1}{\text{Distance}_1} = \frac{\text{Field size at distance}_2}{\text{Distance}_2}$$

In practice the equivalent square of the rectangular field is used in place of the actual field size. For example, if the field size is 20 cm × 10 cm, the equivalent square of 13.0 would be used for the field size. To calculate the given dose using TPR, the following equation is used:

$$\text{Dose}_A = \frac{\text{Dose}_B}{\text{TPR}_B} \times \frac{(\text{SCPD}_B)^2}{(\text{SCPD}_A)^2} \times \text{TPR}_A$$

Where

Dose$_A$ is the dose at point A

Dose$_B$ is the dose at point B

TPR$_A$ is the TPR at point A

TPR$_B$ is the TPR at point B

SCPD$_A$ is the source to calculation point distance for point A

SCPD$_B$ is the source to calculation point distance for point B

Note that ratio of SCPD$_B$ and SCPD$_A$ is the application of the inverse square law. SPCD is found by adding the depth to the SSD for that point. The following table will assist in the organization of data when calculating the dose to points using TAR, TMR, and TPR:

Point	SSD	Depth	SCPD	Equivalent square	TPR	Dose
A						
B						
C						

Part 1. Calculate the dose to points from the anterior field

Point A represents the depth of D$_{max}$ beneath the skin surface. Point B represents the isocentric point, in this case at a depth of 10 cm at mid-plane. Point C represents the depth of the cord beneath the anterior skin surface. The cord depth below the skin surface is found by subtracting the depth of the cord beneath the posterior surface (5 cm) from the patient's total central axis separation. With that we have the following:

Point	SSD	Depth	SCPD	Equivalent square	TPR	Dose
A	90	2.5	92.5			
B	90	10	100	8.0	0.8740	100
C	90	15	105			

With this the equivalent square and TPR for points A and C can be found:

Field size at point A:

$$\frac{\text{Field size at distance}_A}{92.5 \text{ cm}} = \frac{8.0 \text{ cm}}{100 \text{ cm}}, \text{ therefore 7.4 cm}$$

$$\frac{\text{Field size at distance}_A}{92.5 \text{ cm}} = \frac{8.0 \text{ cm}}{100 \text{ cm}}, \text{ therefore 7.4 cm}$$

Now the TPR (2.5, 7.4) can be found. Note that the exact numbers are not directly listed in the tables. Interpolation, as discussed in Chapter 1, can be used to derive the exact numbers. In this case, TPR (2.5, 7.4) = 1.0426.

Field size at point C:

$$\frac{\text{Field size at distance}_c}{105 \text{ cm}} = \frac{8.0 \text{ cm}}{100 \text{ cm}}, \text{ therefore 8.4 cm;}$$

$$\text{TPR (15, 8.4)} = 0.7486.$$

At this point there is enough information to calculate the dose from the anterior field to points A and C.

Dose to point A (from anterior):

$$\text{Dose}_A = \frac{\text{Dose}_B}{\text{TPR}_B} \times \frac{(\text{SCPD}_B)^2}{(\text{SCPD}_A)^2} \times \text{TPR}_A$$

$$\text{Dose}_A = \frac{100 \text{ cGy}}{0.8740} \times \frac{(100 \text{ cm})^2}{(92.5 \text{ cm})^2} \times 1.0426$$

$$\text{Dose}_A = 139.4 \text{ cGy}$$

Dose to point C (from anterior):

$$\text{Dose}_C = \frac{\text{Dose}_B}{\text{TPR}_B} \times \frac{(\text{SCPD}_B)^2}{(\text{SCPD}_C)^2} \times \text{TPR}_C$$

$$\text{Dose}_C = \frac{100 \text{ cGy}}{0.8740} \times \frac{(100 \text{ cm})^2}{(105 \text{ cm})^2} \times 0.7486$$

$$\text{Dose}_C = 77.7 \text{ cGy}$$

At this point the table for the anterior perspective can be completed:

Point	SSD	Depth	SCPD	Equivalent square	TPR	Dose
A	90	2.5	92.5	7.4	1.0426	139.4
B	90	10	100	8.0	0.8740	100
C	90	15	105	8.4	0.7486	77.7

At this point, note the confirmation of trends discussed earlier in the chapter. As the depth of calculation increases, the TPR decreases (because of more attenuation). Also, the dose is greater closer to the skin surface.

Part 2. Calculate the dose to points from the posterior field

Again, point A represents the depth of D_{max} beneath the anterior skin surface. Point B represents the isocentric point, in this case at a depth of 10 cm at mid-plane. Point C represents the depth of the cord beneath the anterior skin surface. However, these points are now measured with respect to the posterior surface. Another grid can be produced:

Point	SSD	Depth	SCPD	Equivalent square	TPR	Dose
A	90	17.5	107.5			
B	90	10	100	8.0	0.8740	100
C	90	5	95			

With this the equivalent square and TPR for points A and C can be found:

Field size at point A (from posterior):

$$\frac{\text{Field size at distance}_A}{107.5 \text{ cm}} = \frac{8.0 \text{ cm}}{100 \text{ cm}}, \text{ therefore } 8.6 \text{ cm}$$

$$\text{TPR (17.5, 8.6)} = 0.6914.$$

Field size at point C (from posterior):

$$\frac{\text{Field size at distance}_c}{95 \text{ cm}} = \frac{8.0 \text{ cm}}{100 \text{ cm}}; \text{ therefore } 7.6 \text{ cm}$$

$$\text{TPR (5, 7.6)} = 1.00.$$

At this point there is enough information to calculate the dose from the posterior field to points A and C.

Dose to point A (from posterior):

$$\text{Dose}_A = \frac{100 \text{ cGy}}{0.8740} \times \frac{(100 \text{ cm})^2}{(10.5 \text{ cm})^2} \times 0.6914$$

$$\text{Dose}_A = 68.5 \text{ cGy}$$

Dose to point C (from posterior):

$$\text{Dose}_C = \frac{100 \text{ cGy}}{0.8740} \times \frac{(100 \text{ cm})^2}{(95 \text{ cm})^2} \times 1.00$$

$$\text{Dose}_C = 125.8 \text{ cGy}$$

At this point the grid from the posterior perspective can be completed:

Point	SSD	Depth	SCPD	Equivalent square	TPR	Dose
A	90	17.5	107.5	8.6	0.6914	68.5
B	90	10	100	8.0	0.8740	100
C	90	5	95	7.6	1.00	126.8

Part 3. Add the doses to the points from the anterior and posterior fields to finalize the problem

Point	Anterior	Posterior	Total
A	139.4	68.5	207.9
B	100	100	200
C	77.7	126.8	204.5

This technique gives a perspective of the doses received at points other than the isocenter for SAD calculations. If cal-culations for several energies were performed for the parameters just given, a pattern would be noted. Lower energies would deposit a higher dose at the peripheral aspects of the treatment volume. In other words the D_{max} doses would be higher for the lower energies, all other parameters remaining the same. Conversely, as energy increases, the superficial doses would be lower. In all cases the dose to isocenter would be the same. The higher energy beams exhibit more skin sparing (less superficial dose) and are therefore better suited for treatment of deep-seated tumors.

UNEQUAL BEAM WEIGHTING

In some cases radiation therapy using parallel opposed or multiple beam arrangements, different doses are delivered to treatment ports. This is commonly done when the tumor volume lies closer to the skin surface but would still benefit from multiportal treatment. The result is a greater dose near the entrance of the favored field and a lower dose in the tissue near the entrance of the opposing field.[1,2] Although uneven doses are administered in the peripheral tissues, the doses to the point of specification should remain consistent with the prescription. In other words, the isocenter in an SAD technique still receives the overall prescribed dose.

Look at the basic dose calculation equation:

$$\text{Treatment setting} = \frac{\text{Dose}}{\text{Dose rate}}$$

The component that is affected directly by the field weighting is the prescribed dose per port. If a prescription is written to deliver 200 cGy through two ports and the fields are equally weighted, each port would deliver 100 cGy to the prescription point. However, if the prescription describes a treatment to be delivered from an AP:PA perspective and specifies that the AP field is to receive twice the amount of the PA field (written as 2 to 1 or 2:1), a different dose must be delivered through each field.

The total dose to be delivered through all ports (in this case two) should be divided by the sum of the weighting. In this case, the weighting sum is three (2 + 1) and the total dose is divided by this number: 200 cGy/3 = 66.7 cGy. This defines the amount of each dose component. Then this component is multiplied by the weighting for each port; this provides the appropriate dosage to be delivered through each port, as follows:

$$\text{AP dose} = 66.7 \times 2 = 133.4$$

$$\text{PA dose} = 66.7 \times 1 = 66.7$$

These numbers would be used in the dose calculation to find the time or monitor unit setting for each treatment port. A quick check for accuracy would be to add the individual port doses; they should equal (or be less due to rounding off numbers) to the original dose prescribed.

This method can be used for any number of treatment ports and beam arrangements and can be used in all treatment calculations. Weighting does not affect the dose rate, only the dose to be administered through each port.

Separation of Adjacent Fields

Many treatment techniques involve the junction of fields with the adjoining margins either abutted or separated depending on various circumstances. Because of rapid "fall off" of the dose near the boundary of the field, a small change in the relative spacing of the field margins can produce a large change in the dose distribution in the junction volume.

The hazard of a "gap" or junction area may either be a dose that:

1. Exceeds normal tissue tolerance
2. Is inadequate to therapeutically treat the tumor

Fields may be abutted or have a gap between them:

1. *Abutted fields**—if the adjacent fields are abutted on the surface, the fields overlap to an increasing degree with depth because of divergence.

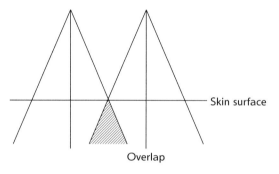

2. *Separated fields*†—the theory behind this is that we can abut the field edges at depth as opposed to on the skin surface. In this way we can spare a tissue at depth an overdose due to overlapping fields. We would have them abut at a desired depth leaving a gap on the skin surface.

*Examples of abutting fields would include lateral head and neck and supraclavicular fossa fields as well as in many breast cases.
†Examples of this would include mantle and abdominal or para-aortic fields, pelvis and para-aortic fields in seminoma cases, and craniospinal irradiation fields.

Methods of Achieving Dose Uniformity Across Field Junctions

1. *Dosimetric isodose matching*—With the availability of computers, separation of fields can easily be planned. The hot and cold spots can be visualized. The accuracy of this method depends upon the accuracy of the individual field isodose curves.
2. *Junction shift*—Fields that abut on the skin surface can be moved during the course of treatment so that any hot or cold spot inherently present can be spread over a distance.
3. *Half-beam blocking*—A shielding block designed to block out one side of a treatment field can be employed to produce a field that has no divergence along one side. Two abutting fields can then be used to match field borders on the phantom surface and have no divergence at depth. Asymmetric jawed field can also accomplish this on modern treatment units.
4. *Geometric*—It is possible to achieve dose uniformity at the junction of two fields at depth from geometric considerations provided that the geometric boundary of the field is defined by the 50% decrement line (at the edge of all fields, the dose to the very edge falls off to 50% of the dose at the central ray).

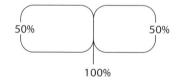

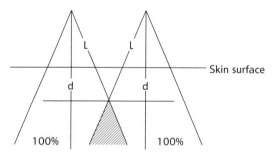

Note: it is possible to have fields at different depths, the important aspect is that the fields abut at a depth and that we can measure what the gap should be on the skin surface with the following equation:

$$\text{Gap} = \left(\frac{L_1}{2} \times \frac{d}{SSD_1}\right) + \left(\frac{L_2}{2} \times \frac{d}{SSD_2}\right)$$

Example 21: A patient is treated using two adjacent fields. The collimator setting for Field 1 is 8 cm width × 12 cm length. The collimator setting for Field 2 is 10 cm width × 20 cm length. Both fields are set up at 100 cm SSD. Calculate the gap on the skin surface for the fields to abut at 5 cm depth.

The geometric gap calculation is based upon the principles of Similar Triangles. A very important consideration when doing a gap calculation is to make sure that the field size (L) is corrected for the SSD. In this example, the field size is defined at the skin surface that is 100 cm SSD. Therefore, the field size is the same as the collimator setting.

A second consideration is that the depth of abutment (d) must be the same for both fields.

$$\text{Gap} = \frac{12 \text{ cm}}{2} \times \frac{5 \text{ cm}}{100 \text{ cm}} + \frac{20 \text{ cm}}{2} \times \frac{5 \text{ cm}}{100 \text{ cm}}$$

$$\text{Gap} = 0.3 \text{ cm} + 0.5 \text{ cm}$$

$$\text{Gap} = 0.8 \text{ cm}$$

The 0.8 cm calculated is the minimal skin gap between the two fields. This means that the distance between the inferior border of Field 1 and superior border of Field 2 must be at least 0.8 cm. Often the gap is made slightly larger to allow for variations in the day-to-day setup.

Example 22: A patient is treated using two adjacent fields. The collimator setting for Field 1 is 8 cm width × 16 cm length. The collimator setting for Field 2 is 10 cm width × 26 cm length. Field 1 is set up at 95 cm SSD and Field 2 is set up at 90 cm SSD. Calculate the gap on the skin surface for the fields to abut at 5 cm depth.

Since the collimator setting is the field size at 100 cm, we must adjust the field sizes to the appropriate SSD. For Field 1 this is 15.2 cm and for Field 2 it is 23.4 cm.

$$\text{Gap} = \frac{15.2 \text{ cm}}{2} \times \frac{5 \text{ cm}}{92.0 \text{ cm}} + \frac{23.4 \text{ cm}}{2} \times \frac{5 \text{ cm}}{90.0 \text{ cm}}$$

$$\text{Gap} = 0.413 \text{ cm} + 0.65 \text{ cm}$$

$$\text{Gap} = 1.063 \text{ cm}$$

Again, 1.063 cm is the minimum gap. Therefore, you would round-up to 1.07 cm.

SUMMARY

We have looked at some basic methods of performing photon beam dose calculations and monitor unit setting calculations. The methods selected in any therapy center will normally be determined by the medical radiation physicists. The calculation presented here represents only a limited perspective of calculation basics. The material here should provide the radiation therapy practitioner with a good basis on which to further explore dosimetry and treatment planning in radiation therapy.

Table 11-3	Reference dose rate	
Treatment machine	**Dose rate specified for**	**Reference dose rate for a 10 cm × 10 cm collimator setting**
Cobalt 60	SSD/PDD	51.7 cGy/min at depth of D_{max}
Cobalt 60	SAD/TAR	50.6 cGy/min in air at 80 cm
6 MV	SSD/PDD	0.993 cGy/MU at depth of D_{max}
6 MV	SAD/TAR	1.000 cGy/MU in air at 100 cm
10 MV	SSD/PDD	0.968 cGy/MU at depth of D_{max}
10 MV	SAD/TAR	1.000 cGy/MU in air at 100 cm
10 MV	SAD/TMR	1.015 cGy/MU at 100 cm at depth D_{max}
18 MV	SSD/PDD	0.944 cGy/MU at depth of D_{max}
18 MV	SAD/TAR	1.000 cGy/MU in air at 100 cm
10 MV	SAD/TPR	1.000 cGy/MU in air at 100 cm

Table 11-4 Output factors

Output factor for PDD calculations (Sc, Sp)

Mach/Eq Sq	4.0	5.0	6.0	7.0	8.0	9.0	10.0	11.0	12.0	13.0	14.0	15.0	16.0	17.0	18.0	19.0	20.0	22.0	24.0	26.0	28.0	30.0	32.0	35.0
Cobalt 60	0.928	0.945	0.962	0.971	0.980	0.990	1.000	1.009	1.019	1.028	1.037	1.046	1.053	1.060	1.067	1.074	1.081	1.089	1.096	1.102	1.105	1.109		
6 MV	0.927	0.940	0.954	0.967	0.979	0.990	1.000	1.007	1.014	1.021	1.028	1.035	1.039	1.044	1.049	1.053	1.058	1.065	1.072	1.079	1.084	1.088	1.092	1.098
10 MV	0.925	0.938	0.953	0.967	0.979	0.990	1.000	1.005	1.011	1.016	1.022	1.027	1.032	1.037	1.041	1.046	1.051	1.058	1.065	1.069	1.071	1.073	1.077	1.081
18 MV	0.904	0.922	0.941	0.961	0.976	0.988	1.000	1.007	1.014	1.021	1.028	1.036	1.041	1.046	1.051	1.056	1.060	1.067	1.073	1.079	1.084	1.087	1.090	1.093

Output factor for TAR calculations (Sc)

Mach/Eq Sq	4.0	5.0	6.0	7.0	8.0	9.0	10.0	11.0	12.0	13.0	14.0	15.0	16.0	17.0	18.0	19.0	20.0	22.0	24.0	26.0	28.0	30.0	32.0	35.0
Cobalt 60	0.946	0.961	0.975	0.981	0.987	0.993	1.000	1.006	1.012	1.018	1.024	1.030	1.035	1.039	1.044	1.048	1.053	1.057	1.061	1.063	1.063	1.063		
6 MV	0.948	0.961	0.970	0.979	0.987	0.994	1.000	1.004	1.008	1.013	1.017	1.021	1.024	1.028	1.031	1.035	1.038	1.041	1.045	1.048	1.051	1.052	1.053	1.055
10 MV	0.938	0.951	0.962	0.973	0.982	0.991	1.000	1.005	1.009	1.014	1.018	1.023	1.026	1.030	1.033	1.037	1.040	1.044	1.048	1.051	1.052	1.054	1.057	1.061
18 MV	0.914	0.931	0.948	0.965	0.978	0.989	1.000	1.006	1.012	1.017	1.023	1.029	1.032	1.036	1.039	1.043	1.046	1.052	1.057	1.063	1.066	1.067	1.069	1.070

Table 11-5 Output factors

Phantom scatter factor for TMR and TPR calculations (Sp)

Mach/Eq Sq	4.0	5.0	6.0	7.0	8.0	9.0	10.0	11.0	12.0	13.0	14.0	15.0	16.0	17.0	18.0	19.0	20.0	22.0	24.0	26.0	28.0	30.0	32.0	35.0
Cobalt 60	0.981	0.983	0.987	0.990	0.993	0.997	1.000	1.003	1.007	1.010	1.013	1.016	1.017	1.020	1.022	1.025	1.027	1.030	1.033	1.037	1.040	1.043		
6 MV	0.978	0.978	0.984	0.988	0.992	0.996	1.000	1.003	1.006	1.008	1.011	1.014	1.015	1.016	1.017	1.017	1.019	1.023	1.026	1.030	1.031	1.034	1.037	1.041
10 MV	0.986	0.986	0.991	0.994	0.997	0.999	1.000	1.000	1.002	1.002	1.004	1.004	1.006	1.007	1.008	1.009	1.011	1.014	1.016	1.017	1.018	1.019	1.019	1.019
18 MV	0.989	0.990	0.993	0.996	0.998	0.999	1.000	1.001	1.002	1.004	1.005	1.007	1.009	1.010	1.012	1.012	1.013	1.014	1.015	1.017	1.017	1.019	1.020	1.021

Table 11-6 Percentage depth dose table cobalt 60 at 80 cm SSD

Depth (cm) \ Eq Sq (cm)	0.0	4.0	5.0	6.0	7.0	8.0	9.0	10.0	11.0	12.0	13.0	14.0	15.0	16.0	17.0	18.0	19.0	20.0	22.0	24.0	26.0	28.0	30.0
0.0	14.9	15.0	17.4	19.8	21.7	23.6	25.5	27.4	28.1	28.8	29.5	30.1	30.8	32.3	33.7	35.2	36.7	38.1	41.2	44.3	47.4	50.4	53.4
0.5	100.0	100.0	100.0	100.0	100.0	100.0	100.0	100.0	100.0	100.0	100.0	100.0	100.0	100.0	100.0	100.0	100.0	100.0	100.0	100.0	100.0	100.0	100.0
1.0	95.6	96.4	96.6	96.8	96.9	97.0	97.0	97.1	97.1	97.1	97.2	97.2	97.2	97.3	97.3	97.4	97.4	97.5	97.7	97.8	98.0	98.1	98.2
2.0	87.4	90.2	90.7	91.3	91.6	92.0	92.3	92.6	92.8	92.9	93.1	93.3	93.5	93.6	93.7	93.8	93.9	94.0	94.1	94.2	94.3	94.4	94.4
3.0	80.1	84.2	85.1	85.8	86.4	87.0	87.4	87.8	88.1	88.5	88.8	89.1	89.3	89.5	89.7	89.9	90.1	90.1	90.2	90.3	90.4	90.5	90.4
4.0	73.2	78.4	79.4	80.4	81.2	81.9	82.6	83.1	83.5	84.0	84.4	84.8	85.1	85.3	85.5	85.8	86.0	86.0	86.1	86.2	86.4	86.5	86.3
5.0	67.1	72.9	74.0	75.1	76.0	76.9	77.7	78.3	78.8	79.4	79.9	80.4	80.7	81.0	81.3	81.6	81.9	81.9	82.0	82.1	82.2	82.3	82.1
6.0	61.4	67.7	68.9	70.1	71.1	72.0	72.9	73.6	74.2	74.8	75.4	76.0	76.3	76.7	77.0	77.3	77.5	77.6	77.7	77.9	78.1	78.2	78.0
7.0	56.2	62.7	64.0	65.3	66.4	67.4	68.3	69.0	69.7	70.3	71.0	71.6	71.9	72.3	72.7	73.1	73.3	73.4	73.6	73.7	73.9	74.0	73.8
8.0	51.5	58.0	59.4	60.7	61.9	62.9	63.9	64.6	65.3	66.1	66.8	67.4	67.8	68.2	68.6	69.1	69.2	69.3	69.5	69.7	69.9	69.9	69.7
9.0	47.3	53.7	55.1	56.4	57.5	58.6	59.6	60.4	61.1	61.9	62.6	63.2	63.6	64.1	64.5	65.0	65.1	65.2	65.4	65.7	65.9	65.9	65.8
10.0	43.3	49.7	51.0	52.3	53.5	54.5	55.6	56.3	57.1	57.9	58.6	59.2	59.7	60.2	60.6	61.1	61.2	61.3	61.6	61.9	62.1	62.1	61.9
11.0	39.8	45.9	47.2	48.5	49.7	50.7	51.7	52.5	53.3	54.1	54.9	55.4	55.9	56.4	56.9	57.3	57.4	57.5	57.8	58.1	58.4	58.4	58.2
12.0	36.4	42.4	43.7	45.0	46.2	47.2	48.1	48.9	49.7	50.5	51.3	51.8	52.3	52.8	53.3	53.6	53.8	53.9	54.3	54.6	55.0	54.8	54.7
13.0	33.4	39.2	40.5	41.5	42.8	43.8	44.7	45.5	46.3	47.1	47.8	48.3	48.8	49.4	49.9	50.1	50.3	50.5	50.9	51.2	51.6	51.4	51.3
14.0	30.7	36.1	37.4	38.5	39.6	40.6	41.5	42.3	43.1	43.9	44.6	45.1	45.6	46.1	46.7	46.8	47.0	47.2	47.6	48.0	48.3	48.1	48.0
15.0	28.1	33.4	34.6	35.7	36.7	37.7	38.5	39.3	40.0	40.8	41.5	42.0	42.5	43.1	43.6	43.8	43.9	44.1	44.6	45.0	45.2	54.1	44.9
16.0	25.9	30.8	31.9	33.0	34.0	34.9	35.7	36.4	37.2	38.0	38.6	39.1	39.6	40.2	40.6	40.8	41.0	41.2	41.6	42.1	42.2	42.1	42.0
17.0	23.8	28.4	29.5	30.5	31.4	32.3	33.1	33.8	34.6	35.3	35.9	36.4	36.9	37.5	37.8	38.0	38.3	38.5	38.9	39.4	39.5	39.3	39.2
18.0	21.8	26.2	27.2	28.2	29.1	30.0	30.7	31.4	32.1	32.8	33.4	33.9	34.4	34.9	35.2	35.4	35.6	35.9	36.3	36.8	36.8	36.7	36.6
19.0	20.0	24.2	25.1	26.0	26.9	27.7	28.4	29.1	29.8	30.5	31.0	31.5	32.0	32.5	32.8	33.0	33.2	33.5	33.9	34.4	34.4	34.3	34.2
20.0	18.4	22.3	23.2	24.1	24.9	25.7	26.3	27.0	27.6	28.3	28.8	29.3	29.8	30.3	30.5	30.7	30.9	31.2	31.7	32.2	32.1	32.0	31.9
21.0	17.0	20.6	21.5	22.3	23.1	23.8	24.4	25.0	25.7	26.3	26.8	27.2	27.7	28.1	28.4	28.6	28.8	29.1	29.6	30.0	29.9	29.8	29.7
22.0	15.6	19.0	19.8	20.6	21.3	22.0	22.6	23.2	23.8	24.3	24.8	25.3	25.7	26.1	26.3	26.6	26.8	27.0	27.5	27.9	27.8	27.7	27.6
23.0	14.3	17.5	18.3	19.0	19.7	20.4	20.9	21.5	22.1	22.6	23.1	23.5	23.9	24.3	24.5	24.7	25.0	25.2	25.7	26.0	25.9	25.8	25.7
24.0	13.1	16.1	16.8	17.5	18.2	18.8	19.3	19.9	20.4	20.9	21.4	21.8	22.2	22.5	22.7	23.0	23.2	23.4	23.9	24.1	24.1	24.0	23.9
25.0	12.1	14.9	15.6	16.2	16.8	17.4	17.9	18.5	19.0	19.5	19.9	20.3	20.7	20.9	21.2	21.4	21.6	21.8	22.3	22.5	22.4	22.3	22.3
26.0	11.1	13.7	14.3	14.9	15.5	16.1	16.6	17.1	17.6	18.0	18.4	18.8	19.2	19.4	19.6	19.8	20.1	20.3	20.8	20.9	20.8	20.7	20.7
27.0	10.2	12.7	13.3	13.8	14.4	14.9	15.4	15.8	16.3	16.7	17.1	17.5	17.8	18.1	18.3	18.5	18.7	18.9	19.4	19.4	19.4	19.3	19.2
28.0	9.4	11.7	12.2	12.8	13.3	13.7	14.2	14.6	15.1	15.5	15.8	16.2	16.5	16.7	17.0	17.2	17.4	17.6	18.0	18.0	18.0	17.9	17.9
29.0	8.7	10.8	11.3	11.8	12.3	12.7	13.1	13.6	14.0	14.4	14.7	15.1	15.4	15.6	15.8	16.0	16.2	16.4	16.8	16.7	16.7	16.6	16.6
30.0	8.0	9.9	10.4	10.9	11.3	11.7	12.1	12.5	12.9	13.3	13.6	13.9	14.2	14.4	14.6	14.8	15.0	15.2	15.6	15.5	15.5	15.4	15.4
BSF/PSF	1.000	1.015	1.018	1.021	1.025	1.028	1.032	1.035	1.038	1.041	1.045	1.048	1.051	1.053	1.056	1.058	1.061	1.063	1.066	1.070	1.073	1.077	1.080

PDD COBLT

Table 11-7 6 MV percentage depth dose at 100 cm SSD

Depth (cm) / Eq Sq	0.0	4.0	5.0	6.0	7.0	8.0	9.0	10.0	11.0	12.0	13.0	14.0	15.0	16.0	17.0	18.0	19.0	20.0	22.0	24.0	26.0	28.0	30.0	32.0	35.0
0.0	19.2	19.2	19.2	20.5	21.8	23.0	24.3	25.6	26.7	27.9	29.1	30.2	31.4	32.6	33.8	35.1	36.3	37.5	39.0	40.4	41.9	43.2	44.5	45.7	47.6
1.0	96.8	96.9	96.9	97.0	97.0	97.0	97.1	97.1	97.2	97.2	97.3	97.3	97.4	97.4	97.5	97.5	97.6	97.6	97.7	97.8	98.0	98.1	98.1	98.2	98.3
1.5	100.0	100.0	100.0	100.0	100.0	100.0	100.0	100.0	100.0	100.0	100.0	100.0	100.0	100.0	100.0	100.0	100.0	100.0	100.0	100.0	100.0	100.0	100.0	100.0	100.0
2.0	97.4	98.2	98.4	98.4	98.5	98.5	98.6	98.6	98.6	98.6	98.6	98.6	98.6	98.6	98.6	98.7	98.7	98.7	98.7	98.7	98.7	98.7	98.7	98.7	98.7
3.0	91.1	93.8	94.4	94.7	94.9	95.0	95.0	95.1	95.1	95.1	95.2	95.2	95.2	95.3	95.3	95.4	95.4	95.5	95.5	95.6	95.6	95.6	95.6	95.6	95.5
4.0	85.3	89.6	90.6	90.9	91.3	91.4	91.5	91.5	91.5	91.6	91.6	91.7	91.7	91.8	91.9	92.0	92.1	92.2	92.2	92.3	92.4	92.3	92.3	92.3	92.2
5.0	79.9	84.5	85.6	86.1	86.6	86.8	87.0	87.1	87.3	87.5	87.7	87.8	87.9	88.1	88.2	88.3	88.5	88.6	88.7	88.8	89.0	89.0	89.0	89.0	88.9
6.0	74.8	79.7	80.9	81.5	82.1	82.4	82.7	83.0	83.2	83.5	83.8	84.0	84.1	84.3	84.5	84.7	84.8	85.0	85.2	85.4	85.6	85.6	85.7	85.8	85.7
7.0	70.1	75.1	76.3	77.1	77.8	78.3	78.7	79.0	79.3	79.6	79.9	80.3	80.4	80.6	80.8	81.0	81.2	81.4	81.7	82.0	82.2	82.3	82.4	82.5	82.3
8.0	65.7	70.8	72.1	72.9	73.7	74.2	74.7	75.1	75.5	75.9	76.2	76.6	76.8	77.0	77.3	77.5	77.8	77.9	78.3	78.6	78.8	78.9	79.0	79.1	79.0
9.0	61.5	66.7	68.0	68.9	69.8	70.4	71.0	71.4	71.8	72.2	72.6	73.0	73.2	73.5	73.8	74.1	74.3	74.5	74.9	75.3	75.5	75.6	75.8	76.0	75.7
10.0	57.7	62.8	64.1	65.1	66.1	66.7	67.4	67.8	68.3	68.8	69.2	69.6	69.8	70.1	70.5	70.8	71.0	71.2	71.6	72.0	72.3	72.5	72.7	72.8	72.6
11.0	54.0	59.2	60.4	61.5	62.4	63.1	63.8	64.2	64.8	65.3	65.8	66.1	66.4	66.8	67.1	67.5	67.7	67.9	68.4	68.8	69.0	69.2	69.4	69.6	69.3
12.0	50.7	55.7	57.0	58.0	58.9	59.7	60.4	60.9	61.4	61.9	62.4	62.8	63.1	63.5	63.9	64.3	64.5	64.8	65.3	65.8	66.0	66.2	66.4	66.5	66.2
13.0	47.5	52.4	53.6	54.6	55.6	56.4	57.2	57.7	58.2	58.8	59.3	59.7	60.0	60.4	60.8	61.2	61.5	61.7	62.2	62.7	63.0	63.2	63.4	63.5	63.3
14.0	44.6	49.4	50.6	51.6	52.5	53.3	54.1	54.6	55.1	55.7	56.3	56.6	57.0	57.4	57.8	58.2	58.5	58.8	59.4	59.9	60.1	60.3	60.6	60.6	60.4
15.0	41.8	46.6	47.8	48.7	49.6	50.5	51.2	51.7	52.3	52.9	53.5	53.9	54.2	54.7	55.1	55.5	55.8	56.1	56.6	57.1	57.4	57.6	57.9	57.8	57.6
16.0	39.2	43.9	45.1	46.0	46.9	47.8	48.5	49.1	49.7	50.3	50.9	51.2	51.6	52.0	52.5	52.8	53.1	53.4	54.0	54.5	54.8	55.1	55.4	55.2	55.1
17.0	36.8	41.4	42.5	43.5	44.3	45.2	45.9	46.4	47.1	47.7	48.2	48.6	49.0	49.4	49.9	50.2	50.6	50.9	51.5	52.0	52.3	52.6	52.9	52.7	52.6
18.0	34.5	39.0	40.1	41.0	41.9	42.7	43.4	44.0	44.6	45.3	45.8	46.2	46.6	47.0	47.5	47.8	48.2	48.5	49.1	49.6	49.9	50.2	50.5	50.3	50.2
19.0	32.4	36.8	37.8	38.7	39.6	40.5	41.1	41.7	42.3	43.0	43.5	43.9	44.3	44.7	45.1	45.5	45.8	46.1	46.8	47.2	47.6	48.0	48.2	48.0	47.9
20.0	30.4	34.6	35.7	36.6	37.4	38.2	38.9	39.5	40.1	40.7	41.2	41.6	42.0	42.5	42.9	43.2	43.6	43.9	44.6	45.0	45.4	45.7	45.9	45.8	45.6
21.0	28.6	32.7	33.7	34.5	35.3	36.1	36.8	37.4	38.0	38.6	39.1	39.5	39.9	40.3	40.7	41.1	41.4	41.8	42.4	42.9	43.2	43.6	43.7	43.6	43.5
22.0	26.8	30.8	31.8	32.6	33.4	34.2	34.8	35.4	36.0	36.9	37.1	37.5	37.9	38.3	38.7	39.1	39.4	39.8	40.4	40.8	41.2	41.6	41.7	41.6	41.5
23.0	25.2	29.1	30.0	30.8	31.6	32.4	33.0	33.6	34.2	34.8	35.2	35.6	36.0	36.4	36.8	37.2	37.5	37.9	38.5	38.9	39.3	39.7	39.8	39.6	39.5
24.0	23.6	27.5	28.4	29.1	29.9	30.6	31.2	31.8	32.4	32.9	33.4	33.7	34.1	34.6	35.0	35.3	35.7	36.0	36.7	37.1	37.5	37.9	37.8	37.7	37.6
25.0	22.2	26.0	26.8	27.6	28.3	29.0	29.6	30.1	30.7	31.3	31.7	32.0	32.4	32.9	33.2	33.6	33.9	34.3	34.9	35.3	35.7	36.1	36.0	35.9	35.8
26.0	20.9	24.5	25.3	26.0	26.7	27.4	27.9	28.5	29.1	29.6	30.0	30.4	30.8	31.2	31.5	31.9	32.2	32.6	33.2	33.6	34.0	34.4	34.3	34.2	34.1
27.0	19.6	23.2	24.0	24.7	25.3	26.0	26.5	27.0	27.6	28.1	28.4	28.8	29.2	29.6	30.0	30.3	30.7	31.0	31.6	32.0	32.4	32.7	32.6	32.6	32.4
28.0	18.4	21.9	22.6	23.3	24.0	24.6	25.1	25.6	26.1	26.6	26.9	27.3	27.7	28.1	28.4	28.8	29.2	29.5	30.1	30.5	30.9	31.1	31.1	31.0	30.9
29.0	17.3	20.7	21.4	22.0	22.7	23.3	23.7	24.2	24.7	25.2	25.6	25.9	26.3	26.7	27.0	27.4	27.7	28.1	28.6	29.0	29.4	29.6	29.5	29.5	29.4
30.0	16.2	19.5	20.2	20.8	21.4	22.0	22.4	22.9	23.4	23.8	24.2	24.6	24.9	25.3	25.7	26.0	26.4	26.7	27.2	27.6	28.0	28.1	28.0	28.0	27.9
PSF	1.000	1.002	1.003	1.007	1.012	1.016	1.021	1.025	1.028	1.031	1.033	1.036	1.039	1.040	1.041	1.043	1.044	1.045	1.048	1.051	1.054	1.057	1.060	1.063	1.067

PDD 6 MV

Table 11-8 Percentage depth dose table 10 MV x-ray at 100 cm SSD

Eq Sq Depth (cm)	0.0	4.0	5.0	6.0	7.0	8.0	9.0	10.0	11.0	12.0	13.0	14.0	15.0	16.0	17.0	18.0	19.0	20.0	22.0	24.0	26.0	28.0	30.0
0.0	10.4	10.5	10.5	11.6	12.6	13.8	14.9	16.1	17.0	17.9	18.8	19.7	20.6	21.4	22.2	23.0	23.8	24.6	25.8	26.9	28.0	29.2	30.4
1.0	77.0	77.0	77.1	78.8	80.6	83.1	86.3	89.1	89.5	89.9	90.2	90.5	90.8	91.1	91.7	91.7	92.0	92.5	92.4	92.5	93.1	93.8	94.4
2.0	94.0	94.0	94.1	94.9	95.6	96.4	97.2	97.9	98.0	98.0	98.1	98.1	98.2	98.2	98.3	98.3	98.4	98.4	98.4	98.5	98.8	99.1	99.3
2.5	100.0	100.0	100.0	100.0	100.0	100.0	100.0	100.0	100.0	100.0	100.0	100.0	100.0	100.0	100.0	100.0	100.0	100.0	100.0	100.0	100.0	100.0	100.0
3.0	96.7	98.0	98.3	98.3	98.3	98.2	98.2	98.2	98.2	98.3	98.3	98.3	98.4	98.3	98.3	98.3	98.3	98.3	98.2	98.2	98.2	98.2	98.2
4.0	91.3	94.7	95.4	95.4	95.5	95.3	95.2	95.1	95.2	95.3	95.5	95.6	95.6	95.6	95.5	95.4	95.4	95.4	95.3	95.3	95.3	95.3	95.3
5.0	86.4	90.3	91.1	91.2	91.4	91.3	91.3	91.4	91.5	91.7	91.8	92.0	92.1	92.0	92.0	92.0	92.0	92.0	92.0	91.9	92.0	92.0	92.0
6.0	81.7	86.0	86.9	87.2	87.5	87.5	87.6	87.1	87.9	88.1	88.3	88.5	88.5	88.6	88.6	88.6	88.7	88.7	88.7	88.7	88.7	88.7	88.7
7.0	77.2	81.9	82.9	83.3	83.7	83.8	83.9	84.1	84.3	84.6	84.8	85.1	85.1	85.2	85.2	85.3	85.3	85.4	85.5	85.5	85.6	85.7	85.7
8.0	73.0	78.1	79.1	79.6	80.1	80.2	80.4	80.7	80.9	81.2	81.5	81.8	81.8	81.9	82.0	82.1	82.1	82.2	82.2	82.3	82.5	82.6	82.6
9.0	69.0	74.1	75.2	75.8	76.3	76.5	76.7	77.0	77.3	77.7	78.0	78.3	78.4	78.5	78.6	78.7	78.8	78.9	79.0	79.1	79.2	79.3	79.3
10.0	65.0	70.5	71.6	72.2	72.8	73.0	73.2	73.5	73.9	74.3	74.7	75.0	75.1	75.2	75.4	75.5	75.6	75.7	75.9	76.0	76.1	76.2	76.2
11.0	61.9	66.9	68.0	68.7	69.3	69.5	69.8	70.2	70.6	71.0	71.4	71.7	71.9	72.1	72.2	72.4	72.5	72.6	72.8	72.9	73.1	73.2	73.2
12.0	58.5	63.6	64.7	65.4	66.0	66.3	66.7	67.0	67.5	67.9	68.3	68.6	68.8	69.0	69.2	69.4	69.5	69.7	69.9	70.0	70.2	70.3	70.3
13.0	55.4	60.3	61.4	62.3	62.9	63.2	63.6	64.0	64.4	64.9	65.3	65.6	65.8	66.0	66.3	66.4	66.6	66.8	67.0	67.2	67.4	67.5	67.4
14.0	52.4	57.3	58.4	59.3	59.9	60.2	60.6	61.0	61.5	62.0	62.5	62.7	63.0	63.2	63.4	63.6	62.8	63.9	64.3	64.4	64.7	64.7	64.7
15.0	49.6	54.3	55.5	56.4	57.0	57.4	57.8	58.3	58.8	59.2	59.7	60.0	60.2	60.5	60.7	60.9	61.1	61.3	61.6	61.8	62.1	62.1	62.0
16.0	47.1	51.6	52.7	53.7	54.3	54.7	55.1	55.6	56.1	56.6	57.1	57.4	57.6	57.9	58.1	58.3	58.5	58.7	59.1	59.3	59.6	59.6	59.5
17.0	44.6	48.9	50.0	50.9	51.5	51.9	52.4	52.9	53.4	53.9	54.4	54.7	55.0	55.2	55.5	55.7	55.9	56.2	56.5	56.8	57.0	57.0	57.0
18.0	42.2	46.4	47.4	48.3	48.9	49.3	49.9	50.4	50.9	51.4	51.9	52.2	52.5	52.7	53.0	53.3	53.5	53.7	54.1	54.4	54.6	54.6	54.6
19.0	40.0	44.0	45.0	45.8	46.3	46.9	47.4	47.9	48.4	49.0	49.4	49.7	50.0	50.3	50.6	50.9	51.1	51.4	51.8	52.1	52.3	52.2	52.2
20.0	37.9	41.7	42.7	43.4	44.0	44.6	45.1	45.6	46.2	46.7	47.1	47.5	47.8	48.1	48.4	48.7	48.9	49.2	49.6	49.9	50.1	50.0	50.0
21.0	35.9	39.6	40.5	41.3	41.8	42.4	42.9	43.4	44.0	44.5	44.9	45.3	45.6	46.0	46.3	46.5	46.9	47.1	47.5	47.8	47.9	47.9	47.9
22.0	34.0	37.6	38.5	39.3	39.9	40.4	41.0	41.5	42.0	42.5	42.9	43.3	43.6	44.0	44.2	44.5	44.8	45.0	45.4	45.8	45.8	45.8	45.8
23.0	32.3	35.8	36.7	37.4	38.0	38.5	39.0	39.5	40.1	40.6	41.0	41.4	41.7	42.1	42.4	42.6	42.9	43.1	43.5	43.9	43.9	43.9	43.8
24.0	30.6	34.0	34.9	35.6	36.1	36.7	37.2	37.7	38.2	38.7	39.1	39.5	39.9	40.2	40.5	40.8	41.0	41.3	41.7	42.0	42.0	42.0	41.9
25.0	29.0	32.7	33.6	34.3	34.8	35.4	35.9	36.4	36.9	37.4	37.8	38.1	38.5	38.9	39.1	39.4	39.7	39.9	40.3	40.6	40.6	40.5	40.5
26.0	27.5	31.4	32.3	33.1	33.6	34.1	34.6	35.1	35.6	36.1	36.5	36.8	37.2	37.5	37.8	38.1	38.3	38.6	38.9	39.2	39.1	39.1	39.1
27.0	26.1	30.3	31.1	31.8	32.3	32.9	33.4	33.8	34.3	34.8	35.2	35.5	35.9	36.2	36.5	36.8	37.1	37.3	37.6	37.9	37.8	37.8	37.8
28.0	24.8	29.2	30.0	30.6	31.2	31.7	32.2	32.7	33.1	33.6	34.0	34.3	34.7	35.0	35.3	35.5	35.8	36.0	36.4	36.5	36.5	36.5	36.5
29.0	23.5	28.1	28.9	29.5	30.0	30.5	31.0	31.5	32.0	32.4	32.8	33.1	33.5	33.8	34.1	34.3	34.6	34.8	35.1	35.3	35.2	35.2	35.2
30.0	22.3	27.0	27.8	28.5	28.9	29.4	29.9	30.4	30.9	31.3	31.6	32.0	32.3	32.6	32.9	33.2	33.5	33.7	33.9	34.0	34.0	34.0	34.0
PSF	1.000	1.001	1.005	1.009	1.012	1.013	1.015	1.016	1.017	1.017	1.018	1.019	1.020	1.021	1.023	1.023	1.024	1.025	1.028	1.031	1.032	1.033	1.034

PDD 10 MV

Table 11-9 18 MV percentage depth dose at 100 cm SSD

Eq Sq	0.0	4.0	5.0	6.0	7.0	8.0	9.0	10.0	11.0	12.0	13.0	14.0	15.0	16.0	17.0	18.0	19.0	20.0	22.0	24.0	26.0	28.0	30.0	32.0
0.0	10.0	10.0	10.1	11.7	13.4	15.4	17.6	19.8	21.3	22.8	24.3	25.8	27.3	28.7	30.1	31.5	32.9	34.4	36.2	38.0	39.3	41.2	42.0	42.9
1.0	77.8	77.8	77.8	78.3	78.7	79.3	80.0	80.6	80.9	81.2	81.6	81.9	82.2	82.7	83.2	83.7	84.2	84.7	85.2	85.7	86.2	86.5	86.8	87.0
2.0	95.4	95.5	95.5	95.6	95.7	95.8	96.0	96.2	96.2	96.2	96.2	96.2	96.3	96.5	96.7	96.9	97.2	97.4	97.5	97.7	97.8	97.9	98.0	98.0
3.0	98.3	98.4	98.4	98.4	98.4	98.5	98.6	98.6	98.6	98.6	98.6	98.6	98.7	98.7	98.8	98.9	99.0	99.0	99.1	99.1	99.2	99.2	99.3	99.3
3.5	100.0	100.0	100.0	100.0	100.0	100.0	100.0	100.0	100.0	100.0	100.0	100.0	100.0	100.0	100.0	100.0	100.0	100.0	100.0	100.0	100.0	100.0	100.0	100.0
4.0	98.1	98.8	98.9	98.9	98.9	98.9	98.9	98.9	98.9	98.8	98.8	98.8	98.8	98.8	98.8	98.8	98.8	98.8	98.8	98.7	98.8	98.7	98.8	98.8
5.0	93.5	95.8	96.3	96.3	96.2	96.2	96.1	96.1	96.1	96.0	96.0	96.0	95.9	95.9	95.9	95.8	95.8	95.7	95.7	95.7	95.7	95.7	95.7	95.8
6.0	89.0	92.8	93.4	93.4	93.4	93.3	93.3	93.3	93.2	93.2	93.2	93.1	93.1	93.0	93.0	92.9	92.9	92.8	92.8	92.8	92.9	92.9	92.9	93.0
7.0	84.9	89.0	89.8	89.8	89.9	89.8	89.8	89.8	89.8	89.8	89.8	89.8	89.8	89.8	89.7	89.7	89.6	89.6	89.6	89.6	89.6	89.7	89.8	89.8
8.0	81.0	85.4	86.2	86.3	86.4	86.4	86.4	86.5	86.5	86.6	86.6	86.7	86.6	86.6	86.5	86.5	86.4	86.4	86.4	86.4	86.5	86.6	86.7	86.8
9.0	77.2	81.8	82.6	82.9	83.1	83.0	83.0	83.1	83.2	83.2	83.3	83.4	83.4	83.4	83.4	83.3	83.3	83.3	83.3	83.4	83.6	83.7	83.8	83.9
10.0	73.6	78.3	79.1	79.5	79.7	79.9	79.7	79.9	80.0	80.1	80.3	80.3	80.3	80.3	80.3	80.3	80.2	80.3	80.3	80.4	80.6	80.8	81.0	81.1
11.0	70.2	74.9	75.7	76.1	76.4	76.5	76.6	76.7	76.9	77.0	77.1	77.2	77.3	77.3	77.3	77.3	77.3	77.3	77.4	77.5	77.7	77.9	78.0	78.1
12.0	67.0	71.7	72.5	72.9	73.2	73.3	73.5	73.6	73.8	73.9	74.1	74.2	74.3	74.3	74.4	74.4	74.4	74.4	74.5	74.6	74.9	75.0	75.2	75.2
13.0	64.0	68.7	69.4	69.8	70.1	70.3	70.5	70.7	70.9	71.0	71.2	71.3	71.4	71.5	71.6	71.6	71.6	71.6	71.7	71.9	72.1	72.3	72.4	72.5
14.0	61.0	65.7	66.4	66.8	67.1	67.4	67.7	67.9	68.0	68.2	68.3	68.5	68.6	68.8	68.9	68.9	68.9	69.0	69.1	69.3	69.5	69.7	69.8	69.8
15.0	58.3	62.8	63.6	64.0	64.4	64.7	64.9	65.1	65.3	65.5	65.7	65.9	66.0	66.2	66.3	66.3	66.3	66.4	66.6	66.8	67.0	67.2	67.4	67.4
16.0	55.6	60.2	60.9	61.4	61.7	62.1	62.4	62.6	62.8	63.0	63.2	63.4	63.5	63.7	63.8	63.8	63.9	64.0	64.2	64.4	64.7	64.9	65.0	65.0
17.0	53.1	57.6	58.3	58.8	59.1	59.5	59.8	60.0	60.3	60.5	60.8	61.0	61.1	61.3	61.4	61.5	61.5	61.6	61.8	62.1	62.3	62.5	62.8	62.7
18.0	50.7	55.1	55.8	56.4	56.7	57.1	57.4	57.7	58.0	58.2	58.5	58.7	58.8	58.9	59.1	59.1	59.2	59.3	59.6	59.8	60.1	60.3	60.5	60.4
19.0	48.4	52.8	53.5	54.0	54.4	54.7	55.0	55.3	55.6	56.0	56.2	56.4	56.6	56.7	56.8	56.9	57.0	57.1	57.3	57.6	57.9	58.2	58.3	58.2
20.0	46.3	50.5	51.2	51.7	52.1	52.4	52.8	53.1	53.4	53.7	54.0	54.2	54.3	54.5	54.6	54.7	54.8	54.9	55.2	55.5	55.9	56.1	56.2	56.1
21.0	44.2	48.3	49.0	49.6	49.9	50.3	50.6	51.0	51.3	51.7	51.9	52.1	52.2	52.4	52.5	52.6	52.7	52.9	53.2	53.5	53.9	54.1	54.2	54.1
22.0	42.3	46.3	46.9	47.5	47.8	48.2	48.6	48.9	49.3	49.6	49.9	50.0	50.2	50.4	50.5	50.6	50.7	50.9	51.3	51.6	51.9	52.2	52.3	52.2
23.0	40.4	44.3	45.0	45.5	45.9	46.3	46.6	47.0	47.3	47.7	47.9	48.1	48.3	48.4	48.5	48.7	48.8	49.0	49.4	49.7	50.0	50.3	50.3	50.2
24.0	38.6	42.4	43.1	43.7	44.0	44.4	44.7	45.1	45.4	45.8	46.0	46.2	46.4	46.6	46.8	46.9	47.0	47.2	47.5	47.8	48.2	48.5	48.4	48.4
25.0	36.9	40.7	41.3	41.9	42.2	42.6	42.9	43.3	43.6	44.0	44.2	44.4	44.6	44.9	45.0	45.1	45.2	45.4	45.8	46.1	46.4	46.7	46.6	46.6
26.0	35.3	38.9	39.6	40.2	40.5	40.9	41.2	41.6	41.9	42.2	42.5	42.7	42.9	43.1	43.2	43.4	43.5	43.7	44.0	44.4	44.7	44.9	44.9	44.8
27.0	33.7	37.3	38.0	38.5	38.9	39.2	39.6	39.9	40.3	40.6	40.8	41.0	41.3	41.5	41.6	41.7	41.9	42.0	42.4	42.7	43.0	43.3	43.2	43.1
28.0	32.2	35.7	36.4	36.9	37.3	37.7	38.0	38.3	38.7	39.0	39.2	39.5	39.7	39.9	40.0	40.1	40.3	40.4	40.8	41.1	41.5	41.6	41.6	41.5
29.0	30.9	34.3	34.9	35.4	35.8	36.1	36.5	36.8	37.1	37.4	37.7	37.9	38.2	38.4	38.5	38.6	38.7	38.7	39.3	39.6	39.9	40.1	40.0	40.0
30.0	29.5	32.9	33.5	34.0	34.3	34.7	35.0	35.3	35.6	35.9	36.2	36.4	36.7	36.9	37.0	37.1	37.3	37.4	37.8	38.1	38.5	38.6	38.5	38.5
PSF	1.000	1.002	1.003	1.006	1.009	1.011	1.012	1.013	1.014	1.015	1.017	1.018	1.019	1.021	1.022	1.024	1.025	1.027	1.028	1.028	1.029	1.030	1.031	1.033

PDD 18 MV

Table 11-10   Cobalt 60 tissue-air ratio

Eq Sq Depth (cm)	0.0	4.0	5.0	6.0	7.0	8.0	9.0	10.0	11.0	12.0	13.0	14.0	15.0	16.0	17.0	18.0	19.0	20.0	22.0	24.0	26.0	28.0	30.0
0.0	0.147	0.150	0.175	0.200	0.220	0.240	0.260	0.280	0.288	0.296	0.304	0.312	0.320	0.336	0.352	0.368	0.384	0.400	0.434	0.468	0.502	0.536	0.570
0.5	1.000	1.015	1.018	1.021	1.025	1.028	1.032	1.035	1.038	1.041	1.045	1.048	1.051	1.053	1.056	1.058	1.061	1.063	1.066	1.070	1.073	1.077	1.080
1.0	0.968	0.990	0.995	1.000	1.005	1.009	1.013	1.017	1.020	1.024	1.027	1.031	1.034	1.037	1.040	1.043	1.046	1.049	1.054	1.059	1.064	1.069	1.074
2.0	0.907	0.949	0.958	0.966	0.973	0.980	0.987	0.993	0.998	1.003	1.008	1.013	1.018	1.022	1.025	1.029	1.032	1.036	1.040	1.045	1.049	1.054	1.058
3.0	0.851	0.907	0.918	0.929	0.939	0.948	0.956	0.964	0.970	0.977	0.983	0.990	0.996	1.000	1.004	1.009	1.013	1.017	1.021	1.025	1.030	1.034	1.038
4.0	0.797	0.864	0.877	0.890	0.902	0.913	0.923	0.933	0.940	0.948	0.955	0.963	0.970	0.975	0.980	0.984	0.989	0.994	0.998	1.002	1.007	1.011	1.015
5.0	0.748	0.821	0.836	0.850	0.863	0.876	0.887	0.898	0.907	0.915	0.924	0.932	0.941	0.946	0.952	0.957	0.963	0.968	0.972	0.976	0.981	0.985	0.989
6.0	0.701	0.779	0.795	0.811	0.825	0.838	0.850	0.862	0.871	0.881	0.890	0.900	0.909	0.915	0.921	0.926	0.932	0.938	0.943	0.947	0.952	0.956	0.961
7.0	0.657	0.737	0.754	0.771	0.786	0.800	0.813	0.826	0.836	0.846	0.855	0.865	0.875	0.881	0.888	0.894	0.901	0.907	0.912	0.917	0.921	0.926	0.931
8.0	0.616	0.697	0.715	0.732	0.747	0.762	0.776	0.789	0.799	0.810	0.820	0.831	0.841	0.848	0.855	0.861	0.868	0.875	0.880	0.885	0.890	0.895	0.900
9.0	0.578	0.659	0.676	0.693	0.709	0.724	0.738	0.752	0.763	0.773	0.784	0.794	0.805	0.812	0.819	0.827	0.834	0.841	0.846	0.852	0.857	0.863	0.868
10.0	0.541	0.622	0.639	0.656	0.672	0.687	0.701	0.715	0.726	0.737	0.748	0.759	0.770	0.777	0.785	0.792	0.800	0.807	0.813	0.819	0.824	0.830	0.836
11.0	0.508	0.586	0.603	0.620	0.636	0.651	0.665	0.679	0.690	0.701	0.713	0.724	0.735	0.743	0.750	0.758	0.765	0.773	0.779	0.785	0.791	0.797	0.803
12.0	0.476	0.552	0.569	0.586	0.602	0.617	0.631	0.644	0.655	0.666	0.678	0.689	0.700	0.708	0.716	0.723	0.731	0.739	0.745	0.752	0.758	0.765	0.771
13.0	0.446	0.520	0.537	0.553	0.568	0.583	0.597	0.610	0.621	0.632	0.644	0.655	0.666	0.674	0.682	0.689	0.697	0.705	0.712	0.719	0.725	0.732	0.739
14.0	0.418	0.489	0.505	0.521	0.536	0.551	0.564	0.577	0.588	0.599	0.611	0.622	0.633	0.641	0.649	0.656	0.664	0.672	0.679	0.686	0.693	0.700	0.707
15.0	0.392	0.460	0.476	0.491	0.506	0.520	0.533	0.546	0.557	0.568	0.578	0.589	0.600	0.608	0.616	0.624	0.632	0.640	0.647	0.654	0.662	0.669	0.676
16.0	0.368	0.433	0.448	0.462	0.476	0.490	0.503	0.515	0.526	0.537	0.547	0.558	0.569	0.577	0.585	0.592	0.600	0.608	0.615	0.623	0.630	0.638	0.645
17.0	0.345	0.406	0.421	0.435	0.449	0.462	0.474	0.486	0.497	0.507	0.518	0.528	0.539	0.547	0.555	0.562	0.570	0.578	0.585	0.593	0.600	0.608	0.615
18.0	0.323	0.382	0.396	0.409	0.422	0.435	0.447	0.459	0.469	0.479	0.490	0.500	0.510	0.518	0.525	0.533	0.540	0.548	0.556	0.563	0.571	0.578	0.586
19.0	0.303	0.359	0.372	0.385	0.397	0.409	0.421	0.432	0.442	0.452	0.462	0.472	0.482	0.490	0.497	0.505	0.512	0.520	0.528	0.535	0.543	0.550	0.558
20.0	0.284	0.337	0.350	0.362	0.374	0.385	0.396	0.407	0.417	0.426	0.436	0.445	0.455	0.462	0.470	0.477	0.485	0.492	0.500	0.508	0.515	0.523	0.531
21.0	0.267	0.317	0.329	0.341	0.352	0.363	0.374	0.384	0.393	0.402	0.412	0.421	0.430	0.437	0.444	0.452	0.459	0.466	0.474	0.482	0.489	0.497	0.505
22.0	0.250	0.297	0.308	0.319	0.330	0.341	0.351	0.361	0.370	0.379	0.387	0.396	0.405	0.412	0.419	0.426	0.433	0.440	0.448	0.456	0.463	0.471	0.479
23.0	0.235	0.279	0.290	0.300	0.311	0.321	0.331	0.340	0.349	0.357	0.366	0.374	0.383	0.389	0.396	0.403	0.410	0.417	0.424	0.432	0.440	0.447	0.455
24.0	0.219	0.261	0.271	0.281	0.291	0.301	0.310	0.319	0.327	0.335	0.344	0.352	0.360	0.367	0.373	0.380	0.386	0.393	0.401	0.408	0.416	0.423	0.431
25.0	0.206	0.245	0.255	0.265	0.274	0.283	0.292	0.301	0.308	0.316	0.324	0.332	0.340	0.346	0.353	0.359	0.365	0.372	0.379	0.387	0.394	0.402	0.409
26.0	0.193	0.230	0.239	0.248	0.257	0.265	0.274	0.282	0.290	0.297	0.305	0.312	0.320	0.326	0.332	0.338	0.344	0.350	0.357	0.365	0.372	0.380	0.387
27.0	0.181	0.216	0.225	0.233	0.241	0.250	0.258	0.266	0.273	0.280	0.287	0.294	0.302	0.307	0.313	0.319	0.325	0.331	0.338	0.345	0.353	0.360	0.367
28.0	0.169	0.202	0.210	0.218	0.226	0.234	0.242	0.249	0.256	0.263	0.269	0.276	0.283	0.289	0.295	0.300	0.306	0.312	0.319	0.326	0.333	0.340	0.347
29.0	0.159	0.190	0.198	0.205	0.213	0.220	0.227	0.234	0.241	0.247	0.254	0.260	0.267	0.272	0.278	0.283	0.289	0.295	0.301	0.308	0.315	0.322	0.329
30.0	0.149	0.178	0.185	0.192	0.199	0.206	0.213	0.219	0.225	0.231	0.238	0.244	0.250	0.255	0.261	0.266	0.272	0.277	0.284	0.290	0.297	0.303	0.310

TAR COBLT

Table 11-11 6 MV tissue-air ratio

Eq Sq / Depth (cm)	0.0	4.0	5.0	6.0	7.0	8.0	9.0	10.0	11.0	12.0	13.0	14.0	15.0	16.0	17.0	18.0	19.0	20.0	22.0	24.0	26.0	28.0	30.0	32.0	35.0
0.0	0.186	0.187	0.187	0.200	0.213	0.227	0.240	0.254	0.266	0.279	0.291	0.304	0.316	0.329	0.342	0.354	0.367	0.380	0.396	0.412	0.428	0.443	0.457	0.471	0.492
1.0	0.957	0.960	0.961	0.965	0.970	0.974	0.979	0.984	0.987	0.990	0.994	0.997	1.000	1.002	1.003	1.005	1.006	1.008	1.012	1.017	1.021	1.025	1.028	1.032	1.037
1.5	1.000	1.002	1.003	1.007	1.012	1.016	1.021	1.025	1.028	1.031	1.033	1.036	1.039	1.040	1.041	1.043	1.044	1.045	1.048	1.051	1.054	1.057	1.060	1.063	1.067
2.0	0.982	0.992	0.994	0.999	1.004	1.009	1.014	1.018	1.021	1.024	1.027	1.030	1.032	1.034	1.035	1.037	1.038	1.039	1.043	1.046	1.049	1.052	1.055	1.057	1.061
3.0	0.936	0.966	0.973	0.979	0.986	0.991	0.996	1.001	1.004	1.007	1.010	1.013	1.016	1.018	1.020	1.021	1.023	1.025	1.028	1.032	1.035	1.038	1.041	1.043	1.047
4.0	0.894	0.940	0.951	0.959	0.966	0.972	0.977	0.982	0.985	0.988	0.991	0.994	0.997	0.999	1.001	1.004	1.006	1.008	1.012	1.015	1.019	1.022	1.025	1.027	1.031
5.0	0.853	0.903	0.915	0.924	0.933	0.941	0.946	0.952	0.956	0.961	0.965	0.970	0.974	0.977	0.979	0.982	0.984	0.987	0.991	0.996	1.000	1.003	1.006	1.009	1.013
6.0	0.814	0.867	0.880	0.890	0.900	0.909	0.916	0.923	0.928	0.933	0.939	0.944	0.949	0.952	0.955	0.958	0.961	0.964	0.969	0.974	0.979	0.984	0.987	0.990	0.995
7.0	0.777	0.831	0.845	0.857	0.868	0.878	0.886	0.894	0.900	0.906	0.911	0.917	0.923	0.926	0.930	0.933	0.937	0.940	0.946	0.951	0.957	0.962	0.965	0.969	0.974
8.0	0.742	0.798	0.812	0.824	0.837	0.847	0.856	0.865	0.871	0.878	0.884	0.891	0.897	0.901	0.905	0.908	0.912	0.916	0.922	0.928	0.934	0.939	0.943	0.946	0.952
9.0	0.708	0.765	0.779	0.792	0.805	0.817	0.826	0.836	0.843	0.850	0.856	0.863	0.870	0.874	0.878	0.883	0.887	0.891	0.898	0.904	0.911	0.916	0.920	0.924	0.930
10.0	0.676	0.733	0.747	0.761	0.775	0.787	0.798	0.808	0.815	0.822	0.830	0.837	0.844	0.848	0.853	0.857	0.862	0.866	0.873	0.880	0.887	0.892	0.897	0.901	0.908
11.0	0.645	0.702	0.716	0.730	0.744	0.756	0.767	0.778	0.786	0.793	0.801	0.808	0.816	0.821	0.826	0.830	0.835	0.840	0.847	0.854	0.861	0.867	0.872	0.876	0.883
12.0	0.616	0.672	0.686	0.700	0.714	0.727	0.738	0.749	0.757	0.765	0.772	0.780	0.788	0.793	0.798	0.804	0.809	0.814	0.822	0.829	0.837	0.843	0.848	0.852	0.859
13.0	0.588	0.643	0.657	0.671	0.684	0.697	0.709	0.721	0.729	0.737	0.745	0.753	0.761	0.766	0.772	0.777	0.783	0.788	0.796	0.804	0.812	0.818	0.823	0.828	0.835
14.0	0.561	0.616	0.630	0.643	0.656	0.669	0.681	0.693	0.701	0.709	0.718	0.726	0.734	0.740	0.745	0.751	0.756	0.762	0.771	0.779	0.788	0.794	0.799	0.804	0.811
15.0	0.536	0.590	0.604	0.617	0.630	0.642	0.655	0.667	0.675	0.684	0.692	0.701	0.709	0.715	0.721	0.726	0.732	0.738	0.747	0.755	0.764	0.771	0.776	0.781	0.788
16.0	0.511	0.565	0.579	0.592	0.605	0.617	0.630	0.642	0.651	0.659	0.668	0.676	0.685	0.691	0.697	0.702	0.708	0.714	0.723	0.732	0.741	0.748	0.753	0.758	0.766
17.0	0.488	0.542	0.555	0.568	0.581	0.593	0.605	0.617	0.626	0.634	0.643	0.651	0.660	0.666	0.672	0.678	0.684	0.690	0.699	0.708	0.717	0.725	0.730	0.736	0.744
18.0	0.466	0.518	0.531	0.544	0.557	0.569	0.581	0.593	0.602	0.611	0.619	0.628	0.637	0.643	0.649	0.655	0.661	0.667	0.676	0.686	0.695	0.703	0.708	0.714	0.722
19.0	0.445	0.496	0.509	0.521	0.534	0.546	0.558	0.570	0.579	0.588	0.596	0.605	0.614	0.620	0.626	0.632	0.638	0.644	0.653	0.663	0.672	0.680	0.686	0.692	0.701
20.0	0.424	0.474	0.478	0.499	0.512	0.524	0.535	0.547	0.556	0.565	0.573	0.582	0.591	0.597	0.603	0.609	0.615	0.621	0.631	0.640	0.650	0.658	0.664	0.670	0.679
21.0	0.405	0.455	0.467	0.479	0.490	0.502	0.513	0.525	0.534	0.543	0.551	0.560	0.569	0.575	0.581	0.587	0.593	0.599	0.609	0.618	0.628	0.636	0.642	0.649	0.658
22.0	0.387	0.435	0.447	0.459	0.470	0.482	0.493	0.504	0.513	0.522	0.530	0.539	0.548	0.554	0.560	0.566	0.572	0.578	0.588	0.597	0.607	0.615	0.622	0.628	0.638
23.0	0.370	0.417	0.429	0.440	0.451	0.463	0.474	0.485	0.493	0.502	0.510	0.519	0.528	0.534	0.539	0.546	0.552	0.558	0.567	0.577	0.587	0.595	0.602	0.608	0.618
24.0	0.352	0.399	0.411	0.422	0.433	0.443	0.454	0.465	0.473	0.482	0.490	0.499	0.507	0.513	0.519	0.525	0.531	0.537	0.547	0.557	0.567	0.575	0.582	0.588	0.598
25.0	0.337	0.383	0.394	0.405	0.415	0.426	0.436	0.447	0.455	0.463	0.471	0.480	0.488	0.494	0.500	0.506	0.512	0.518	0.528	0.538	0.548	0.556	0.562	0.569	0.579
26.0	0.321	0.366	0.377	0.387	0.398	0.408	0.418	0.428	0.436	0.444	0.453	0.461	0.469	0.475	0.481	0.486	0.492	0.498	0.508	0.518	0.528	0.536	0.543	0.549	0.559
27.0	0.307	0.351	0.362	0.372	0.382	0.392	0.402	0.412	0.419	0.427	0.435	0.443	0.451	0.457	0.462	0.468	0.474	0.480	0.490	0.500	0.510	0.518	0.525	0.531	0.541
28.0	0.292	0.336	0.347	0.357	0.366	0.376	0.385	0.395	0.403	0.410	0.418	0.425	0.433	0.439	0.444	0.450	0.455	0.461	0.471	0.482	0.492	0.500	0.507	0.513	0.523
29.0	0.279	0.322	0.333	0.342	0.351	0.361	0.370	0.379	0.386	0.394	0.401	0.409	0.416	0.422	0.427	0.433	0.438	0.444	0.454	0.464	0.474	0.483	0.489	0.495	0.505
30.0	0.266	0.308	0.318	0.327	0.336	0.345	0.354	0.363	0.370	0.377	0.385	0.392	0.399	0.405	0.410	0.416	0.421	0.427	0.437	0.447	0.457	0.465	0.471	0.478	0.487

6 MV TAR

Table 11-12 10 MV tissue-air ratio

Eq Sq Depth (cm)	0.0	4.0	5.0	6.0	7.0	8.0	9.0	10.0	11.0	12.0	13.0	14.0	15.0	16.0	17.0	18.0	19.0	20.0	22.0	24.0	26.0	28.0	30.0
0.0	0.099	0.100	0.100	0.111	0.122	0.133	0.144	0.156	0.165	0.174	0.182	0.191	0.200	0.208	0.216	0.225	0.233	0.241	0.253	0.264	0.276	0.288	0.300
1.0	0.749	0.750	0.750	0.770	0.790	0.816	0.848	0.880	0.884	0.888	0.892	0.896	0.900	0.904	0.908	0.912	0.916	0.920	0.924	0.928	0.934	0.942	0.950
2.0	0.933	0.934	0.934	0.945	0.956	0.967	0.976	0.986	0.987	0.989	0.990	0.991	0.993	0.994	0.996	0.997	0.999	1.001	1.004	1.007	1.011	1.015	1.019
2.5	1.000	1.001	1.001	1.005	1.009	1.012	1.013	1.015	1.016	1.017	1.017	1.018	1.019	1.020	1.021	1.023	1.024	1.025	1.028	1.031	1.032	1.033	1.034
3.0	0.978	0.992	0.995	0.999	1.003	1.006	1.007	1.008	1.009	1.010	1.012	1.013	1.014	1.015	1.016	1.017	1.018	1.019	1.021	1.024	1.025	1.026	1.027
4.0	0.942	0.976	0.985	0.989	0.993	0.995	0.995	0.995	0.997	0.999	1.001	1.003	1.005	1.006	1.006	1.007	1.007	1.008	1.010	1.013	1.014	1.015	1.016
5.0	0.908	0.948	0.958	0.963	0.968	0.972	0.973	0.974	0.976	0.979	0.981	0.984	0.986	0.987	0.988	0.989	0.990	0.991	0.993	0.996	0.998	0.999	1.000
6.0	0.875	0.920	0.931	0.937	0.944	0.949	0.950	0.952	0.955	0.958	0.960	0.963	0.966	0.967	0.969	0.970	0.972	0.973	0.976	0.979	0.981	0.982	0.983
7.0	0.843	0.892	0.904	0.912	0.919	0.924	0.927	0.930	0.933	0.936	0.940	0.943	0.946	0.948	0.949	0.951	0.952	0.954	0.957	0.960	0.963	0.965	0.967
8.0	0.812	0.868	0.876	0.886	0.895	0.901	0.904	0.908	0.912	0.915	0.919	0.922	0.926	0.928	0.930	0.931	0.933	0.935	0.938	0.941	0.944	0.947	0.950
9.0	0.782	0.836	0.849	0.858	0.867	0.874	0.878	0.882	0.886	0.890	0.895	0.899	0.903	0.905	0.907	0.909	0.911	0.913	0.917	0.921	0.924	0.927	0.929
10.0	0.754	0.808	0.822	0.832	0.842	0.849	0.853	0.857	0.862	0.866	0.871	0.875	0.880	0.882	0.885	0.887	0.890	0.892	0.896	0.900	0.903	0.906	0.909
11.0	0.727	0.781	0.794	0.805	0.816	0.823	0.828	0.832	0.837	0.842	0.847	0.852	0.857	0.860	0.862	0.865	0.867	0.870	0.874	0.879	0.883	0.886	0.889
12.0	0.700	0.754	0.768	0.779	0.790	0.798	0.803	0.808	0.813	0.818	0.824	0.829	0.834	0.837	0.840	0.843	0.846	0.849	0.854	0.859	0.863	0.866	0.869
13.0	0.675	0.728	0.741	0.752	0.765	0.774	0.779	0.784	0.789	0.795	0.800	0.806	0.811	0.814	0.817	0.821	0.824	0.827	0.832	0.837	0.842	0.845	0.849
14.0	0.650	0.703	0.716	0.728	0.741	0.750	0.755	0.760	0.766	0.772	0.777	0.783	0.789	0.792	0.795	0.799	0.802	0.805	0.811	0.816	0.821	0.825	0.829
15.0	0.626	0.678	0.691	0.704	0.717	0.726	0.731	0.737	0.743	0.749	0.755	0.761	0.767	0.770	0.774	0.777	0.781	0.784	0.790	0.796	0.801	0.805	0.809
16.0	0.604	0.654	0.667	0.680	0.693	0.703	0.708	0.714	0.720	0.727	0.773	0.740	0.746	0.749	0.753	0.756	0.760	0.763	0.769	0.776	0.781	0.786	0.790
17.0	0.582	0.631	0.643	0.655	0.668	0.677	0.684	0.690	0.696	0.703	0.709	0.716	0.722	0.726	0.730	0.733	0.737	0.741	0.747	0.754	0.759	0.764	0.769
18.0	0.560	0.608	0.620	0.632	0.644	0.653	0.660	0.667	0.674	0.680	0.687	0.693	0.700	0.704	0.708	0.711	0.715	0.719	0.726	0.733	0.739	0.744	0.749
19.0	0.540	0.586	0.597	0.609	0.620	0.630	0.637	0.644	0.651	0.657	0.664	0.670	0.677	0.681	0.685	0.690	0.694	0.698	0.705	0.712	0.719	0.724	0.729
20.0	0.520	0.565	0.576	0.587	0.598	0.607	0.615	0.623	0.630	0.636	0.643	0.649	0.656	0.660	0.665	0.669	0.674	0.678	0.685	0.692	0.699	0.704	0.710
21.0	0.501	0.544	0.555	0.566	0.577	0.586	0.594	0.602	0.609	0.615	0.622	0.628	0.635	0.640	0.644	0.649	0.653	0.658	0.666	0.673	0.680	0.685	0.691
22.0	0.483	0.525	0.536	0.547	0.558	0.567	0.575	0.583	0.590	0.596	0.603	0.609	0.616	0.621	0.625	0.630	0.634	0.639	0.647	0.654	0.661	0.666	0.672
23.0	0.466	0.507	0.518	0.528	0.539	0.548	0.556	0.564	0.571	0.577	0.584	0.590	0.597	0.602	0.607	0.611	0.616	0.621	0.629	0.636	0.643	0.648	0.654
24.0	0.449	0.489	0.499	0.510	0.521	0.530	0.537	0.545	0.552	0.558	0.565	0.571	0.578	0.583	0.588	0.593	0.598	0.603	0.611	0.618	0.625	0.630	0.636
25.0	0.433	0.477	0.488	0.498	0.509	0.518	0.526	0.534	0.540	0.547	0.553	0.560	0.567	0.571	0.576	0.581	0.586	0.591	0.599	0.607	0.613	0.619	0.624
26.0	0.416	0.464	0.476	0.487	0.498	0.507	0.514	0.522	0.529	0.535	0.542	0.548	0.555	0.560	0.565	0.569	0.574	0.579	0.587	0.595	0.602	0.607	0.612
27.0	0.402	0.453	0.466	0.476	0.486	0.495	0.503	0.511	0.518	0.524	0.531	0.537	0.544	0.548	0.553	0.558	0.563	0.568	0.576	0.584	0.590	0.595	0.601
28.0	0.387	0.441	0.455	0.465	0.475	0.484	0.492	0.500	0.506	0.513	0.519	0.526	0.532	0.537	0.542	0.546	0.551	0.556	0.564	0.572	0.579	0.584	0.589
29.0	0.373	0.430	0.444	0.454	0.464	0.473	0.481	0.488	0.495	0.502	0.508	0.515	0.521	0.526	0.530	0.535	0.540	0.545	0.553	0.561	0.568	0.573	0.578
30.0	0.359	0.418	0.433	0.443	0.454	0.463	0.470	0.477	0.484	0.490	0.497	0.503	0.510	0.515	0.519	0.524	0.528	0.533	0.541	0.550	0.556	0.561	0.566

10 MV TAR

Table 11-13 18 MV tissue-air ratio

Eq Sq Depth (cm)	0.0	4.0	5.0	6.0	7.0	8.0	9.0	10.0	11.0	12.0	13.0	14.0	15.0	16.0	17.0	18.0	19.0	20.0	22.0	24.0	26.0	28.0	30.0	32.0	35.0
0.0	0.093	0.094	0.094	0.110	0.126	0.145	0.166	0.187	0.201	0.216	0.230	0.245	0.259	0.273	0.287	0.301	0.315	0.329	0.347	0.364	0.382	0.395	0.404	0.413	0.426
1.0	0.739	0.741	0.742	0.748	0.755	0.762	0.769	0.776	0.780	0.784	0.788	0.792	0.796	0.802	0.808	0.814	0.820	0.826	0.831	0.837	0.842	0.847	0.851	0.854	0.860
2.0	0.925	0.928	0.929	0.932	0.935	0.939	0.942	0.945	0.946	0.947	0.949	0.950	0.951	0.955	0.958	0.962	0.965	0.969	0.971	0.976	0.975	0.977	0.979	0.982	0.985
3.0	0.972	0.975	0.975	0.978	0.981	0.984	0.986	0.988	0.989	0.990	0.991	0.992	0.994	0.996	0.998	1.001	1.003	1.005	1.006	1.007	1.009	1.010	1.012	1.014	1.016
3.5	1.000	1.002	1.003	1.006	1.009	1.011	1.012	1.013	1.014	1.015	1.017	1.018	1.019	1.021	1.022	1.024	1.025	1.027	1.028	1.028	1.029	1.030	1.031	1.033	1.035
4.0	0.989	0.998	1.000	1.003	1.005	1.007	1.008	1.009	1.010	1.011	1.013	1.014	1.015	1.016	1.018	1.019	1.021	1.022	1.023	1.023	1.024	1.025	1.026	1.028	1.030
5.0	0.960	0.986	0.992	0.994	0.997	0.998	0.999	1.000	1.001	1.002	1.002	1.003	1.004	1.005	1.006	1.008	1.009	1.010	1.010	1.011	1.011	1.012	1.014	1.015	1.018
6.0	0.932	0.971	0.981	0.983	0.986	0.987	0.988	0.990	0.990	0.991	0.991	0.992	0.993	0.994	0.995	0.996	0.997	0.998	0.998	0.999	0.999	1.000	1.002	1.004	1.007
7.0	0.906	0.949	0.960	0.963	0.966	0.968	0.969	0.970	0.971	0.972	0.974	0.975	0.976	0.977	0.978	0.979	0.980	0.981	0.982	0.982	0.983	0.984	0.986	0.988	0.991
8.0	0.880	0.926	0.938	0.942	0.946	0.949	0.950	0.951	0.953	0.954	0.956	0.957	0.959	0.960	0.961	0.962	0.963	0.964	0.965	0.965	0.966	0.967	0.970	0.972	0.976
9.0	0.855	0.903	0.915	0.920	0.925	0.928	0.929	0.930	0.932	0.934	0.936	0.938	0.940	0.941	0.942	0.944	0.945	0.946	0.947	0.948	0.949	0.951	0.954	0.956	0.960
10.0	0.830	0.880	0.892	0.898	0.904	0.908	0.909	0.910	0.912	0.915	0.917	0.920	0.922	0.923	0.924	0.926	0.927	0.928	0.929	0.931	0.932	0.935	0.938	0.941	0.945
11.0	0.806	0.856	0.869	0.875	0.881	0.885	0.888	0.890	0.892	0.895	0.897	0.900	0.902	0.904	0.905	0.907	0.908	0.910	0.911	0.913	0.914	0.917	0.920	0.923	0.927
12.0	0.783	0.834	0.847	0.853	0.859	0.863	0.866	0.869	0.872	0.874	0.877	0.879	0.882	0.884	0.886	0.887	0.889	0.891	0.893	0.894	0.896	0.899	0.902	0.905	0.909
13.0	0.761	0.812	0.825	0.831	0.837	0.842	0.845	0.849	0.852	0.854	0.857	0.859	0.862	0.864	0.866	0.869	0.871	0.873	0.875	0.876	0.878	0.881	0.884	0.887	0.891
14.0	0.739	0.790	0.803	0.809	0.815	0.820	0.825	0.829	0.832	0.834	0.837	0.839	0.842	0.845	0.847	0.850	0.852	0.855	0.857	0.859	0.861	0.864	0.867	0.870	0.874
15.0	0.718	0.768	0.781	0.788	0.795	0.800	0.805	0.809	0.812	0.815	0.818	0.821	0.824	0.827	0.829	0.832	0.834	0.837	0.839	0.842	0.844	0.847	0.850	0.853	0.858
16.0	0.697	0.748	0.761	0.768	0.775	0.780	0.785	0.790	0.793	0.796	0.800	0.803	0.806	0.809	0.811	0.814	0.816	0.819	0.822	0.825	0.828	0.831	0.834	0.837	0.842
17.0	0.677	0.727	0.740	0.747	0.754	0.760	0.765	0.770	0.774	0.777	0.781	0.784	0.788	0.791	0.794	0.796	0.799	0.802	0.805	0.808	0.811	0.814	0.817	0.821	0.826
18.0	0.658	0.708	0.720	0.728	0.735	0.741	0.746	0.751	0.755	0.759	0.763	0.767	0.771	0.774	0.776	0.779	0.781	0.784	0.787	0.791	0.794	0.798	0.801	0.805	0.810
19.0	0.639	0.689	0.701	0.709	0.716	0.722	0.727	0.732	0.736	0.740	0.745	0.749	0.753	0.759	0.759	0.761	0.764	0.767	0.770	0.774	0.777	0.781	0.785	0.788	0.794
20.0	0.621	0.670	0.682	0.690	0.697	0.703	0.708	0.713	0.717	0.722	0.726	0.731	0.735	0.738	0.741	0.743	0.746	0.749	0.753	0.757	0.761	0.765	0.769	0.772	0.778
21.0	0.603	0.651	0.663	0.671	0.679	0.685	0.690	0.695	0.700	0.704	0.709	0.713	0.718	0.721	0.724	0.726	0.729	0.732	0.736	0.741	0.745	0.749	0.753	0.757	0.763
22.0	0.586	0.633	0.645	0.653	0.660	0.667	0.672	0.677	0.682	0.687	0.691	0.696	0.701	0.704	0.707	0.709	0.712	0.715	0.720	0.724	0.729	0.733	0.737	0.742	0.748
23.0	0.569	0.605	0.627	0.635	0.643	0.650	0.655	0.660	0.665	0.670	0.674	0.679	0.684	0.687	0.690	0.692	0.695	0.698	0.703	0.708	0.713	0.717	0.721	0.726	0.732
24.0	0.553	0.599	0.610	0.618	0.626	0.633	0.638	0.643	0.648	0.653	0.657	0.662	0.667	0.670	0.673	0.677	0.680	0.683	0.688	0.692	0.697	0.701	0.705	0.710	0.716
25.0	0.538	0.582	0.594	0.602	0.610	0.617	0.622	0.627	0.632	0.636	0.641	0.646	0.651	0.654	0.657	0.660	0.664	0.667	0.672	0.676	0.681	0.686	0.690	0.694	0.701
26.0	0.522	0.556	0.577	0.585	0.594	0.601	0.606	0.611	0.616	0.620	0.625	0.629	0.634	0.637	0.641	0.644	0.648	0.651	0.656	0.661	0.666	0.670	0.674	0.679	0.685
27.0	0.507	0.551	0.565	0.570	0.578	0.585	0.590	0.596	0.600	0.605	0.609	0.614	0.619	0.622	0.626	0.629	0.633	0.636	0.641	0.645	0.650	0.655	0.659	0.663	0.670
28.0	0.492	0.535	0.546	0.554	0.562	0.569	0.574	0.580	0.585	0.589	0.594	0.598	0.603	0.607	0.610	0.614	0.617	0.621	0.626	0.630	0.635	0.639	0.644	0.648	0.655
29.0	0.479	0.521	0.532	0.540	0.548	0.554	0.560	0.565	0.570	0.574	0.579	0.583	0.588	0.591	0.595	0.599	0.602	0.606	0.611	0.615	0.620	0.625	0.629	0.634	0.641
30.0	0.465	0.507	0.517	0.525	0.533	0.540	0.545	0.550	0.554	0.559	0.563	0.568	0.572	0.576	0.580	0.583	0.587	0.591	0.596	0.601	0.606	0.610	0.615	0.619	0.626

Table 11-14   6 MV tissue maximum ratio

Eq Sq Depth (cm)	0.0	4.0	5.0	6.0	7.0	8.0	9.0	10.0	11.0	12.0	13.0	14.0	15.0	16.0	17.0	18.0	19.0	20.0	22.0	24.0	26.0	28.0	30.0	32.0	35.0
0.0	0.186	0.187	0.186	0.199	0.210	0.223	0.235	0.248	0.259	0.271	0.282	0.293	0.304	0.316	0.329	0.339	0.352	0.364	0.378	0.392	0.406	0.419	0.431	0.443	0.461
1.0	0.957	0.958	0.958	0.958	0.958	0.959	0.959	0.960	0.960	0.960	0.962	0.962	0.962	0.963	0.963	0.964	0.964	0.965	0.966	0.968	0.969	0.970	0.970	0.971	0.972
1.5	1.000	1.000	1.000	1.000	1.000	1.000	1.000	1.000	1.000	1.000	1.000	1.000	1.000	1.000	1.000	1.000	1.000	1.000	1.000	1.000	1.000	1.000	1.000	1.000	1.000
2.0	0.982	0.990	0.991	0.992	0.992	0.993	0.993	0.993	0.993	0.993	0.994	0.994	0.993	7.692	0.994	0.994	0.994	0.994	0.995	0.995	0.995	0.995	0.995	0.994	0.994
3.0	0.936	0.964	0.970	0.972	0.974	0.975	0.976	0.977	0.977	0.977	0.978	0.978	0.978	7.692	0.980	0.979	0.980	0.981	0.981	0.982	0.982	0.982	0.982	0.981	0.981
4.0	0.894	0.938	0.948	0.952	0.955	0.957	0.957	0.958	0.958	0.958	0.959	0.959	0.960	7.692	0.962	0.963	0.964	0.965	0.966	0.966	0.967	0.967	0.967	0.966	0.966
5.0	0.853	0.901	0.912	0.918	0.922	0.926	0.927	0.929	0.930	0.932	0.934	0.936	0.937	7.692	0.940	0.942	0.943	0.944	0.946	0.948	0.949	0.949	0.949	0.949	0.949
6.0	0.814	0.865	0.877	0.884	0.889	0.895	0.897	0.900	0.903	0.905	0.909	0.911	0.913	7.692	0.917	0.556	0.920	0.922	0.925	0.927	0.929	0.931	0.931	0.931	0.933
7.0	0.777	0.829	0.842	0.851	0.858	0.864	0.868	0.872	0.875	0.879	0.882	0.885	0.888	7.692	0.893	0.895	0.898	0.900	0.903	0.905	0.908	0.910	0.910	0.912	0.913
8.0	0.742	0.796	0.810	0.818	0.827	0.834	0.838	0.844	0.847	0.852	0.856	0.860	0.863	7.692	0.869	0.871	0.874	0.877	0.880	0.883	0.886	0.888	0.890	0.890	0.892
9.0	0.708	0.763	0.777	0.786	0.795	0.804	0.809	0.816	0.820	0.824	0.829	0.833	0.837	7.692	0.843	0.847	0.850	0.853	0.857	0.860	0.864	0.867	0.868	0.869	0.872
10.0	0.676	0.732	0.745	0.756	0.766	0.775	0.782	0.788	0.793	0.797	0.803	0.808	0.812	7.692	0.819	0.822	0.826	0.829	0.833	0.837	0.842	0.844	0.846	0.848	0.851
11.0	0.645	0.701	0.714	0.725	0.735	0.744	0.751	0.759	0.765	0.769	0.775	0.780	0.785	7.692	0.793	0.796	0.800	0.804	0.808	0.813	0.817	0.820	0.823	0.824	0.828
12.0	0.616	0.671	0.684	0.695	0.706	0.716	0.723	0.731	0.736	0.742	0.747	0.753	0.758	7.692	0.767	0.771	0.775	0.779	0.784	0.789	0.794	0.798	0.800	0.802	0.805
13.0	0.588	0.642	0.655	0.666	0.676	0.686	0.694	0.703	0.709	0.715	0.721	0.727	0.732	7.692	0.742	0.745	0.750	0.754	0.760	0.765	0.770	0.774	0.776	0.779	0.783
14.0	0.561	0.615	0.628	0.639	0.648	0.658	0.667	0.676	0.682	0.688	0.695	0.701	0.706	7.692	0.716	0.720	0.724	0.729	0.736	0.741	0.748	0.751	0.754	0.756	0.760
15.0	0.536	0.589	0.602	0.613	0.623	0.620	0.642	0.651	0.657	0.663	0.670	0.677	0.682	7.692	0.693	0.696	0.701	0.706	0.713	0.718	0.725	0.729	0.732	0.735	0.739
16.0	0.511	0.564	0.577	0.588	0.598	0.607	0.617	0.626	0.633	0.639	0.647	0.653	0.659	7.692	0.670	0.673	0.678	0.683	0.690	0.696	0.703	0.708	0.710	0.713	0.718
17.0	0.488	0.541	0.553	0.564	0.574	0.584	0.593	0.602	0.609	0.615	0.622	0.628	0.635	7.692	0.646	0.650	0.655	0.660	0.667	0.674	0.680	0.686	0.689	0.692	0.697
18.0	0.466	0.517	0.529	0.540	0.550	0.560	0.569	0.579	0.586	0.593	0.599	0.606	0.613	7.692	0.623	0.628	0.633	0.638	0.645	0.653	0.659	0.665	0.668	0.672	0.677
19.0	0.445	0.495	0.507	0.517	0.528	0.537	0.547	0.556	0.563	0.570	0.577	0.584	0.591	7.692	0.601	0.606	0.611	0.616	0.623	0.631	0.638	0.643	0.647	0.651	0.657
20.0	0.424	0.473	0.486	0.496	0.506	0.515	0.524	0.534	0.541	0.548	0.555	0.562	0.569	7.692	0.579	0.584	0.589	0.594	0.602	0.609	0.617	0.623	0.626	0.630	0.636
21.0	0.405	0.454	0.466	0.476	0.484	0.494	0.502	0.512	0.519	0.527	0.533	0.541	0.548	7.692	0.558	0.563	0.568	0.573	0.581	0.588	0.596	0.602	0.606	0.611	0.616
22.0	0.387	0.434	0.446	0.456	0.464	0.474	0.483	0.492	0.499	0.506	0.513	0.520	0.527	7.692	0.538	0.543	0.548	0.553	0.561	0.568	0.576	0.582	0.587	0.591	0.598
23.0	0.370	0.416	0.428	0.437	0.446	0.455	0.464	0.473	0.480	0.487	0.494	0.501	0.508	7.692	0.518	0.523	0.529	0.534	0.541	0.549	0.557	0.563	0.568	0.572	0.579
24.0	0.352	0.398	0.410	0.419	0.428	0.436	0.445	0.454	0.460	0.468	0.474	0.482	0.488	7.692	0.499	0.503	0.509	0.514	0.522	0.530	0.538	0.544	0.549	0.553	0.560
25.0	0.337	0.382	0.393	0.402	0.410	0.419	0.427	0.436	0.443	0.449	0.456	0.463	0.470	7.692	0.480	0.485	0.490	0.496	0.504	0.512	0.520	0.526	0.530	0.535	0.543
26.0	0.321	0.365	0.376	0.384	0.393	0.402	0.409	0.418	0.424	0.431	0.439	0.445	0.451	7.692	0.462	0.466	0.471	0.477	0.485	0.493	0.501	0.507	0.512	0.516	0.524
27.0	0.307	0.350	0.361	0.369	0.377	0.386	0.394	0.402	0.408	0.414	0.421	0.428	0.434	7.692	0.444	0.449	0.454	0.459	0.468	0.476	0.484	0.490	0.495	0.500	0.507
28.0	0.292	0.335	0.346	0.355	0.362	0.370	0.377	0.385	0.392	0.398	0.405	0.410	0.417	7.692	0.427	0.431	0.436	0.441	0.449	0.459	0.467	0.473	0.478	0.483	0.490
29.0	0.279	0.321	0.332	0.340	0.344	0.355	0.362	0.370	0.375	0.382	0.388	0.395	0.400	7.692	0.410	0.415	0.420	0.425	0.433	0.441	0.450	0.457	0.461	0.466	0.473
30.0	0.266	0.307	0.317	0.325	0.332	0.340	0.347	0.354	0.360	0.366	0.373	0.378	0.384	7.692	0.394	0.399	0.403	0.409	0.417	0.425	0.434	0.440	0.444	0.450	0.456

Table 11-15 10 MV tissue maximum ratio

Eq Sq Depth (cm)	0.0	4.0	5.0	6.0	7.0	8.0	9.0	10.0	11.0	12.0	13.0	14.0	15.0	16.0	17.0	18.0	19.0	20.0	22.0	24.0	26.0	28.0	30.0
0.0	0.099	0.100	0.100	0.111	0.122	0.133	0.144	0.156	0.165	0.174	0.182	0.191	0.200	0.208	0.216	0.225	0.233	0.241	0.253	0.264	0.276	0.288	0.300
1.0	0.749	0.750	0.750	0.770	0.790	0.816	0.848	0.880	0.884	0.888	0.892	0.896	0.900	0.904	0.908	0.912	0.916	0.920	0.924	0.928	0.934	0.942	0.950
2.0	0.933	0.934	0.934	0.945	0.956	0.967	0.976	0.986	0.987	0.989	0.990	0.991	0.993	0.994	0.996	0.997	0.999	1.001	1.004	1.007	1.011	1.015	1.019
2.5	1.000	1.001	1.001	1.005	1.009	1.012	1.013	1.015	1.016	1.017	1.017	1.018	1.019	1.020	1.021	1.023	1.024	1.025	1.028	1.031	1.032	1.033	1.034
3.0	0.978	0.992	0.995	0.999	1.003	1.006	1.007	1.008	1.009	1.010	1.012	1.013	1.014	1.015	1.016	1.017	1.018	1.019	1.021	1.024	1.025	1.026	1.027
4.0	0.942	0.976	0.985	0.989	0.993	0.995	0.995	0.995	0.997	0.999	1.001	1.003	1.005	1.006	1.006	1.007	1.007	1.008	1.010	1.013	1.014	1.015	1.016
5.0	0.908	0.948	0.958	0.963	0.968	0.972	0.973	0.974	0.976	0.979	0.981	0.984	0.986	0.987	0.988	0.989	0.990	0.991	0.993	0.996	0.998	0.999	1.000
6.0	0.875	0.920	0.931	0.937	0.944	0.949	0.950	0.952	0.955	0.958	0.960	0.963	0.966	0.967	0.969	0.970	0.972	0.973	0.976	0.979	0.981	0.982	0.983
7.0	0.843	0.892	0.904	0.912	0.919	0.924	0.927	0.930	0.933	0.936	0.940	0.943	0.946	0.948	0.949	0.951	0.952	0.954	0.957	0.960	0.963	0.965	0.967
8.0	0.812	0.864	0.878	0.886	0.895	0.901	0.904	0.908	0.912	0.915	0.919	0.922	0.926	0.928	0.930	0.931	0.933	0.935	0.938	0.941	0.944	0.947	0.950
9.0	0.782	0.836	0.849	0.858	0.867	0.874	0.878	0.882	0.886	0.890	0.895	0.899	0.903	0.905	0.907	0.909	0.911	0.913	0.917	0.921	0.924	0.927	0.929
10.0	0.754	0.808	0.822	0.832	0.842	0.849	0.853	0.857	0.862	0.866	0.871	0.875	0.880	0.882	0.885	0.887	0.890	0.892	0.896	0.900	0.903	0.906	0.909
11.0	0.727	0.781	0.794	0.805	0.816	0.823	0.828	0.832	0.837	0.842	0.847	0.852	0.857	0.860	0.862	0.865	0.867	0.870	0.874	0.879	0.883	0.886	0.889
12.0	0.700	0.754	0.768	0.779	0.790	0.798	0.803	0.808	0.813	0.818	0.824	0.829	0.834	0.837	0.840	0.843	0.846	0.849	0.854	0.859	0.863	0.866	0.869
13.0	0.675	0.728	0.741	0.752	0.765	0.774	0.779	0.784	0.789	0.795	0.800	0.806	0.811	0.814	0.817	0.821	0.824	0.827	0.832	0.837	0.842	0.845	0.849
14.0	0.650	0.703	0.716	0.728	0.741	0.750	0.755	0.760	0.766	0.772	0.777	0.783	0.789	0.792	0.795	0.799	0.802	0.805	0.811	0.816	0.821	0.825	0.829
15.0	0.626	0.678	0.691	0.704	0.717	0.726	0.731	0.737	0.743	0.749	0.755	0.761	0.767	0.770	0.774	0.777	0.781	0.784	0.790	0.796	0.801	0.805	0.809
16.0	0.604	0.654	0.667	0.680	0.693	0.703	0.708	0.714	0.720	0.727	0.733	0.740	0.746	0.749	0.753	0.756	0.760	0.763	0.769	0.776	0.781	0.786	0.790
17.0	0.582	0.631	0.643	0.655	0.668	0.677	0.684	0.690	0.696	0.703	0.709	0.716	0.722	0.726	0.730	0.733	0.737	0.741	0.747	0.754	0.759	0.764	0.769
18.0	0.560	0.608	0.620	0.632	0.644	0.653	0.660	0.667	0.674	0.680	0.687	0.693	0.700	0.704	0.708	0.711	0.715	0.719	0.726	0.733	0.739	0.744	0.749
19.0	0.540	0.586	0.597	0.609	0.620	0.630	0.637	0.644	0.651	0.657	0.664	0.670	0.677	0.681	0.685	0.690	0.694	0.698	0.705	0.712	0.719	0.724	0.729
20.0	0.520	0.565	0.576	0.587	0.598	0.607	0.615	0.623	0.630	0.636	0.643	0.649	0.656	0.660	0.665	0.669	0.674	0.678	0.685	0.692	0.699	0.704	0.710
21.0	0.501	0.544	0.555	0.566	0.577	0.586	0.594	0.602	0.609	0.615	0.622	0.628	0.635	0.640	0.644	0.649	0.653	0.658	0.666	0.673	0.680	0.685	0.691
22.0	0.483	0.525	0.536	0.547	0.558	0.567	0.575	0.583	0.590	0.596	0.603	0.609	0.616	0.621	0.625	0.630	0.634	0.639	0.647	0.654	0.661	0.666	0.672
23.0	0.466	0.507	0.518	0.528	0.539	0.548	0.556	0.564	0.571	0.577	0.584	0.590	0.597	0.602	0.607	0.611	0.616	0.621	0.629	0.636	0.643	0.648	0.654
24.0	0.449	0.489	0.499	0.510	0.521	0.530	0.537	0.545	0.552	0.558	0.565	0.571	0.578	0.583	0.588	0.593	0.598	0.603	0.611	0.618	0.625	0.630	0.636
25.0	0.433	0.477	0.488	0.498	0.509	0.518	0.526	0.534	0.540	0.547	0.553	0.560	0.567	0.571	0.576	0.581	0.586	0.591	0.599	0.607	0.613	0.619	0.624
26.0	0.416	0.464	0.476	0.487	0.498	0.507	0.514	0.522	0.529	0.535	0.542	0.548	0.555	0.560	0.565	0.569	0.574	0.579	0.587	0.595	0.602	0.607	0.612
27.0	0.402	0.453	0.466	0.476	0.486	0.495	0.503	0.511	0.518	0.524	0.531	0.537	0.544	0.548	0.553	0.558	0.563	0.568	0.576	0.584	0.590	0.595	0.601
28.0	0.387	0.441	0.455	0.465	0.475	0.484	0.492	0.500	0.506	0.513	0.519	0.526	0.532	0.537	0.542	0.546	0.551	0.556	0.564	0.572	0.579	0.584	0.589
29.0	0.373	0.430	0.444	0.454	0.464	0.473	0.481	0.488	0.495	0.502	0.508	0.515	0.521	0.526	0.530	0.535	0.540	0.545	0.553	0.561	0.568	0.573	0.578
30.0	0.359	0.418	0.433	0.443	0.454	0.463	0.470	0.477	0.484	0.490	0.497	0.503	0.510	0.515	0.519	0.524	0.528	0.533	0.541	0.550	0.556	0.561	0.566

Table 11-16 10 MV tissue phantom ratio

Eq Sq Depth (cm)	0.0	4.0	5.0	6.0	7.0	8.0	9.0	10.0	11.0	12.0	13.0	14.0	15.0	16.0	17.0	18.0	19.0	20.0	22.0	24.0	26.0	28.0	30.0
0.0	0.109	0.105	0.104	0.127	0.126	0.137	0.148	0.160	0.169	0.168	0.185	0.194	0.203	0.211	0.219	0.227	0.235	0.243	0.255	0.265	0.277	0.288	0.300
1.0	0.825	0.791	0.783	0.821	0.816	0.840	0.871	0.903	0.905	0.903	0.909	0.910	0.912	0.916	0.919	0.922	0.925	0.928	0.930	0.932	0.936	0.943	0.950
2.0	1.028	0.985	0.975	0.993	0.988	0.995	1.003	1.012	1.011	1.008	1.009	1.007	1.007	1.007	1.008	1.008	1.009	1.010	1.011	1.011	1.013	1.016	1.019
2.5	1.101	1.056	1.045	1.044	1.043	1.042	1.041	1.042	1.041	1.038	1.036	1.034	1.033	1.033	1.033	1.034	1.034	1.034	1.035	1.035	1.034	1.034	1.034
3.0	1.077	1.046	1.039	1.038	1.037	1.035	1.034	1.034	1.033	1.031	1.031	1.029	1.028	1.028	1.028	1.028	1.028	1.028	1.028	1.028	1.027	1.027	1.027
4.0	1.037	1.030	1.028	1.027	1.026	1.024	1.022	1.021	1.021	1.020	1.020	1.019	1.019	1.019	1.018	1.018	1.017	1.017	1.017	1.017	1.016	1.016	1.016
5.0	1.000	1.000	1.000	1.000	1.000	1.000	1.000	1.000	1.000	1.000	1.000	1.000	1.000	1.000	1.000	1.000	1.000	1.000	1.000	1.000	1.000	1.000	1.000
6.0	0.964	0.971	0.972	0.973	0.976	0.977	0.976	0.977	0.978	0.978	0.978	0.978	0.979	0.979	0.980	0.981	0.982	0.982	0.983	0.983	0.983	0.983	0.983
7.0	0.928	0.941	0.944	0.947	0.950	0.951	0.952	0.954	0.956	0.956	0.958	0.958	0.959	0.960	0.960	0.961	0.961	0.962	0.964	0.964	0.965	0.966	0.967
8.0	0.894	0.911	0.917	0.920	0.925	0.927	0.929	0.932	0.934	0.934	0.936	0.937	0.939	0.940	0.941	0.941	0.942	0.943	0.945	0.945	0.946	0.948	0.950
9.0	0.861	0.882	0.886	0.891	0.896	0.900	0.902	0.905	0.907	0.909	0.912	0.913	0.915	0.917	0.918	0.919	0.920	0.921	0.923	0.925	0.926	0.928	0.929
10.0	0.830	0.852	0.858	0.864	0.870	0.874	0.876	0.880	0.883	0.884	0.888	0.889	0.892	0.893	0.895	0.897	0.899	0.900	0.902	0.904	0.905	0.907	0.909
11.0	0.801	0.824	0.829	0.836	0.843	0.847	0.851	0.854	0.857	0.860	0.863	0.865	0.869	0.871	0.872	0.874	0.876	0.878	0.880	0.883	0.885	0.887	0.889
12.0	0.771	0.795	0.802	0.809	0.816	0.821	0.825	0.829	0.833	0.835	0.840	0.842	0.846	0.848	0.850	0.852	0.854	0.857	0.860	0.862	0.865	0.867	0.869
13.0	0.743	0.768	0.774	0.781	0.791	0.797	0.800	0.805	0.808	0.812	0.815	0.819	0.822	0.824	0.827	0.830	0.832	0.834	0.838	0.840	0.844	0.846	0.849
14.0	0.716	0.742	0.747	0.756	0.766	0.772	0.776	0.780	0.785	0.788	0.792	0.795	0.800	0.802	0.804	0.808	0.810	0.812	0.817	0.819	0.823	0.826	0.829
15.0	0.689	0.715	0.721	0.731	0.741	0.747	0.751	0.756	0.761	0.765	0.769	0.773	0.778	0.780	0.783	0.785	0.789	0.791	0.796	0.799	0.803	0.806	0.809
16.0	0.665	0.690	0.696	0.706	0.716	0.724	0.727	0.733	0.737	0.742	0.748	0.752	0.756	0.759	0.762	0.764	0.768	0.770	0.774	0.779	0.783	0.787	0.790
17.0	0.641	0.666	0.671	0.680	0.690	0.697	0.703	0.708	0.713	0.718	0.722	0.727	0.732	0.735	0.739	0.741	0.744	0.748	0.752	0.757	0.761	0.765	0.769
18.0	0.617	0.641	0.647	0.656	0.666	0.672	0.680	0.685	0.690	0.694	0.700	0.704	0.710	0.713	0.716	0.719	0.722	0.725	0.731	0.736	0.741	0.745	0.749
19.0	0.595	0.618	0.623	0.633	0.641	0.648	0.654	0.661	0.667	0.671	0.677	0.681	0.686	0.690	0.693	0.698	0.701	0.704	0.710	0.715	0.720	0.725	0.729
20.0	0.573	0.596	0.601	0.610	0.618	0.625	0.632	0.639	0.645	0.649	0.655	0.659	0.665	0.668	0.673	0.676	0.681	0.684	0.690	0.695	0.700	0.705	0.710
21.0	0.552	0.574	0.579	0.588	0.596	0.603	0.610	0.618	0.624	0.628	0.634	0.638	0.644	0.648	0.652	0.656	0.659	0.664	0.671	0.676	0.681	0.686	0.691
22.0	0.532	0.554	0.560	0.568	0.577	0.584	0.591	0.598	0.604	0.609	0.614	0.619	0.624	0.629	0.632	0.637	0.640	0.645	0.652	0.657	0.662	0.667	0.672
23.0	0.513	0.535	0.541	0.548	0.557	0.564	0.571	0.579	0.585	0.589	0.595	0.599	0.605	0.610	0.614	0.618	0.622	0.627	0.633	0.639	0.644	0.649	0.654
24.0	0.494	0.516	0.521	0.530	0.538	0.546	0.552	0.559	0.565	0.570	0.576	0.580	0.586	0.590	0.595	0.599	0.603	0.608	0.615	0.621	0.626	0.631	0.636
25.0	0.477	0.503	0.509	0.517	0.526	0.533	0.540	0.548	0.553	0.559	0.563	0.569	0.575	0.578	0.583	0.587	0.592	0.596	0.603	0.609	0.614	0.620	0.624
26.0	0.458	0.489	0.497	0.506	0.515	0.522	0.528	0.536	0.542	0.546	0.552	0.557	0.563	0.567	0.572	0.575	0.580	0.584	0.591	0.597	0.603	0.608	0.612
27.0	0.443	0.478	0.486	0.494	0.502	0.510	0.517	0.524	0.531	0.535	0.541	0.546	0.552	0.555	0.560	0.564	0.569	0.573	0.580	0.586	0.591	0.596	0.601
28.0	0.426	0.465	0.475	0.483	0.491	0.498	0.505	0.513	0.518	0.524	0.529	0.534	0.539	0.544	0.548	0.552	0.556	0.561	0.568	0.574	0.580	0.585	0.589
29.0	0.411	0.454	0.463	0.472	0.480	0.487	0.494	0.501	0.507	0.513	0.518	0.523	0.528	0.533	0.536	0.541	0.545	0.550	0.557	0.563	0.569	0.574	0.578
30.0	0.395	0.441	0.452	0.460	0.469	0.477	0.483	0.490	0.496	0.500	0.506	0.511	0.517	0.522	0.525	0.530	0.533	0.538	0.545	0.552	0.557	0.562	0.566

	Tray	Factor	Wedge	Factor	Brass compensator	Factor
Table 11-17	Tray wedge and compensator factors					
Cobalt 60	5 mm solid	0.96	15 degree	0.828	1 mm	0.956
	5 mm slotted	0.97	30 degree	0.744	2 mm	0.914
			45 degree	0.653	3 mm	0.874
			60 degree	0.424	4 mm	0.835
6 MV	5 mm solid	0.97	15 degree	0.828	1 mm	0.965
	5 mm slotted	0.98	30 degree	0.714	2 mm	0.931
			45 degree	0.580	3 mm	0.899
			60 degree	0.424	4 mm	0.867
10 MV	5 mm solid	0.97	15 degree	0.895	1 mm	0.971
	5 mm slotted	0.98	30 degree	0.802	2 mm	0.943
			45 degree	0.702	3 mm	0.916
			60 degree	0.513	4 mm	0.889
18 MV	5 mm solid	0.98	15 degree	0.866	1 mm	0.927
	5 mm slotted	0.99	30 degree	0.775	2 mm	0.945
			45 degree	0.656	3 mm	0.918
			60 degree	0.449	4 mm	0.892

Review Questions

Multiple Choice

1. Percentage depth dose increases with increasing:
   I. Energy
   II. Depth
   III. Field size
   a. I and II
   b. I and III
   c. II and III
   d. I, II, and III

2. Tissue air ratio decreases with decreasing:
   I. Field size
   II. Depth
   III. SSD
   a. I
   b. II
   c. III
   d. I, II, and III

3. When blocking is used in a treatment calculation, the area of the collimator is used in determining:
   I. TMR
   II. OF
   III. PDD
   a. I
   b. II
   c. III
   d. I, II, and III

4. Which of the following central axis depth dose quantities would most likely be used to compute an accurate monitor unit setting on an 18 MV unit for an isocentric treatment?
   a. Percentage depth dose
   b. Backscatter factor
   c. Tissue-maximum ratio
   d. All of the above

5. Two parallel opposed equally weighted cobalt 60 fields are separated by 20 cm of tissue and treated with an SSD technique. The maximum dose will occur:
   a. Directly on the skin surface
   b. At the midline of the patient
   c. 0.5 cm under skin surface
   d. 5 cm under the skin surface

6. The advantages of using parallel opposed isocentric fields for treatment delivery are (compared to nonisocentric):
   a. Less opportunity for movement error
   b. Less overall dose to the skin surface
   c. Both A and B
   d. Neither A nor B

7. A wedge filter _____ the output of the beam and must thus be taken into account in the treatment calculations:
   a. Increases
   b. Decreases
   c. Does not affect
   d. Not enough information given
8. Mayneord's factor is used to convert
   a. PDD with a change in SSD from the standard
   b. TAR with a change in SSD from the standard
   c. Exposure rate with a change in SSD from the standard
   d. An exposure in roentgens to rads

True or False

9. Any time an object is placed in the path of a therapeutic beam of radiation, it must be corrected for in the dose calculation to account for beam absorption.
   True _____   False _____

Questions to Ponder

1. Analyze how the collimator or field size can affect the output of a linear accelerator.
2. Describe how the source to skin distance causes percentage depth dose to vary.
3. A patient's larynx is to be treated using an isocentric technique on a cobalt 60 unit; the patient's separation at the central axis (CAX) is 9 cm and will be treated to midplane. The treatment will use parallel opposed right and left lateral fields. The isocenter of the machine is established at 80 cm.
   a. What is the SSD on the patient's skin?
   b. If a field size of 6 cm × 6 cm is set on the collimator, what is the field size on the skin surface?
4. Explain the relationship between beam quality (energy) and TMR.
5. A 20 cm thick patient is to be treated on a cobalt unit at 80 cm SAD. Two opposed 15 cm × 15 cm ports are used to deliver a treatment dose of 180 rads per day to the midline (mid-plane). Determine the treatment time per port.
6. A patient is to receive 5040 rads to his lung in 28 fractions. The treatment will use 15 cm × 11 cm opposed 10 MV photons to mid plane at 100 cm SAD. The separation is 21 cm. The field is blocked to a 11 cm × 11 cm equivalent field. A 5 mm solid tray is used to support the blocks. Find the MU for each port each day.
7. Calculate the MU setting to deliver 300 rads to a depth of 12 cm on a 6 MV unit using a single beam at 100 cm SSD using a field size of 15 cm × 8 cm. Using this information, determine what the dose would be at a depth of 6 cm.

8. Compare and contrast the factors that influence percentage depth dose and tissue phantom ratio.
9. Look up the percentage depth dose at 80 cm SSD and 7 cm depth for a cobalt unit with a 10 cm × 10 cm field size. Determine the percentage depth dose for the same field size and depth at 100 cm SSD.
10. Two opposing 10 cm × 10 cm cobalt 60 fields at an SSD of 80 cm are used with a separation of 20 cm. If the given dose is 100 cGy from each field, what is the dose at midline?

REFERENCES

1. Bentel GC: *Radiation therapy planning*, ed 2. New York, 1996, McGraw-Hill.
2. Bentel GC, Nelson CE, Noell KT: *Treatment planning and dose calculations in radiation oncology*, ed 4. Elmsford, NY, 1989, Pergamon Press.
3. Johns H, Cunningham J: *The physics of radiology*, ed 4. Springfield, IL, 1983, Charles C Thomas.
4. Kahn FM: *The physics of radiation therapy*, ed 2. Baltimore, 1994, Williams & Wilkins.
5. Levitt SH et al: *Levitt and Tapley's technological basis of radiation therapy: practical clinical applications*, ed 2. Malvern, PA, 1992, Lea & Febiger.
6. Mizer S et al: *Radiation therapy simulation workbook*. Elmsford, NY, 1986, Pergamon Press.
7. Selman J: *The basic physics of radiation therapy*, ed 3. Springfield, IL, 1990, Charles C Thomas.
8. Shahabi S: *Blackburn's introduction to clinical radiation therapy physics*. Madison, WI, 1989, Medical Physics Publishing.
9. Stanton R, Stinson D: *An introduction to radiation oncology physics*. Madison, WI, 1992, Medical Physics Publishing.

Dose Distribution

Teresa L. Bruno

Outline

Key terms

Algorithms
Attenuation
Beam block
Beam profiles
Bolus
Bremsstrahlung
Compensating filter
Depth dose profile
Effective SSD method
Equivalent depth
Field size
Flatness

Inhomogeneities
Inverse square law method
Isodose chart
Isodose curve
Isodose shift method
Normalization
Off-axis effect
Penumbra
Symmetry
TAR or TMR ratio method
Wedge filter

 Literally speaking, dosimetry in radiation therapy is the measurement of radiation dose, or the quantity of radiation deposited in tissue. There are different methods for directly and indirectly measuring quantities of radiation: calorimetry, chemical, TLD, and ion chambers connected to electrometers.[5] Radiobiologists have been able to document the amount of radiation necessary to kill different tumor cells grown in culture. Before we can determine if the same amount of radiation will destroy tumor cells in a living host, we need to be able to determine how much radiation dose is actually being deposited in the tissue.

The measurement techniques just listed are not well suited to measurement of radiation in patient tissue. Physicists and mathematicians have developed mathematical models, **algorithms**, to calculate the dose to specified depths within the patient. The application of some of these mathematical models is discussed in the chapter that follows. Dosimetrists use these to develop treatment plans and calculate the dose to targeted tumor areas and to dose-limiting critical structures.

PHOTON DOSE DISTRIBUTIONS
Beam profiles

The optimum radiation beam delivers the desired dose to a patient's tumor while giving minimal dose to normal tissue. While understanding that there is no "perfect" beam that delivers its full dose to tumor tissue exclusively, treatments may be tailored to each individual patient by knowing the relative dose distributions for different radiation beams.

In the process of producing a useful beam from a linear accelerator, a stream of high energy x-rays emerges from the linear accelerator's target. This stream of x-rays is forward-peaked in intensity, with higher energy x-rays along the central ray of the beam.[7] A conical flattening filter is placed in the center of this stream of x-rays to give the beam flatness at treatment depth.[10] The average energy of the beam is still somewhat lower on the periphery compared to the central axis. **Flatness** changes with depth because of this and because of differences in scatter.[10] For a photon beam, flatness is usually measured at a depth of 10 cm. Adequate flatness is specified as within ±3%, over 80% of the field at this depth. The plane of measurement is perpendicular to the central axis. Isodose lines close to D_{max} depth may be very uneven, with "horns" on either side of the central ray in order to be flat at 10 cm depth. The **depth dose profile** used for flatness and symmetry measurements is a very useful beam profile, showing the variation of dose across the field at the selected depth. This curve generally shows the maximum dose within the field as 100% and the dose measured across the field as it relates to the maximum dose.[2,7,10]

A beam may meet flatness specifications but not meet specifications for **symmetry**. Beam symmetry is sameness from side to side. Usual symmetry specifications are within ±2% from side to side, over 80% of the beam width at a depth of 10 cm. Beam flatness profiles may also be used to determine symmetry by comparing the profile from side to side (Fig. 12-1).[7,10]

Isodose curves

An electrometer may be used to measure the collected charge caused by ionizations at a given point within a medium to determine the dose delivered at the point, or doses of radiation may be calculated mathematically. This gives information only for that one point in space. The measured data for points in several different planes are useful in radiation therapy. One of the most frequently used tools that shows the dose distribution in a plane is the isodose chart.[7,10] An **isodose chart** consists of information useful for determining doses at different depths within tissue for a specific beam. This means that the isodose chart must be for one specific beam type and energy for one particular machine. There are some standard charts published for a given beam type and energy showing average data from many machines with the same construction, that is, the same manufacturer with the same beam specifications. These averaged charts may be used for general information purposes but should not be used for patient calculations.[2] Isodose curves on the chart show where the same dose is delivered, across the width of the beam, at different depths, for a specific beam size and source-to-skin distance (SSD). Isodose curve charts are usually set up with 100% showing the maximum dose within the treatment field. The other lines show percents of that maximum. A number of important beam properties may be found by studying the isodose curve chart (Fig. 12-1).[2]

Scattered radiation from all sides increases the absorbed dose at the center of the field. Farther away from the center

there is less scatter available, and the isodose values decrease. The light field is made to coincide with the isodose line where the dose decreases to 50% of the central axis (CAX) dose. Therefore the **field size** is defined as the distance between the 50% isodose lines on each side of the beam at the standard source-to-axis distance (SAD) for the machine.[2,7,9,10] Because one component of the dose is the primary beam and the other component is scattered radiation, the dose drops off near the edges of the field, as the scatter component decreases.[7] The area between the 20% isodose line on the outside and the 90% on the inside is the **penumbra** region.[9,10] For lower energy beams the radiation is more easily deflected to the side and the penumbra region is wider. Higher energy beams have a narrower penumbra because the scatter will be more forward directed.[7] Electrons have a much higher probability of interacting with other atoms because of their mass and charge. The lower electron isodose lines especially tend to bulge below the surface. Different terms used to describe this effect are mushrooming and ballooning of the lower percentage isodose curves.[10] Probably the easiest to see and one of the most important is how the depth of penetration increases with increasing energy (Fig. 12-3).

Off-axis effect and irregularly shaped fields

X-rays produced by linear accelerators radiate out in a sphere. Shielding material inside and outside the head of the machine shapes the beam to match the area to be treated. A third beam profile is a "beam's eye view" profile, which shows the relative doses parallel to the beam across the field at a particular depth.[7] Because the corners of the shaped treatment field are actually farther from the relatively small radiation source and because the scatter component of the beam decreases, the isodose lines in this plane are rounded at the corners of the field. The radiation therapy treatment planning computer should be able to account for the changes across the width and length of the field.[2,7]

The highest dose is at the CAX of the beam, and the dose decreases with greater distance from the CAX. This **off-axis effect** is one of the reasons that the field size should be a bit larger than the tumor.[7] When dose-limiting critical structures or tumor tissue lies away from the CAX, special calculations are done to determine exactly what dose is delivered. One way to compensate for the nonuniformity across a large field is to give additional dose to the high risk areas. Another is to use a field size larger than the target volume, so that no high risk tissue is in the lower dose areas. The beam also may be modified using a compensator to flatten the beam, or to flatten the beam and also compensate for sloping skin surface.

The dose delivered to a particular point within the treatment volume, a point of interest such as the spinal cord or involved lymph nodes, is determined by a number of factors. The physical characteristics of the treatment unit are the first consideration. Any information used in calculations must be for that particular machine, not just the beam type, energy, and manufacturer. Calculations for beam on time or monitor

A

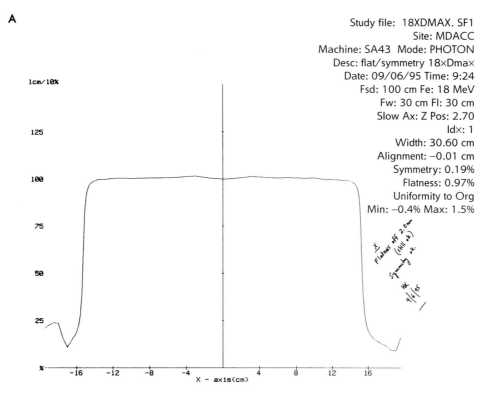

Study file: 18XDMAX. SF1
Site: MDACC
Machine: SA43 Mode: PHOTON
Desc: flat/symmetry 18×Dmax
Date: 09/06/95 Time: 9:24
Fsd: 100 cm Fe: 18 MeV
Fw: 30 cm Fl: 30 cm
Slow Ax: Z Pos: 2.70
Idx: 1
Width: 30.60 cm
Alignment: −0.01 cm
Symmetry: 0.19%
Flatness: 0.97%
Uniformity to Org
Min: −0.4% Max: 1.5%

B

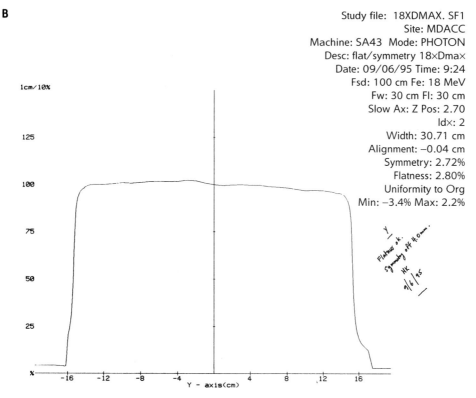

Study file: 18XDMAX. SF1
Site: MDACC
Machine: SA43 Mode: PHOTON
Desc: flat/symmetry 18×Dmax
Date: 09/06/95 Time: 9:24
Fsd: 100 cm Fe: 18 MeV
Fw: 30 cm Fl: 30 cm
Slow Ax: Z Pos: 2.70
Idx: 2
Width: 30.71 cm
Alignment: −0.04 cm
Symmetry: 2.72%
Flatness: 2.80%
Uniformity to Org
Min: −3.4% Max: 2.2%

Fig. 12-1 Beam flatness and symmetry profile for an 18 MV photon beam. **A**, *x*-Axis with both flatness and symmetry within acceptable range. **B**, The same beam, *y*-axis, with acceptable flatness, but with symmetry out of range.

A   Target pr-4j21.0205 release 1.0.4 2:33 pm on 6 September 1995

Patient name   : Block Phantom
Patient code   : 090695
Plan number   : 3
Plan comment   : cobalt 60
Outline set   : 1
Slice   : 1 at off-axis distance 0 mm
Plan units   : Percent
Magnification   : 100%

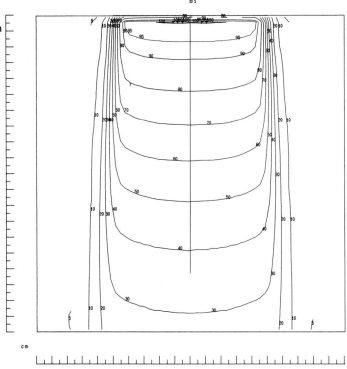

B   Target pr-4j21.0205 release 1.0.4 2:31pm on 6 September 1995

Patient name   : Block Phantom
Patient code   : 090695
Plan number   : WARNING: unsaved plan!
Plan comment   : Single 6 MV beam
Outline set   : 1
Slice   : 1 at off-axis distance 0 mm
Normalized to   : 100%
Plan units   : Percent
Magnification   : 100%

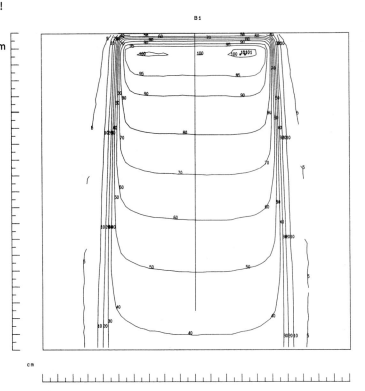

Fig. 12-2 For legend see opposite page.

C Patient name   : Block Phantom
   Patient code   : 090695
   Plan number   : 2
   Plan comment : 18 MV c12100c18
   Outline set   : 1
   Slice   : 1 at off-axis distance 0 mm
   Normalized to : 100%
   Plan units   : Percent
   Magnification : 100%

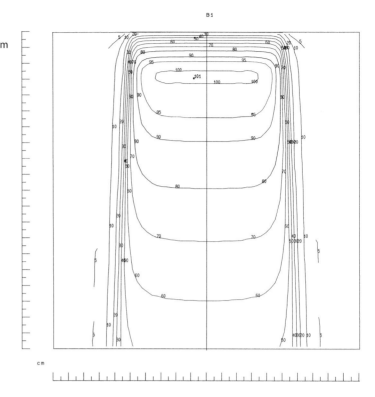

Fig. 12-2, cont'd Three photon beam isodose charts shown normalized to D_{max}. The 100% isodose line is at the depth of maximum dose along the central ray. **A**, Cobalt 60 beam, 10 × 10 cm², 80 cm SSD. **B**, 6 MV photon beam, 10 × 10 cm², 100 cm SSD. **C**, 18 MV beam, 10 × 10 cm², 100 cm SSD.

unit settings are based on the data for the machine along the central ray of the beam. Everything else is relative to the dose calculated here. The point for which the beam on time or monitor units are calculated is the reference point. To find the dose to the point of interest, we then account for (1) increased or decreased SSD, (2) location of the point of interest relative to the CAX (*x* and *y* coordinates), (3) location of the point of interest relative to beam-shaping blocks, and (4) increase or decrease of depth in tissue compared to the reference point.[2,7]

Early in the clinical use of radiation as cancer therapy, Clarkson developed the scatter function calculation method for irregularly shaped fields. The primary and scatter radiation contributions to a point are calculated separately. The irregularly shaped field is divided into sectors. Then the scatter dose contributed by individual sectors may be summed and added to the primary dose.[2,7,10]

A representation of the treatment port, either a simulator radiograph or a tracing from the simulator radiograph, is marked with the locations of the reference point and any points of interest. This gives the *x* and *y* coordinates for the points of interest to be used in calculating the off-axis factor. Measurements are taken at these coordinates on the patient. A separation, or diameter, is measured along with the SSD at each location. The information may be entered into a treatment planning computer, which quickly calculates the percent of the prescribed dose delivered to the points of interest. Early planning systems took longer to perform these calculations than an experienced dosimetrist required to calculate the doses using a set of scatter rulers and scatter curves for various depths. The data used by the treatment planning computer are entered by the medical physicist. Even though experienced radiation oncologists, physicists, and dosimetrists may recognize that doses are not within a predictable range, it is still important to be able to verify the computer calculation with a manual calculation method (Fig. 12-4).

A fairly simple manual method for calculating the percent depth dose for a point not along the central ray has been presented by Day. Using the off-axis point as the "center," the field is divided into four quadrants. The percent depth dose for each quadrant is found using four times the quadrant size as the field size, then reading the percent depth dose for this square field size from a table. One fourth this value is added to one fourth the percent depth dose value for each of the other quadrants (finding the value for the square field size four

A   Target pr-4j21.0205 release 1.0.4 2:38 pm on 6 September 1995

Patient name   : Block Phantom
Patient code   : 090695
Plan number   : 5
Plan comment   : 6 MeV EB
Outline set   : 1
Slice   : 1 at off-axis distance 0 mm
Normalized to   : 98%
Plan units   : Percent
Magnification   : 100%

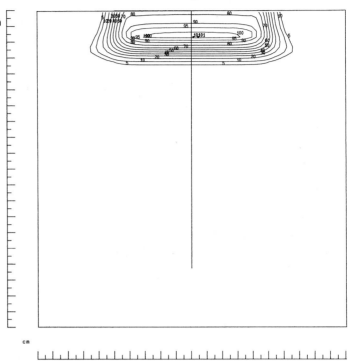

B   Target pr-4j21.0205 release 1.0.4 2:36 pm on 6 September 1995

Patient name   : Block Phantom
Patient code   : 090695
Plan number   : 4
Plan comment   : 16 MeV EB
Outline set   : 1
Slice   : 1 at off-axis distance 0 mm
Normalized to   : 100%
Plan units   : Percent
Magnification   : 100%

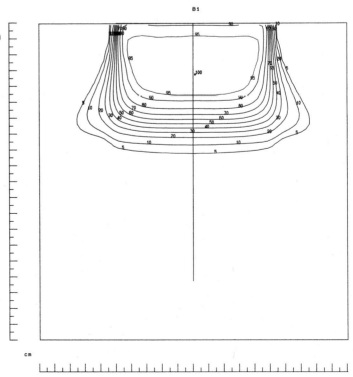

Fig. 12-3 For legend see opposite page.

C   Target pr-4j21.0205 release 1.0.4 2:39 pm on 6 September 1995

Patient name   : Block Phantom
Patient code   : 090695
Plan number   : 6
Plan comment   : 20 MeV EB
Outline set   : 1
Slice   : 1 at off-axis distance 0 mm
Normalized to   : 98%
Plan units   : Percent
Magnification   : 100%

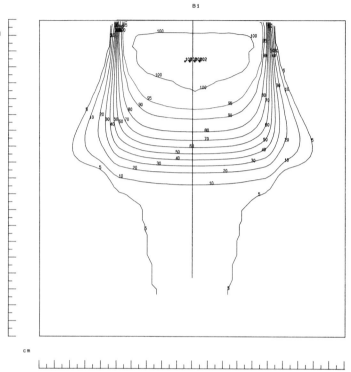

Fig. 12-3, cont'd Three electron beam isodose curve charts. **A**, 6 MeV, 10 × 10 cm², 100 cm SSD. **B**, 16 MeV, 10 × 10 cm², 100 cm SSD. **C**, 20 MeV, 10 × 10 cm², 100 cm SSD.

times the quadrant size). The following example shows the percent depth dose for a point 5 cm lateral and 4 cm superior to the CAX of a 16 cm (L) × 20 cm (W) field (Fig. 12-5)[7]:

$$(0.25)(PDD_{(5 \times 4)}) + (0.25)(PDD_{(15 \times 4)}) + (0.25)(PDD_{(15 \times 12)}) + (0.25)(PDD_{(5 \times 12)}) = PDD \text{ at } {}^{+}4 \text{ cm } y, {}^{-}5 \text{ cm } x$$

CORRECTIONS FOR TISSUE DIFFERENCES
Sloping skin surface

As alluded to earlier, a sloping skin surface has an effect on how the dose is distributed. Thinking in terms of the inverse square law, the areas closer to the source will receive a higher dose than the areas farther away from the source, over the same amount of time. Therefore the isodose curves will somewhat follow the slope of the skin surface. A standard isodose curve for the machine, field size, and energy may be modified using the **inverse square law method**, also known as the **effective SSD method**. A corrected isodose curve is created by sliding the isodose chart down to match the surface at intervals, perpendicular to the central ray of the beam, then correcting the percent depth dose lines at that distance from the CAX[2,7,10]:

$$PDD_{corrected} = PDD_{original}\left(\frac{SSD_{CAX} + d_{max}}{SSD_{CAX} + gap + d_{max}}\right)^2$$

A second method of correcting for a sloping skin surface uses the tissue-air ratio (TAR) or tissue-maximum ratio (TMR), which are independent of SSD. The standard isodose chart is corrected by a factor using a ratio of the TAR or TMR for the depth in tissue using the field size as projected to that depth over the TAR or TMR at the depth plus the difference in SSD, using the same field size. This is appropriately called the **TAR or TMR ratio method**[7,10]:

$$Correction = \frac{TAR_{(d,FS@d)}}{TAR_{(d + gap,FS@d)}}$$

or

$$Correction = \frac{TMR_{(d,FS@d)}}{TMR_{(d + gap,FS@d)}}$$

The third common method is the **isodose shift method**. This method requires less calculating and is therefore faster, but the isodoses obtained are approximate values. The surface contour is traced onto a sheet of paper. The central ray

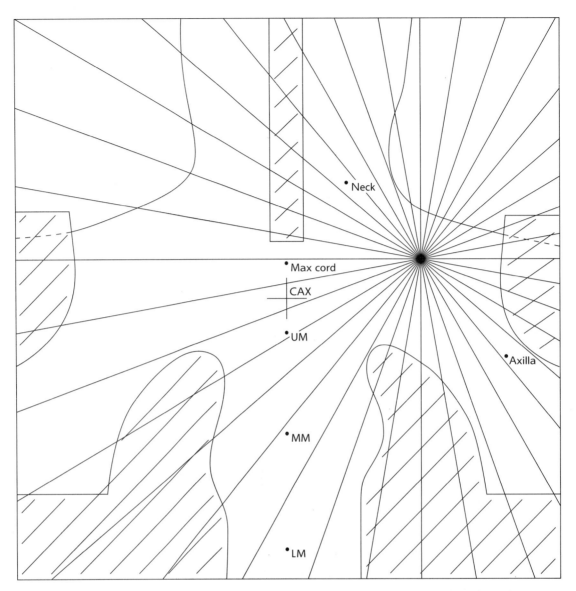

Fig. 12-4 A tracing from a simulator film. Note the location of Cerrobend blocks and skin surfaces along the neck and shoulder. Radii have been drawn at 10-degree increments radiating out from the location of the point of supraclavicular dose measurement. (From Fletcher GH: Textbook of radiotherapy, Baltimore, 1980, Williams and Wilkins.)

of the beam is drawn, along with lines parallel to the central ray, at intervals of 1 cm. This paper is laid over a standard isodose curve. At each interval the isodose chart is shifted toward the skin surface by a percentage of the difference in SSD. The percentage of shift depends on the beam energy. The two-thirds shift method refers to cobalt 60 because the shift is 70% times the difference in SSD for that energy (Fig. 12-6).[2,4,7,10] Table 12-1 on p. 255 shows the percentage shift for photon energies used in the therapeutic range.

Correcting for tissue inhomogeneities

Up to this point, isodose curves and beam data for radiation interacting with water have been used. This is close to the radiation interaction with soft tissue. The calculation is com-

plicated by the fact that irradiated tissue volumes rarely contain only soft tissue. To make an accurate assessment of the dose in volumes comprising different tissue types, we must know how the interactions compare with those in water, a medium in which measurements can easily be taken. Even though the probability of ionizations caused by radiation in a given material (medium) may be calculated and these probabilities used to calculate how much radiation of a particular type needs to be used to attain the desired absorbed dose, the method of calculating in three dimensions is very complex and has not been fully developed. Simply put, the currently used methods for calculating dose through different mediums assign a correction factor for tissue types based on their electron density, ρ_e. It is probably easiest to see this by using an

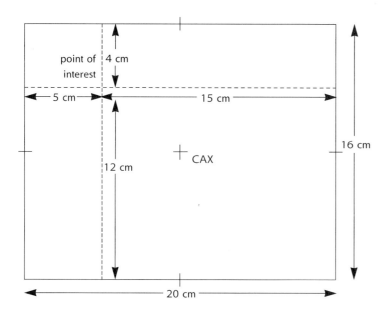

$(.25) \ (\%dd_{(5\times4)})$

$(.25) \ (\%dd_{(15\times4)})$

$(.25) \ (\%dd_{(15\times12)})$

$\underline{+ \ (.25) \ (\%dd_{(5\times12)})}$

%dd for point of interest @ +4cm y and -5cm x

Fig. 12-5 The Day method of calculating dose to a point away from the central ray of the beam.

example. If we are calculating the dose to a point beyond bone (~ 1.3 times as dense as soft tissue), we will measure the thickness of soft tissue in centimeters before the bone, multiply this by 1.0, add to this the thickness of bone in centimeters multiplied by 1.3, then add the remaining soft tissue thickness multiplied by 1.0. The resulting number is the **equivalent depth** in tissue. Electron density for bone depends on how compact the bone is; spongy bone may have an electron density only 1.1 times that of water, and very compact bone's density is up to 1.65 times the density of water (Fig. 12-7).[2,7]

Similarly, if the beam passes through tissue less dense than water, such as lung, or through an air cavity, the thickness of this tissue is multiplied by a number less than 1.0, and the resulting equivalent depth is less than the actual depth.

As stated earlier, this is a very simplified version of what happens when radiation passes through inhomogeneous tissue. It does not take into account the effects seen at the interface between tissues of differing densities. This effect is especially important when dealing with high linear energy transfer (LET) radiations.[7]

BEAM-MODIFYING DEVICES

Several factors contributing to uneven dose distributions have been discussed. Now we will look at some beam modification devices that help tailor the radiation beam to the specific needs for each case. Three of these—wedge filters, compensating filters, and shielding blocks—are placed at least 15 cm away from the patient to decrease the skin dose caused by electron contamination. The fourth factor—bolus—is in contact with the patient's skin, so the skin-sparing effect is lost.[7,8]

Wedges

A **wedge filter** is designed to progressively attenuate the beam across the width of the field. Usually the wedge is made from a dense material, such as copper, brass, or steel, and placed on a tray near the machine collimators. Originally the wedge angle was defined as the angle of the 50% isodose line as it crosses the central ray of the beam. This is not a concrete definition, however, because physicists disagree on the practicality of this definition, especially as it applies to higher energy beams. Also, wedges are usually used for tumors close to the surface. To simplify the designation, 10 cm is the depth at which the wedge isodose angle is specified (Fig. 12-8).[2,5,7,10]

Any beam modification device placed between the source and the patient not only modifies the dose distribution in tissue, it also absorbs some of the useful beam. Early treatment units had substantially lower output rates (mu [monitor units]/min) than the linear accelerators currently in use. Since the **attenuation** (absorption) of radiation by the wedge will always require more monitor units to deliver the same dose in tissue without a wedge in place, an individualized wedge system was commonly used. Its design allowed the thin edge of the wedge to be aligned with the treatment field edge. This permits the least possible attenuation and therefore the least increase in treatment time. Using an individualized wedge system the wedge transmission factor for calculating monitor units may vary greatly with field size, increasing the risk of calculation error. A separate wedge for each beam width also complicates the treatment setup.[2,5,7]

The universal wedge system uses one wedge for all field sizes. The center of the wedge is aligned with the central ray of the beam. Even though the wedge factor actually still

A Target pr-4j21.0205 release 1.0.4 2:52 pm on 6 September 1995

Patient name : Sloping surface
Patient code : 0906952
Plan number : 6
Plan comment : Cobalt 60
Outline set : 1
Slice : 1 at off-axis distance 0 mm
Normalized to : 100%
Plan units : Percent
Magnification : 100%

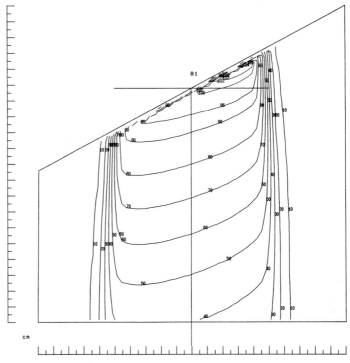

B Target pr-4j21.0205 release 1.0.4 2:51 pm on 6 September 1995

Patient name : Sloping surface
Patient code : 0906952
Plan number : 5
Plan comment : 6 MV photons
Outline set : 1
Slice : 1 at off-axis distance 0 mm
Normalized to : 100%
Plan units : Percent
Magnification : 100%

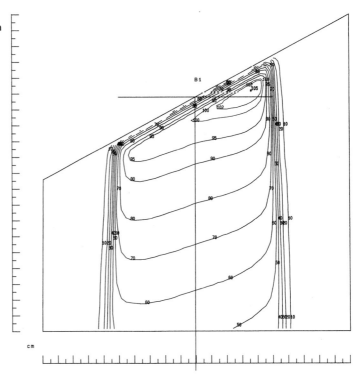

Fig. 12-6 For legend see opposite page.

C   Target pr-4j21.0205 release 1.0.4 2:50 pm on 6 September 1995

Patient name   : Sloping surface
Patient code   : 0906952
Plan number   : 4
Plan comment   : 18 MV photons
Outline set   : 1
Slice   : 1 at off-axis distance 0 mm
Normalized to : 100%
Plan units   : Percent
Magnification : 100%

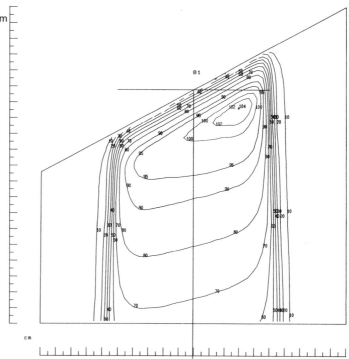

cm

Fig. 12-6, cont'd Computer-generated isodose distributions. Note the effect of sloping skin surface on the dose at depth in tissue. These are the same beams as shown in Fig. 12-2. **A,** Cobalt 60 beam, 10 × 10 cm², 80 cm SSD. **B,** 6 MV photon beam, 10 × 10 cm², 100 cm SSD. **C,** 18 MV beam, 10 × 10 cm², 100 cm SSD.

Table 12-1	Isodose shift method for sloping skin surfaces

Photon energy (Mv)	Percent shift
Up to 1	80%
Cobalt 60 to 5	70%
5 to 15	60%
15 to 30	50%
Above 30	40%

varies slightly with field size and depth with the universal wedge system, the use of a single factor for all field sizes is often acceptable.[7]

A third system is the dynamic wedge, where the linear accelerator itself will decrease beam intensity across the field width as specified. Two important considerations using the traditional wedges are (1) correctly including the wedge transmission factor in the output (the attenuation through the

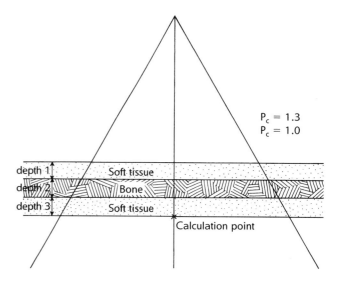

Fig. 12-7 Simplified version of calculating equivalent depth in tissue when the calculation point is beyond a tissue with a different ρ_e.

Target pr-4j21.0205 release 1.0.4 3:48 pm on 6 September 1995

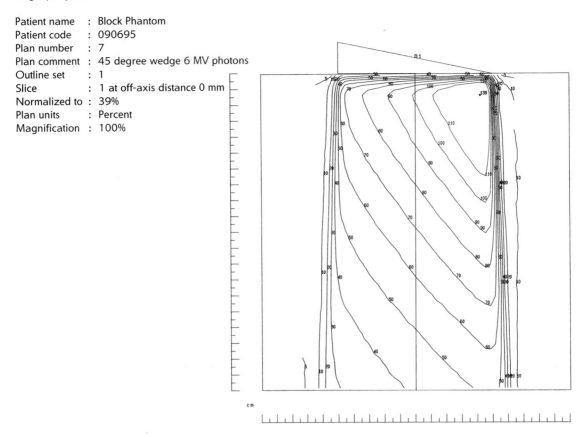

Patient name   : Block Phantom
Patient code   : 090695
Plan number   : 7
Plan comment   : 45 degree wedge 6 MV photons
Outline set   : 1
Slice   : 1 at off-axis distance 0 mm
Normalized to   : 39%
Plan units   : Percent
Magnification   : 100%

Fig. 12-8 Isodose distribution for a 45-degree wedge filter (6 MV beam, field size = 10 × 10 cm², 100 cm SSD, normalized to depth of d_{max} along the central ray of the beam).

wedge is sometimes around 50%) and (2) allowing for the effect on the quality of the beam caused by its attenuation. The wedge may have the effect of hardening the beam by completely stopping lower energy x-rays, or an almost opposite effect of decreasing the overall energy because of the Compton interactions.[2,5,7,10]

Compensating filters

In some cases the correction for irregular skin surfaces may be accomplished using a **compensating filter**. Two-dimensional transmission blocks may be poured from a low melting point alloy, constructed using sheets of lead, or machined either from one block of acrylic resin (Lucite) or stacking Lucite plates. Three-dimensional compensators are constructed using the moiré camera, magnetic digitizers, or computed tomography (CT)–based computer software. Early compensator information was collected using apparatus such as the rod box. Still relatively in a research and development stage is a truly three-dimensional system, which will take into account the surface irregularities as well as tissue heterogeneities. Other materials may be used to construct the filters, such as aluminum blocks and milled wax. The impor-

tant consideration is matching the thickness of the compensator to attenuate the beam exactly the amount required by the tissue deficit. Compensating filters allow an even dose distribution at one depth within the patient.[1,2,7,10]

Bolus

Another means of compensating for missing tissue is the use of tissue-equivalent material placed directly on the skin. This is called **bolus**. Often bolus is used to fill a cavity in the surface or internal anatomy caused by a surgical defect. The purpose of the bolus in this case is to increase the dose on the surface, whether internally or externally. In cases where the tumor is close to a critical structure or when the tumor margin is closer than it was thought to be, there is a need to counteract the skin-sparing effect of high energy x-rays while still providing the penetration required. In either case the dose distribution in the tissue is not going to resemble the even isodose curves obtained in a water phantom. In the first case, using compensating filters, the isodose line at a selected depth is even. Using tissue-equivalent bolus a sheet of bolus material may be used across the entire field; then you will still have the effect of the uneven surface, but all isodose lines are closer to the surface, or you have different thicknesses of bolus custom-made for the patient to selectively increase or decrease the surface dose and cause changes in the underlying tissue.[2,7,9]

Shielding materials

A fourth type of beam modification device that affects the isodose distribution is the **beam block**, including asymmetrical, or independent, collimator jaws. Beam blocks are mentioned here because they have an effect not only on the penumbra region but also on all the isodose curves. Custom blocks should be constructed following the beam divergence so that all areas that appear to be blocked, that is, where the light field is blocked, are blocked by the full thickness of the shielding material.[7,10] Cerrobend is the brand name for Lipowitz metal, which is made of bismuth (50%), lead (26.7%), tin (13.3%), and cadmium (10%). Cadmium-free Cerrobend is also available.[7,9]

Independent jaws may have some unexpected effects on the isodose distribution. When the field is blocked to the CAX, the loss of scatter contribution may actually decrease the penetration along the central ray and therefore cause a relative increase in the dose distribution away from the central ray. Cases where the jaw is closed beyond the CAX of the beam require that special measurements be taken to determine the machine output in the treatment volume because data for beam on time and monitor unit calculations are taken along the CAX, and the horns on a linear accelerator may cause a very different output at the area to be treated, which corresponds neither to d_{max} nor to the isocenter.[7]

COMBINING ISODOSE LINES
Hand-drawn model

Since the time that radiation was found to be effective in killing cancer cells, improvements have been made in the dose distribution. Even when orthovoltage was the modern form of treatment, attempts were made to decrease the dose to normal tissue by using more than one treatment port. The dose contribution from one port to a point in tissue at a specified depth may be calculated, then added to the dose contribution from any other ports. As with single beam calculations, this will tell you only the dose at that point. Following are instructions for a manual method of finding the dose throughout the treatment volume:

- First, overlay the patient contour on the isodose curves for one beam.
- Trace the isodose lines onto the contour using one color.
- Using a different color, do the same for each beam.
- Where the isodose lines intersect, add the percentages for each.
- Connect the points where the values are the same to create a combined isodose distribution.

To improve the accuracy of your combined isodose line, find where like values are located between lines using inter-polation. For example, where two 90% isodose lines intersect, the resulting value is 180%. Where an 85% and a 95% isodose line would intersect, the resulting value is also 180%. Even if the values are not on the original chart, you can measure the distance between values that are shown and interpolate to find where the desired value falls.

The combination isodose percentages may be used to show the dose distribution just as they are added, or **normalization** may be used to show the dose distribution as percents of the dose at a particular point, usually the isocenter. Whatever the value is at the isocenter becomes 100%, and the other values are shown as percentages of this. For example, if the value at the isocenter is 150%, it becomes 100% and the 165% line will become the 110% line. Some physicians prefer to see the highest dose (hot spot) as the reference point for normalization. Whatever the highest value is within the combined isodose percentages becomes 100%, and all other values will be shown as they relate to this value (Fig. 12-9).[2,5,7,10]

Reading through these instructions and practicing the combination of isodose curves for two fields in a water phantom, you can easily see what a tedious chore this will quickly become. Consider the factors previously discussed—sloping skin surface and tissue inhomogeneities—and hope that your instructor will not ask you to combine isodose distributions on a contour from a CT slice of the thorax and correct for obliquity and heterogeneities. That is when the treatment planning computer is appreciated as a miracle of modern technology.

Computer programs

In a matter of seconds a treatment planning system retrieves data on the beams selected and displays combined isodose distributions that include corrections for irregular skin surfaces, tissue inhomogeneities, off-axis effects, and beam-modifying devices on multiple CT slices. Three minimum requirements for a treatment planning system include: (1) external beam program, (2) irregular field calculation routine, and (3) brachytherapy planning capabilities. Institutions with programmers on site may choose to develop their own software for performing these functions.[2,4,7]

The Milan-Bentley algorithm for the external beam treatment planning computer uses a matrix model for beam data. It requires matrix points from 47 fan lines at specified depths. Data are put into the computer for the CAX and 23 fan lines on each side of the CAX. CAX percent depth dose data are input for 17 equally spaced depths from d_{max} to the maximum depth chosen for each beam. Beam profiles in the CAX plane for each of the other 46 fan lines are required at five equally spaced depths, from the d_{max} (CAX) depth to the maximum entered for the CAX. For points in a field size not entered, the algorithm does a linear interpolation. So the more field sizes entered, the more accurate is the calculation. Using a scanning water phantom, data may be quickly read for many field sizes. The information for all points is then either manually entered into the computer or down loaded

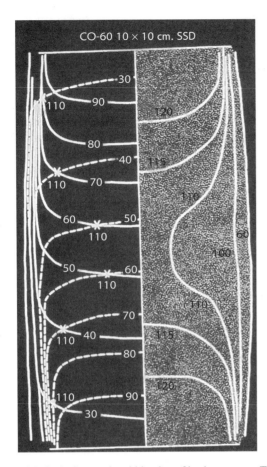

Fig. 12-9 Method of manual combination of isodose curves. The left side of the central axis shows the individual isodose curve orientation on a patient contour. The intersection of the two curves showing a combined percentage of 100 is indicated. Other values would be similarly found and the resultant complete combination is shown on the right side of the central axis. (From Fletcher GH: *Textbook of Radiotherapy*, Baltimore, 1980, Williams & Wilkins.)

directly into the system. The dose at any point in the principal plane is expressed as the CAX percent depth dose times the off-axis factor. For planes parallel to the CAX plane, for example, those located superior or inferior to the CAX plane, this value is then multiplied by the off-axis factor for the distance in that direction.[4]

Horton shows the Milan-Bentley dose written as follows:

$$D_{(d,x)} = PDD_{(d)}f_{(d,x)}$$

where d is depth, x is off-axis distance, and $PDD_{(d)}$ is CAX percent depth dose at depth d. The off-central plane calculation is expressed as follows:

$$D_{(d,x,y)} = PDD_{(d)}f_{(d,x)}g_{(d,y)}$$

where y is the distance off the central plane and $g_{(d,y)}$ is the off-axis factor in the perpendicular plane. Other models have been developed that use either mathematical calculations or curve fitting to determine doses. The Clarkson technique,

with elaboration by Cunningham, separates the radiation beam into primary and scatter components. The primary component is written as follows:

$$D_{prim} = D_{a(d)}f_{(x,y)}TAR_{(d,0)}$$

where $D_{a(d)}$ is the dose in air for a given field size at d, $TAR_{(d,0)}$ is the TAR for zero area field size at depth d, and $f_{(x,y)}$ is a function dependent on the penumbra, collimator transmission, source size, and type of filter.

The scatter dose is determined by the following equation:

$$SAR_{(d,r)} = TAR_{(d,r)} - TAR_{(d,0)}$$

where $SAR_{(d,r)}$ is the scatter air ratio at depth d and distance r from the edge of the beam, $TAR_{(d,r)}$ is the tissue air ratio at depth d for field size of radius r, and $TAR_{(d,0)}$ is the TAR for zero area field size at depth d.

As you can see, the calculation method used by the treatment planning computer is similar to that derived in the earlier discussion of calculating point doses for irregularly shaped fields and looking at doses off the central ray of the beam. The computer can more quickly and accurately perform these calculations while also calculating the effects of many other factors that influence dose distribution. Each year advances are made in computer systems that allow more data storage, so the computer can perform more complex calculations in less time. Many programs currently used were unheard of 5 years ago. The basic principles of physics, however, have not changed, although we are now better able to mimic these interactions with our calculation systems and document these calculations on paper to store in the patient's chart. Progress is also being made toward electronically storing patient data so that radiographs and treatment plans may be viewed along with the patient's treatment record.

ELECTRON BEAMS
Dose distributions

In some cases the radiation oncologist may choose to use electrons for radiation therapy. Some situations where electrons may be used are treatment of the postmastectomy chest wall, superficial tumors such as skin lesions, total skin irradiation, and boost volumes for areas at higher risk for recurrence.[3,6,7]

An electron is a subatomic particle with a negative charge that orbits around the positively charged nucleus. The two properties of an electron mentioned in the previous statement are the properties that give therapeutic electron beams their most unique characteristics. Electrons, having a negative charge, are directly ionizing. They will therefore be more likely to interact with any atoms between the radiation source and the tumor. This includes the treatment machine, beam modifying devices (blocks), and air. Because of the charge and the mass (it is a particle) of an electron, energy is more likely to be deposited along a given path length. The linear energy transfer (LET) of an electron beam is therefore higher than the LET of a photon beam of the same energy.[3,6,7]

Treatment planning

The single most important property of an electron beam, making it the radiation type of choice for superficial lesions, is the abrupt fall-off in depth dose resulting from the LET of these negatively charged particles. A high dose may be delivered close to the surface with minimal dose distal to the target area. The depth where the radiation dose falls off to about 5% is called the practical range of the electron beam (R_p). A useful rule of thumb for estimating the R_p is that the R_p is about 1 cm for each 2 MeV of electron energy. Therefore the practical range, in centimeters, is one-half the energy in MeV. As with photon beams, the target volume will be assured of the prescribed dose if it lies within a selected isodose line. Usually 80% to 90% is chosen for electrons. Another useful rule of thumb for electron beams is that the depth, in centimeters, to 80% along the CAX is one-third the energy in MeV. Using 15 MeV electrons as an example, the depth to 80% is approximately 5.0 cm, and the practical range 7.5 cm. Within the 2.5 cm beyond the 80% line the dose drops to approximately 5%. The dose does not fall to 0% because of x-ray contamination of the electron beam (Fig. 12-10).[3,6,7]

Remembering the basic physics interactions of therapeutic radiation, high energy electrons striking material with a high atomic number (Z) produce **bremsstrahlung** x-rays. The electrons interacting with the high Z components of the treatment machine, such as the collimators and scattering foils, will produce the bremsstrahlung tail on an electron depth dose profile.[3,6-8]

The isodose curve for this electron beam demonstrates some of the other differences in dose distribution for electrons compared to photon dose distributions. The 10% to 40% isodose curves balloon outward deeper in the tissue, contributing dose beyond the geometrical field edge. This effect is of particular concern when the treatment area is

large enough to require two abutting fields. There may be an area of overlap, causing a line of overdose that could result in fibrosis. To prevent this occurrence the field edges may be moved at intervals during the course of radiation therapy so as to feather the junction, which spreads the overlap so no one area receives the higher dose throughout treatment. Leaving a gap between the fields may leave a cold spot in the target volume.[3,7]

There are other differences in the electron beam dose distribution that influence treatment planning. Electron beam production differs from photon beam production. A photon beam basically radiates out in all directions from a central position. Electron beams begin as a pencil-thin stream of electrons that are either scanned across a selected field size or scattered using a scattering foil and then a cone to shape the field. The electron beam therefore only appears to diverge from a point. The point from which the electrons appear to diverge is called the virtual source position. The electrons actually travel to the skin surface in a pattern resembling many individual pencil-thin beams, which must be considered individually by a treatment planning computer to accurately represent the dose distribution.[3,6-8]

One of the effects of an increased SSD is a decrease in the overall energy of the electron beam as it has more interactions with air molecules before reaching the tissue. Two changes in the dose distribution in the patient are (1) a widening of the penumbra and (2) constriction of the 80% and 90% isodose lines, similar to what is seen at a deeper depth in the tissue.[3]

These effects are also seen in the dose distribution for a sloping surface because of the increased SSD for a portion of the field. An even greater effect is caused by the beam intercepting the skin surface at an angle. Oblique incidence generally should be avoided to ensure a more homogeneous dose distribution and to prevent dose beyond the intended target volume (Fig. 12-11).[3,7]

As mentioned earlier, bolus may be used for several reasons in the electron field. If only a portion of the field is covered with bolus, the edge of the bolus that lies within the treatment area may greatly disrupt the dose homogeneity. An abrupt change in SSD within the field results in a lower dose just inside the bolused surface and a higher dose just inside the nonbolused surface. Using a beveled edge greatly decreases the dose gradient at the edge of the bolus (Fig. 12-12).[3,7,10]

An area where similar conditions occur is in a treatment volume containing tissue of different densities. Electron fields are very useful in the head and neck region because the dose gradient allows the treatment of superficial lesions with little dose to underlying critical structures such as the spinal cord. One complication of calculating head and neck dose distributions is the presence of high density bones mixed with low density air cavities and soft tissue. The areas next to and beyond the higher and lower density tissues receive very different doses than they would receive if the tissue were of homogeneous density (Fig. 12-13).[3,7]

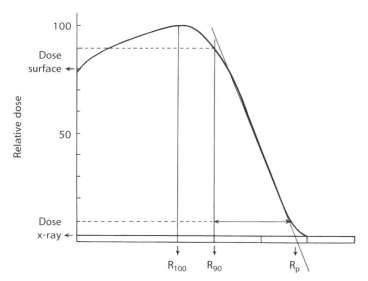

Fig. 12-10 Depth dose profile for a 15 MeV electron beam.

A   Target pr-4j21.0205 release 1.0.4 2:45 pm on 6 September 1995

Patient name   : Sloping surface
Patient code   : 0906952
Plan number   : 1
Plan comment   : 6 MeV EB
Outline set   : 1
Slice   : 1 at off-axis distance 0 mm
Normalized to : 100%
Plan units   : Percent
Magnification : 100%

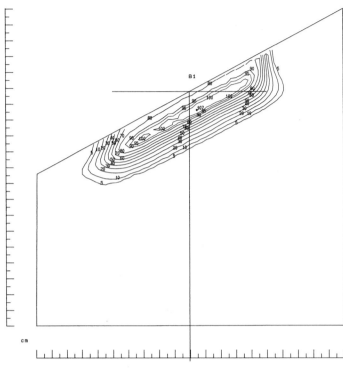

B   Target pr-4j21.0205 release 1.0.4 2:47 pm on 6 September 1995

Patient name   : Sloping surface
Patient code   : 0906952
Plan number   : 2
Plan comment   : 16 MeV EB
Outline set   : 1
Slice   : 1 at off-axis distance 0 mm
Normalized to : 100%
Plan units   : Percent
Magnification : 100%

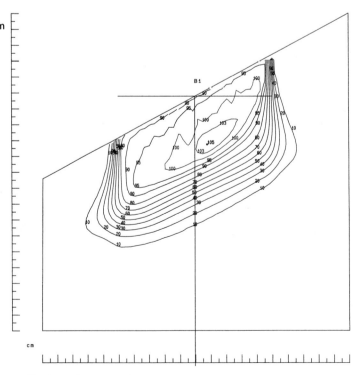

Fig. 12-11 For legend see opposite page.

C   Target pr-4j21.0205 release 1.0.4 2:49 pm on 6 September 1995

Patient name   : Sloping surface
Patient code   : 0906952
Plan number   : 3
Plan comment   : 20 MeV EB
Outline set   : 1
Slice   : 1 at off-axis distance 0 mm
Normalized to : 100%
Plan units   : Percent
Magnification : 100%

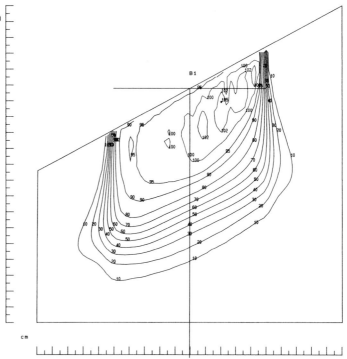

Fig. 12-11, cont'd Computer-generated isodose distributions for the three electron beams shown on a sloping surface. The beams are the same as in Fig. 12-3. **A**, 6 MeV, 10 × 10 cm², 100 cm SSD. **B**, 16 MeV, 10 × 10 cm², 100 cm SSD. **C**, 20 MeV, 10 × 10 cm², 100 cm SSD.

A useful tool for improving electron beam dose distribution is the use of skin collimation. This involves shielding material, usually lead, placed directly on the patient's skin surface. The field edges are defined by the lead, while the machine collimator or cone opening is larger. The penumbra region is then being blocked, allowing an improved coverage of the target area within the 90% isodose line. Adjacent critical structures also receive less scattered dose. Use of skin collimation is especially important when the field is very small and when bolus or scatter plates are being used. These cause scatter dose outside the treatment port as defined by the light field (Fig. 12-14).[3]

SUMMARY

The tremendous advances made in the types and energies of beams available for radiation therapy, combined with the use of beam modification devices and improved treatment planning techniques, allow us to tailor radiation treatment to accurately encompass the tumor while avoiding dose to normal tissue. This has made possible increased doses to tumor cells with improved prognosis for our patients. With the continuing improvement in dose delivery, radiation therapy has maintained its place as a viable modality in the treatment of patients with cancer.

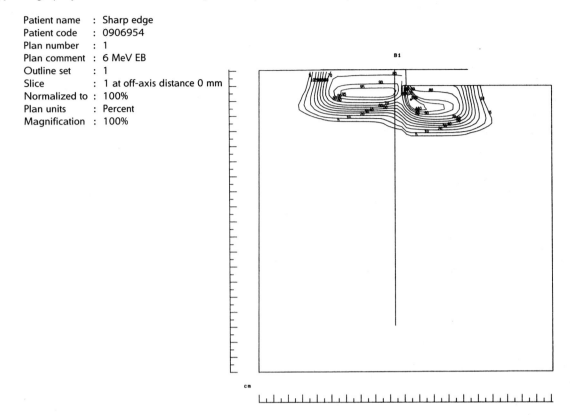

A   Target pr-4j21.0205 release 1.0.4 3:10 pm on 6 September 1995

Patient name   : Sharp edge
Patient code   : 0906954
Plan number   : 1
Plan comment   : 6 MeV EB
Outline set   : 1
Slice   : 1 at off-axis distance 0 mm
Normalized to   : 100%
Plan units   : Percent
Magnification   : 100%

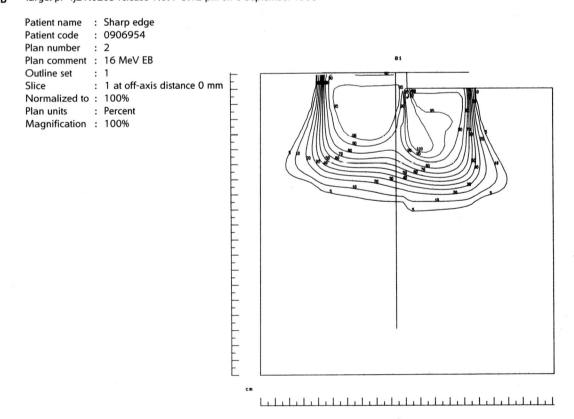

B   Target pr-4j21.0205 release 1.0.4 3:12 pm on 6 September 1995

Patient name   : Sharp edge
Patient code   : 0906954
Plan number   : 2
Plan comment   : 16 MeV EB
Outline set   : 1
Slice   : 1 at off-axis distance 0 mm
Normalized to   : 100%
Plan units   : Percent
Magnification   : 100%

Fig. 12-12 Dose distributions shown for three electron beams (10×10 cm^2, 100 cm SSD, with a sharp edge in the field and with a beveled edge in the field). **A**, 6 MeV beam—sharp edge. **B**, 16 MeV beam—sharp edge.

C   Target pr-4j21.0205 release 1.0.4 3:13 pm on 6 September 1995

Patient name   : Sharp edge
Patient code   : 0906954
Plan number   : 3
Plan comment   : 20 MeV EB
Outline set   : 1
Slice   : 1 at off-axis distance 0 mm
Normalized to : 100%
Plan units   : Percent
Magnification : 100%

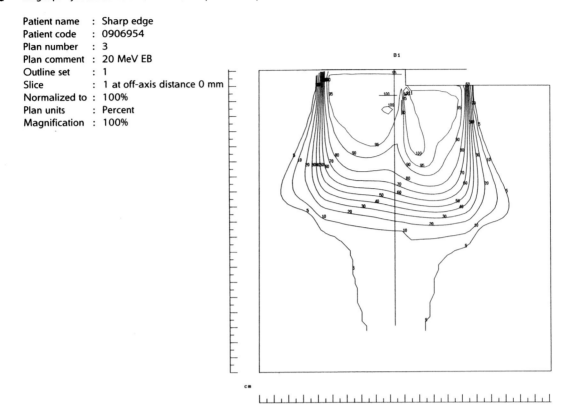

D   Target pr-4j21.0205 release 1.0.4 3:01 pm on 6 September 1995

Patient name   : Bevel
Patient code   : 0906953
Plan number   : 2
Plan comment   : 6 MeV e
Outline set   : 1
Slice   : 1 at off-axis distance 0 mm
Normalized to : 100%
Plan units   : Percent
Magnification : 100%

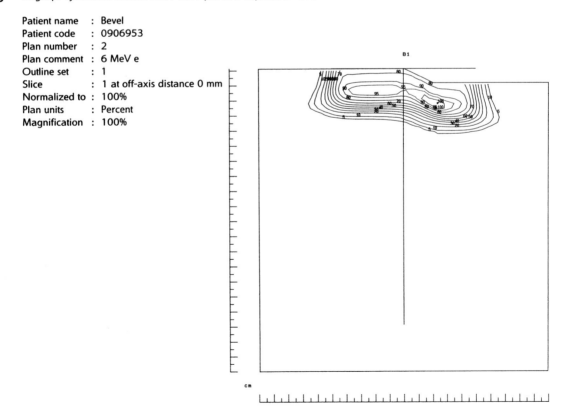

Fig. 12-12, cont'd C, 20 MeV beam—sharp edge. **D**, 6 MeV beam with bevel.

E   Target pr-4j21.0205 release 1.0.4 3:00 pm on 6 September 1995

Patient name   : Bevel
Patient code   : 0906953
Plan number   : 1 -
Plan comment : 16 MeV EB
Outline set   : 1
Slice   : 1 at off-axis distance 0 mm
Normalized to : 100%
Plan units   : Percent
Magnification : 100%

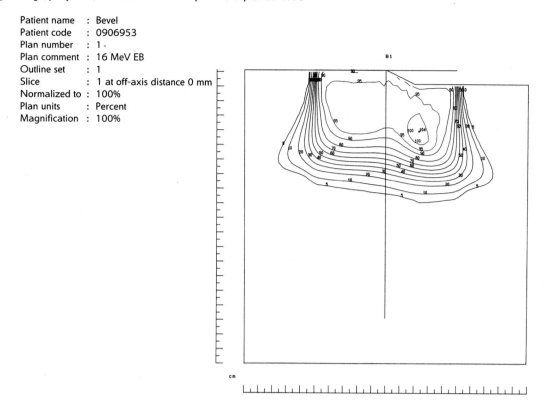

F   Target pr-4j21.0205 release 1.0.4 3:01 pm on 6 September 1995

Patient name   : Bevel
Patient code   : 0906953
Plan number   : 3
Plan comment : 20 MeV EB
Outline set   : 1
Slice   : 1 at off-axis distance 0 mm
Normalized to : 100%
Plan units   : Percent
Magnification : 100%

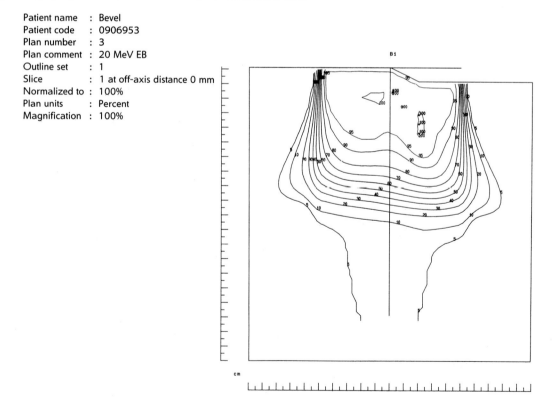

Fig. 12-12, cont'd E, 16 MeV beam with bevel. **F,** 20 MeV beam with bevel.

A   Target pr-4j21.0205 release 1.0.4 3:23 pm on 6 September 1995

Patient name   : Phantom with air cavity
Patient code   : 0906955
Plan number   : 1
Plan comment : 16 MeV
Outline set   : 1
Slice   : 1 at off-axis distance 0 mm
Normalized to : 99%
Plan units   : Percent
Magnification : 100%

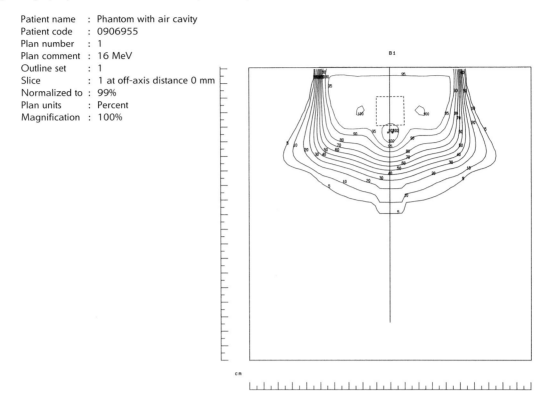

B   Target pr-4j21.0205 release 1.0.4 3:44 pm on 6 September 1995

Patient name   : Bone in phantom
Patient code   : 0906956
Plan number   : 1
Plan comment : 16 MeV
Outline set   : 1
Slice   : 1 at off-axis distance 0 mm
Normalized to : 100%
Plan units   : Percent
Magnification : 100%

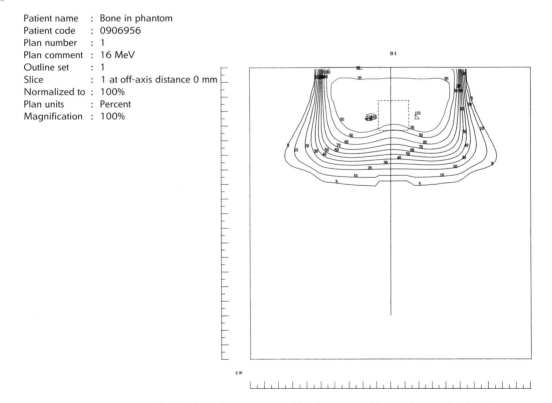

Fig. 12-13 Changes in dose distribution. These are caused by, **A**, an area of lower electron density, air, within the field and, **B**, an area of higher electron density, bone, within the field. Beam shown is 16 MeV electrons. The heterogeneity is represented by the *dashed lines*.

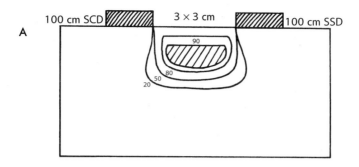

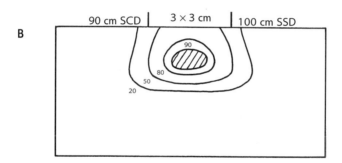

Fig. 12-14 How skin collimation improves the coverage of the 90% isodose line for very small fields. **A,** With lead skin collimation and the light field opened beyond the treatment field by the penumbra width on all sides of the beam. **B,** Electron cone at 10 cm from the patient's skin surface, light field opened to fit the treatment field.

Review Questions

Multiple Choice

1. Which of the following are properties of field flatness?
   a. Measured from a depth dose profile
   b. Defined across 80% of the field
   c. Changes with depth for linear accelerators
   d. All of the above are correct

2. Which of the following statements is *not* true of isodose charts?
   a. Usually set up with 100% of the maximum dose within the treatment field
   b. May be used interchangeably for different machines with the same photon energy
   c. Contain curves of connected points where the same dose is being delivered
   d. Show doses at depths within tissue for a specific beam

3. Which of the following are part of the calculation of dose to points not along the central ray of the beam, using the Clarkson irregular field calculation?
   I. Off-axis factors for the x and y coordinates of the points of interest
   II. Source to surface distances for all points being calculated
   III. Field shaping information—depiction of the beam blocks in use
   IV. Percent depth dose data for the beam used for treatment
   a. I, II, and III only are correct
   b. II and IV only are correct
   c. IV only is correct
   d. All of the above are correct

4. Which of these beam modification devices results in loss of the skin-sparing effect?
   I. Cerrobend block
   II. Compensating filter
   III. Wedge filter
   IV. Bolus
   a. I, II, and II only are correct
   b. II and IV only are correct
   c. IV only is correct
   d. All of the above are correct

5. Which of the following is **not a requirement** for a treatment planning system?
   a. External beam program
   b. Irregular field calculation routine
   c. Brachytherapy planning capability
   d. Three-dimensional planning software

6. The practical range for a 12 MeV electron beam is:
   a. 3.6 cm
   b. 4.0 cm
   c. 5.0 cm
   d. 6.0 cm

7. Normalization means assigning _____ to a selected reference point.
   a. A dose
   b. Maximum value
   c. A minimum allowed dose
   d. 100%

True or False

8. The penumbra region is wider for lower energy radiation beams.
   True _____ False _____

9. The universal wedge system allows for the minimum attenuation of the radiation beam by always placing the thinnest edge of the filter at the field edge.
   True _____ False _____

10. The use of skin collimation with electron beam therapy improves the dose distribution by decreasing the penumbra width.
    True _____ False _____

Questions to Ponder

1. Explain the difference between using bolus and using a compensating filter to correct for an uneven skin surface.
2. What are some of the radiation beam properties that require the treatment port to be larger than the tumor?
3. How can the dose overlap of adjacent electron fields be decreased?
4. Which type of radiation has the most skin sparing effect: low LET or high LET? Why?
5. Explain how beam flatness and symmetry are attained for linear accelerator photons.

REFERENCES

1. Boyer AL: Compensating filters for high energy x-rays. *Med Physics* 9(3):429-433, 1982.
2. Hendee WR: *Radiation therapy physics.* Chicago, 1981, Year Book.
3. Hogstrom KR: Treatment planning in electron beam therapy. In Vaeth JM, Meyer JL, editors: *Frontiers of radiation therapy and oncology, vol 25. The role of high energy electrons in the treatment of cancer.* Basel, 1991, Karger.
4. Horton JL: *Handbook of radiation therapy physics.* Englewood Cliffs, NJ, 1987, Prentice-Hall.
5. Johns HE, Cunningham JR: *The physics of radiology,* ed 3. Springfield, IL, 1969, Charles C Thomas.
6. Khan FM: Basic physics of electron beam therapy. In Vaeth JM, Meyer JL, editors: *Frontiers of radiation therapy and oncology, vol 25: The role of high energy electrons in the treatment of cancer.* Basel, 1991, Karger.
7. Khan FM: *The physics of radiation therapy,* ed 2. Baltimore, 1994, Williams & Wilkins.
8. Klevenhagen SC: *Medical physics handbooks #13: physics of electron beam therapy.* Bristol, 1985, Adam Higer.
9. Mould RF: *Medical physics handbooks #7: radiotherapy treatment planning.* Bristol, 1981, Adam Higer.
10. Stanton R, Stinson D (edited by S Shahabi, PhD): *An introduction to radiation oncology physics.* Madison, WI, 1992, Medical Physics.

Electron Beams in Radiation Therapy

Adam F. Kempa

Outline

Key terms

The goal of this chapter is to provide an accurate overview of electron beam therapy at the student level. To accomplish this goal, concepts dealing with the physics of electrons and electron beams will be dealt with in a general manner. Often important issues become obscured by intricacy and detail. A more detailed treatment of electron beam therapy may be found in the references listed at the end of the chapter.

The art of radiation therapy treatment planning may be described as making use of the unique physical properties of various sources of radiation to optimize and individualize a patient's treatment. Electron beams are a good example of this concept. Selection of the energy of an electron beam allows the choice of depth of treatment and the dose to tissues deep to the treatment volume. Basic rules of thumb may be used to understand how the energy of an electron beam is defined and to provide a basis for the selection of an electron beam energy for treatment.

REVIEW OF THE PHYSICS OF ELECTRON BEAMS
Interactions of electron beams with matter

Before a meaningful discussion of electron beam dosimetry can take place, the physical differences between electron beams and photon beams must be considered. A photon has no charge or mass. An electron has a negative charge and a mass approximately 2000 times smaller than that of a proton.

Electron beams' interactions with matter differ from those of photon beams largely because of these two characteristics.

Since the electron has mass, the probability of an interaction between the electron and an atom is greater than that of a photon, which has no mass. Similarly, the probability of a negatively charged electron interacting with an atom's coulomb forces is greater than that of a photon with no charge.

Collisional and radiation interactions

Electron beams interact with matter by a combination of collisional processes and radiation processes.[4] The energy loss of these two processes is expressed in terms of mass stopping powers. The **mass stopping power** (S/p) is the rate of energy loss per unit length (S), divided by the density of the medium (p).[4] The total mass stopping power is the sum of all energy losses. This includes both losses caused by collisions of electrons with atomic electrons $(S/p)_{col}$ and radiation losses or bremsstrahlung production $(S/p)_{rad}$. The expression for the total mass stopping power $(S/p)_{tot}$ is as follows[4]:

$$(S/p)_{tot} = (S/p)_{col} + (S/p)_{rad}$$

The contribution of each of these processes is affected by the energy of the electron beam and the atomic (Z) number of the irradiated material.[8]

A refinement of the total mass stopping power is the restricted mass collisional stopping power. The **restricted mass collisional stopping power** better describes the absorbed dose by accounting for energy transferred by delta rays. Delta rays are electrons scattered with enough energy to cause further ionization and excitations in other atoms.[1] All of the energy loss due to the interactions of the delta rays may not be deposited locally. Energy transfer by collisions of delta rays is restricted by specification of an energy below which energy losses are counted as part of the restricted collisional mass stopping power.[14] Energy losses considered as part of the restricted collisional mass stopping power relate to local absorption of dose.[14] Above this specified energy the energy losses are not counted as part of the restricted collisional mass stopping power.[14] By this mechanism a more accurate representation of absorbed dose is obtained.

In collisional losses the predominate interaction may be described as an incident electron interacting with the electron of an atom. Low Z number materials have a greater **electron density** (number of electrons per unit mass) than high Z number materials.[14] As one would expect, collisional interactions are the predominant process by which electrons lose energy in low Z number materials. Radiation or **bremsstrahlung** losses occur when an incident electron interacts with the coulomb forces of the nucleus of an atom.[14] The probability of the occurrence of energy loss due to the radiation process increases with increasing energy or increasing Z number of the absorbing material.[8]

Energy dependence of electron interactions

"For water, energy loss by collision is approximately 2 MeV/cm in the energy range of 1 to 100 MeV."[14] Radiation losses vary from 0.01 to 0.4 MeV/cm in the 1 to 20 MeV

energy range.[14] A crude comparison of these values demonstrates that collisional interactions occur several times more often than radiation interactions in low Z number materials. In clinical radiation therapy in the energy range from 1 to 20 MeV, the predominant mechanism by which an electron beam loses energy is by collisional interactions in tissues because of the low Z number of tissue.[8]

Electron beam energy spectrum dependence on depth

An electron beam emerges from the accelerator guide of the linear accelerator at a point called the "accelerator window." Before the electron beam moves through the accelerator window the energy spectrum is very narrow.[4] The electron beam then moves through various components of the linear accelerator, the accelerator window, scattering foils, ionization monitor chambers, and the air between the patient and treatment machine to the patient surface. The spectrum of the beam at the patient surface is decreased and broadened in energy because of interactions with the accelerator components.[4] As the electron beam passes into the patient, it undergoes a decrease in energy and broadening of the energy spectrum.[8] The energy spectrum of the electron beam in the patient depends on the depth in the patient and the energy spectrum at the surface of the patient.[4]

Production of clinically useful electron beams

Electron beams are most commonly produced by linear accelerators in current practice. There are several modifications of the linear accelerator required for electron beam production. The first is to remove the "target" and flattening filter used to produce x-rays from the path of the electron beam. The second is to decrease the "electron gun" current to lower the dose rate of the electron beam to clinically acceptable ranges. The reason for the reduction in the current becomes apparent when one considers the amount of current used in x-ray mode compared to that used in electron mode. "In normal electron therapy mode operation, the beam current through the electron window is on the order of 1/1000 of the beam current at the x-ray target for x-ray therapy mode."[5] Without a reduction of the current at the electron gun window, unwieldy dose rates in the thousands of centigrays per second could result.[5] A narrow electron beam commonly referred to as a "pencil beam" is produced by the linear accelerator. This pencil beam of electrons may be widened for clinical use by two methods: the use of a scattering foil or the use of a scanning electron beam.

Scattering foils

The most common method of producing a beam wide enough for clinical use is to use a scattering foil.[5] A **scattering foil** is a thin sheet of a material that has a high Z number placed in the path of the "pencil beam" of electrons. A second scattering foil may be added to create a "dual scattering foil" arrangement. The first scattering foil is used to widen the beam; the second is used to improve the flatness of the beam.[5] Often the x-ray field flattening filter and scattering foil are mounted on a carousel arrangement (Fig. 13-1). This allows for a simple switch from photon to electron mode of operation.

Scanning beams

Scanning electron beams are the second way a beam wide enough for clinical purposes may be produced. The narrow "pencil beam" of electrons is scanned by magnetic fields across the treatment area. This constantly moving pencil beam distributes the dose evenly throughout the field. **Scanning beams** are especially useful above 25 MeV, where the thickness of the required scattering foils would result in difficulties with their mechanical size and also would cause problems with electron contamination.[5]

Advantages and disadvantages of scattering foils versus scanning beams

A drawback of the use of scattering foils is the production of bremsstrahlung contamination by the electron beam's interaction with the scattering foil. An advantage of the use of scattering foils is that they are relatively simple and reliable when compared to the scanning beam method. An advantage of the scanning beam method is that there is none of the bremsstrahlung contamination caused by the interaction of the electron beam and the scattering foil. However, x-ray contamination from the collimators, ionization chambers,

and the intervening air is still present.[5] A disadvantage of the scanning beam method is the maintenance of complex electronic systems. Failures of the scanning beam mechanism could allow the entire dose to be delivered in one small area of the patient with disastrous results.[14]

CHARACTERISTICS OF THERAPEUTIC ELECTRON BEAMS
Dosage gradients of clinically useful electron beams

Electron beam therapy offers the ability to treat superficially located lesions with almost no dose to the deep underlying tissues. This is illustrated by Fig. 13-2, *A*. The darkened high dose area is followed by a narrow lighter low dose area and a white area indicating negligible dose. The implication for treatment planning is that organs and structures deep to the darkened area will receive minimal dose. This results from rapid fall off of percent depth dose with increasing depth and is characteristic of electron beams below 15 MeV.[12]

Fig. 13-2, *B*, numerically demonstrates this rapid fall off of dose with depth. The rate of change of a value (dose) with a change in position is termed a **gradient**. While the relative distances between the surface to 80% and from 80% to 10% isodose curves are approximately equal, the rates of change of isodose values are not. In the first half of the distance there is a 20% change, compared to a 70% change in isodose values in the second half of the distance. This advantageous

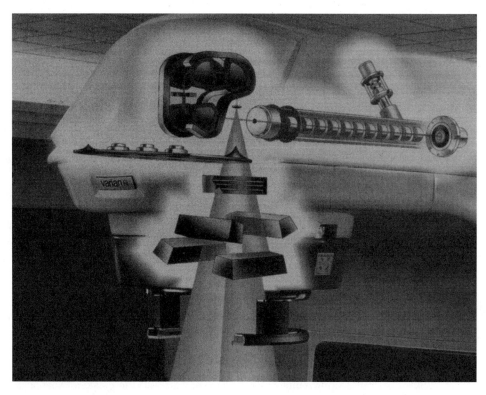

Fig. 13-1 Three scattering foils mounted in a "carousel" arrangement within the head of a modern linear accelerator. (Courtesy Varian Associates.)

A

B

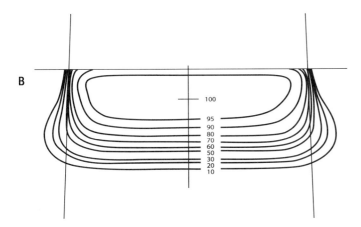

Fig. 13-2 **A,** Film of a 12 MeV 14 × 8 cm electron beam used for obtaining isodose curves. **B,** Isodensity curves from the 12 MeV electron beam. (From Khan F: *The physics of radiation therapy.* Baltimore, 1984, Williams & Wilkins.)

Table 13-1	Comparison of percent depth dose data for varying electron beam energies		
Nominal beam energy (MeV)	**Percent depth dose/depth (cm)**		
10.6	100%/1.9	80%/3.5	10%/5.2
15	100%/2.9	80%/4.9	10%/7.1
30	100%/3.7	80%/8.7	10%/14.6

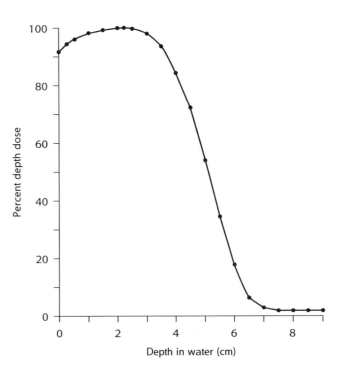

Fig. 13-3 Central axis depth dose distribution measured in water. Incident energy, 13 MeV; 8 × 10 cm cone; effective SSD = 68 cm. (From Khan F: *The physics of radiation therapy.* Baltimore, 1984, Williams & Wilkins.)

dosage gradient may be manipulated by varying the energy of the electron beam. This may be demonstrated by a comparison of percent depth dose data in the following example (Table 13-1). The 80% isodose value is commonly used to describe the treatment depth of an electron beam. As the nominal energy of the electron beam is increased, the depth of the 80% isodose value increases from 3.5 cm at 10.6 MeV to 4.9 cm at 15 MeV. At the nominal energy of 30 MeV the rapid fall off of dose with increasing depth is greatly diminished. The 80% isodose value is at a depth of 9 cm, and at approximately 15 cm, 10% of the dose remains. "The clinically advantageous shape cut-off to the percentage depth dose achieved with low-energy electron beams of 10-15 MeV is lost at very high energies, and that consequently there is no real clinical advantage in using electron beams of energies higher than about 20 MeV."[12] Restated simply, high energy electron beams begin to approximate the depth dose characteristics of low energy photon beams with the disadvantage of having no "true" skin-sparing effect.

Shape of the plot of percent depth dose versus depth

The characteristic shape of the plot of dose versus depth for an electron beam is demonstrated in Fig. 13-3. The dose at the surface begins at approximately 85% of maximum and builds up to 100% in the first few centimeters below the surface. Beyond the 80% to 90% depth dose in Fig. 13-3, the fall off

dose with increasing depth is rapid. The curve does not reach 0 but "flattens out" at a value of a few percent. The dose in this end region is composed of bremsstrahlung-produced x-ray contamination from the interaction of the electron beam with scattering foils, ionization chambers, collimators, and the air between the patient and the treatment unit.[4] While this dose is clinically insignificant in most cases, caution is warranted when large areas are treated, as in total body electron treatments for mycosis fungoides (cutaneous T-cell lymphoma).[8] An interesting use of this x-ray contamination has been to obtain port film radiographs of electron beam treatments.[2]

Shape of electron beam isodose curves

Electron beam isodose curves have a characteristic shape, which is described as a lateral bulge or ballooning of the isodose curves. "As the beam penetrates a medium, the beam expands rapidly below the surface due to scattering."[14] This is evident in Fig. 13-2, *B*, where the 10%, 20%, 30%, and 50% isodose curves balloon or bulge beyond the edge of the field. The lateral scattering or ballooning of electron beam decreases with increasing electron beam energy.[8]

TREATMENT PLANNING OF ELECTRON BEAM THERAPY
Electron beam rules of thumb

Treatment planning using electron beams may be explained using several relationships or rules of thumb. The resulting information gained by application of the rules of thumb clarify the use of a particular electron beam for a specific treatment application.

The first of these relationships is used to determine the energy of an electron beam. As an electron beam passes through matter, it decreases both in intensity and in energy with increasing depth. For this reason the measurement of an electron beam's energy depends on the depth of the electron beam in the phantom or patient. While there are several methods of determining the energy of an electron beam, one method is widely used because of its practicality in the clinical setting. Simply stated, the depth of the 50% dose in centimeters (R_{50}) is multiplied by a constant (C_4). The resulting product is the mean energy of the electron (E_o) beam stated in MeV at the phantom surface,[7] as follows:

$$E_o = C_4 R_{50}$$

The value of the constant C_4 has varied slightly from 2.33 MeV in American Association of Physicists in Medicine (AAPM) Task Group 21 to 2.4 MeV in Task Group 25.[7] There is little difference between the final value determined by the use of either number for the constant C_4. For this reason, it is recommended that physicists select one of the two values along with other parameters and use it consistently in the calibration protocol.[7]

The second of these relationships deals with the reduction of the energy of an electron beam as it moves through matter. The energy of an electron beam at a given depth in water may be approximated based on the following relationship. The rate at which an electron beam loses energy is approximately 2 MeV/cm in water.[1] For example, an electron beam with an energy of 10 MeV incident on the phantom surface will have an energy of 6 MeV at a depth of 2 cm in water.

The third relationship deals with the practical range (E_r) in centimeters of an electron beam in tissue. The practical range of an electron beam is determined by dividing the energy of the electron beam in MeV by 2, as follows

$$E_r = MeV/2$$

Past the practical range within the patient, dosage drops off quickly with depth to a value of several percent. The dosage does not reach zero because of the bremsstrahlung radiation produced by the interaction of the beam with collimators, the intervening air, and the patient.

The practical range is a helpful guide in treatment planning. This simple relationship demonstrates clearly that a lesion at a depth of 4 cm is beyond the range of a 7 MeV electron beam. In a similar manner this relationship can be used in the selection of the energy of an electron beam so that critical structures receive a minimal dose.

The fourth relationship is directly related to the choice of an electron beam energy for a specific treatment depth. The depth of the 80% isodose value is often specified as treatment depth. Treatment depth may be determined by dividing the energy of the electron beam in MeV by 3, as follows:

$$80\% \text{ isodose} = MeV/3$$

In a similar manner, the depth of the 90% isodose curve may be found by dividing the energy of the electron beam in MeV by 4, as follows:

$$90\% \text{ isodose} = MeV/4$$

Use of these simple relationships gives insight into a particular treatment. For example, a patient treated with a 10 MeV electron beam will have the following: an 80% isodose at a depth of 3.3 cm, a 90% isodose line as a depth of 2.5 cm, and a range within the patient of approximately 5 cm. Structures deeper than 5 cm deep receive a minimal dose.

The relationships for the depth of the 80% and 90% isodose lines and the dose to deep structures are for homogeneous treatment volumes of tissue-equivalent material. If the treatment area overlies an air cavity such as a lung, the choice of the isodose line for treatment must take into account the increased transmission through the lung tissue. Selection of the isodose line for treatment may vary from the 70% to the 80% isodose line in an attempt to minimize the dose to the lung.[9]

Electron beam characteristics at the surface

Megavoltage electron beams in the 6 to 20 MeV energy range have varying degrees of dose reduction at the skin surface. Variables that affect the surface dose include the scattering system, atomic number of the absorber, beam energy, field size, and beam collimation. Of these variables, only the last three may be manipulated for treatment planning purposes.

"The actual absorbed dose at the surface of a water equivalent medium usually is about 0.85 of the maximum in the absence of contamination of the beam."[4] Difficulties in measuring the dose at the phantom's surface have caused AAPM Task Group 25 to specify the surface dose as the dose at 0.5 cm on the central axis of the electron beam.[7] Surface dose values for electron beams in the 6 to 20 MeV range vary from 80% to 100%. In megavoltage photon beams, increased energy of the treatment beam results in a decrease in surface dose. With electron beams the reverse is true. "As the energy of the electron beam increases, the surface dose and percent depth dose also increase."[6]

There is little effect of field size on both surface dose and percent depth dose of electron beams, provided the fields are of sufficient size.[4] The rule is that the electron beam's diameter (field size) in centimeters should not be less than the practical range. This rule is extended to include field sizes that are less than the practical range in either dimension.[14] For example, a 10 MeV electron beam's percent depth dose characteristics will not vary significantly as long as the diameter (field size) is 5 cm or greater ($R_p = 10$ MeV/2 = 5). "The field size dependence of the depth dose curves increases as the energy of the electron beam increases."[15] The surface dose depends on the field size in a similar manner. In general, "the smaller the diameter the larger the surface dose."[15] Increased dose produced by increasing field size continues until the diameter of the electron beam equals the practical range of the electron beam. Additional increases in field size where the diameter of the field is greater than the practical range of the electrons will not result in a significant change in dose.[16]

Electron beam characteristics in the build-up region

The region from the surface to the depth of maximum dose is at risk for being underdosed in many clinical situations. This is most true for lower energy electron beams (less than 12 MeV). A bolus may be used to increase the dose to the surface, much as in megavoltage beams. However, the use of bolus materials in electron beam therapy is somewhat more complicated than in photon beams. It is possible to decrease the dose in an electron beam setup by use of a bolus. For this reason, "A partial bolus should never be used with electrons."[13] The dose under a small (1 × 1 cm) bolus placed in the middle of a small treatment field may decrease the surface dose by 10% to 15%.[13] Another problem, sometimes called an "edge effect," results from the use of a large bolus with an edge perpendicular to the surface, across a portion of a treatment field. Areas of increased dose and decreased dose of 20% to 30% may be produced.[3] Near the border between bolused and unbolused portions of the field, areas under the bolus have decreased dose and the unbolused areas have increased dose. In an attempt to reduce the areas of increased and decreased dose, the edge of the partial bolus may be beveled so that it forms a 45% angle with the surface. While this eliminates the area of decreased dose near the surface, the area of increased dose remains.[13]

The use of bolus materials in electron beam therapy is not limited to increasing the dose to the surface. Hogstrom identifies two other uses for bolus material in electron beam therapy: as a tissue compensator for irregular surfaces or air cavities, and to shape isodose distributions to better conform to the treatment volume or decrease the dose to critical structures at depth.[3] "A simple rule of thumb for bolus—that utilization of bolus to make the patient anatomy present itself as a water phantom results in a more uniform dose distribution."[3]

Energy dependence of the width of the 80% isodose curve

With increasing electron beam energy, the ballooning of the isodose lines decreases. "At approximately 15 MeV, the phenomenon of lateral constriction of the higher isodose values, such as at the 80% line, occurs."[14] To cover an area at depth with the 80% isodose line, a larger area must be treated on the skin surface.[13] "A good standard is to leave a margin of at least 1 cm between the lateral edge of the target volume and the projected edge of the collimator."[3] As always, this should be based on a careful evaluation of measured data specific to the treatment machine, beam energy, and treatment cone used. It should also be noted that there is a similar constriction of the 90% isodose line for electron beams in this energy range.

Distance correction factors for electron beam treatments

Anatomical restrictions most often require the use of electron beams at an extended SSD.[7] In the AAPM Task Group 25 report, "extended SSD" is defined as treatments that are not more than 15 cm beyond standard SSD. This constraint will apply to the following discussion of extended SSD treatments.[7] "The use of an extended treatment distance has only minimal effect on the central-axis depth dose and the off-axis ratios."[7] For this reason it is suggested that the use of standard depth-dose curves will give an approximation that is within a millimeter at extended distances.[7] However, factors such as the output of an electron beam and the beam penumbra change dramatically with a change in treatment distance.[7]

Clinical electron beams are created by scanning a narrow pencil-width beam across the treatment area or by use of a scattering foil. In either case there is no simple point source of the electron beam from which changes in distance may be calculated. This may be resolved in two different ways: by determining an "effective point source" or by determining the position of the "virtual source." Two methods of correction of the output of electron beams relate to these methods.

Effective point source method

The effective point source is defined "such that the dose varies in accordance with the inverse square law with distance from this source."[6] This method allows for use of an inverse square correction factor with the following factors[7]:

D'_{max} = The dose to D_{max} at extended distance

D_{max} = The dose to D_{max} at nominal or normal distance

SSD = Nominal or normal SSD

SSD' = Extended SSD

SSD_{eff} = Effective SSD

d_{max} = Depth of maximum dose on central axis

g = Difference between the extended SSD and the nominal SSD (SSD' − SSD)

The formula is as follows:

$$D'_{max} = \frac{D_{max} (SSD_{eff} + d_{max})^2}{(SSD_{eff} + g + d_{max})^2}$$

Conditions such as large air gaps, small treatment field sizes, or low energy beams may require additional modification of this formula or a new calibration measurement specific for the individual set of treatment conditions.

Virtual source method

One method of finding the position of a virtual point source is by "back-projection" of the 50% width of the beam profiles from several distances.[6] The point at which these back-projections intersect is termed the virtual source position.[6] The parameters for the virtual SSD output correction factor are identical to those of the effective point source method, with the following exceptions:

$$SSD_{vir} = \text{Virtual SSD for calibration}$$

$$f_{air} = \text{Air gap correction factor}$$

$$D'_{max} = (D_{max}) \frac{(SSD_{vir} + d_{max})^2}{(f_{air}) (SSD_{vir} + g + d_{max})^2}$$

In the virtual SSD method the variation in the inverse square law for small field sizes, low beam energy, and large air gaps is corrected by the factor f_{air}. "The factor (f_{air}) depends on the energy, field size and extent of the air gap."[6]

IRREGULAR FIELDS AND ELECTRON BEAMS
Shielding dependence on electron beam energy

Various methods have been used to shape electron beams for clinical purposes. These include lead strips, cutouts, or masks placed directly on the patient's skin or at the end of the treatment cone or collimator. Low melting point shields that insert into the end of the treatment cone (Fig. 13-4) have also been used. The thickness of the shielding material required increases with increasing beam energy and field size. In the measurement of the transmission of shielding material, two approaches are used to address the effect of field size on the thickness of material needed. The first approach is to measure the transmission with large field sizes; this will provide a shield thickness that is appropriate to any smaller fields used.[7] A second method relates to the use of internal shields where the thickness of the shielding device is limited by the internal space available within the patient. In the case of internal shielding devices a calibration measurement under actual conditions specific to the individual patient's treatment is recommended.[7]

A rule of thumb may be used to approximate the thickness of shielding material needed in external beam treatments. "The thickness of lead in millimeters required for shielding is approximately given by the energy in MeV divided by two,"[7] as follows:

$$\text{MeV/2} = \text{Shield thickness in millimeters of lead}$$

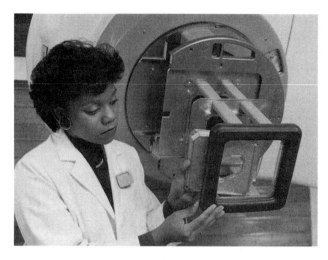

Fig. 13-4 Inserting a custom shielding device into a treatment cone. (Courtesy Varian Associates.)

Khan suggests that an additional millimeter of lead be added to the amount indicated by the rule of thumb method to provide an "extra safety margin."[9] Use of lead or alloys for shielding may result in an increase in dose if the thickness of the shielding material is not sufficient to reduce the dose to less than 5% of the total dose.[8] The thickness of Lipowitz alloy (Cerrobend) required may be obtained by multiplying the thickness in lead indicated by the rule of thumb by 1.2.[7]

Internal shielding

In some cases it is appropriate to place shielding devices within the oral cavity or under the eyelids. The objective is to shield the electron beam as it exits from the volume of tissue to be treated before it reaches normal tissue. A danger in the use of internal shielding devices is that the dose to the tissues directly in front of the shield may be increased by 30% to 70% because of the electron backscatter from the shield.[8] This problem may be minimized by placing a low Z number material between the shield and the tissue. Caution should be used in the selection of the thickness of low Z number material, which should be greater than the range of the backscattered electrons. Dental acrylic is commonly used to surround the lead shield, separating it from the oral cavity and reducing electron backscatter.[8] In the case of internal eye shields, there may not be sufficient space to allow adequate thickness of both lead and low atomic Z number material to absorb the electron backscatter produced by the lead shield.[8] Lead shields thick enough to reduce dosage to "acceptable levels" may be coated "with a thin film of wax or dental acrylic (to absorb very low energy electrons)."[8]

Effects of irregularly shaped electron fields on dose

An in-depth discussion of the calculation of irregular electron fields is beyond the scope of this chapter. However, situations that result in changes of dose will be identified. "Field shaping affects the output factor as well as depth dose distribution in a complex manner."[8] Variables encountered in field shaping that affect dose include the field size, the thickness of shielding material, the amount of blocking, and the treatment distance.[8] The dose rate or output factor of a clinical electron beam has a greater dependence upon field size than that of a clinical photon beam.[11] The dose at any point in the patient is composed of primary and scattered radiation. The greater dependence on field size of clinical electron beams than that of photon beams results from the amount of scattered radiation that contributes to the total dose. In photon beams, approximately 10% to 30% of the dose results from scattered radiation. In electron beams, almost all the absorbed dose results from electrons that have been scattered.[11] Lateral equilibrium of these scattered electrons is an important feature in electron beam dosimetry. Lateral equilibrium is reached when the number of electrons entering an area equals the number of electrons leaving the area. This condition is met when the diameter of the field size exceeds that of the practical range of the electron beam.[11] When the diameter of the electron beam field is less than the practical range, there is a decrease in dose. The smaller the diameter of the electron beam, the greater the change in the dose because of the lack of electronic equilibrium. For this reason, changes in dose associated with irregularly shaped electron fields may be anticipated if the dimensions of any portion of the treatment field are less than the practical range (MeV/2) of the electron beam.[16] Field shaping or blocking causes changes in the output of an electron beam. The size of the change in output depends on the percentage of the area of the total treatment field that is shielded or blocked. The higher the percentage of the field that is blocked, the greater the change in output. If greater than 25% of the treatment area is blocked, measurement of the output factor for that specific treatment is recommended.[8] The effect of the electron beam energy on the output factor increases with increasing electron beam energy when blocking is used.[13] For example, at extended treatment distances (110 cm SSD), field blocking causes a large change in the output of an electron beam, which may also require measurement of the output.[13] Olch states that "for SSD at 110 cm, almost any blockage severely changes the output factor."[8]

The use of irregularly shaped electron beams should be approached with caution. While it has been suggested that the output factor, depth dose, and isodose distribution should be measured for any irregularly shaped electron field, this is not practical.[8] A more reasonable approach is to investigate cases of irregularly shaped electron fields in which the field edges are not greater than the practical range.[3] Computerized treatment planning of irregularly shaped electron fields by pencil-beam algorithms may resolve the uncertainties in their use. It has been demonstrated that by using treatment planning computers with CT scans, both irregular fields at non-standard air gaps and dosage behind inhomogeneities may be calculated that are in agreement with measured data.[3] However, Hogstrom[3] indicates that careful evaluation of treatment planning computer programs used to calculate irregularly shaped electron fields is necessary. It should be noted that the treatment planning computer represents only half of the tools required.[16] CT scans of the treatment area with the patient in treatment position can be used to obtain calculation data that are not otherwise readily available.

Tissue heterogeneities and their effects on electron beams

"The sensitivity of high-energy electron dose distribution to the presence of tissue heterogeneities makes it essential to consider these effects in treatment planning and selection of technique."[7] The change in the dose distribution "depends on the shape, size, electron density (number of electrons/cm^3) and the effective atomic number of the heterogeneity."[10] The methods of calculating dose distributions are beyond the scope of this chapter; however, changes in the dose distributions as the result of tissue heterogeneity will be described.

Small heterogeneities cause local disturbances in the dose distribution.[8] Difficulties in determining the dose distribution around small heterogeneities result from enhanced scattering effects.[10] The dose to tissues behind small bones is decreased, as might be expected, because of the shielding effect of the bone. The dose to tissues lateral to the bone is increased because of lateral scattering of the electron beam.[10] The effect of a small air cavity surrounded by tissues is somewhat different. As might be expected, the dose to tissues beyond the air cavity is increased as a result of decreased scattering of the electrons as they pass through the air cavity. Similarly, the dose to tissues lateral to the air cavity is not increased, as in the case of a bone surrounded by tissue. This results from the decreased scattering of the electrons when passing through the air cavity. The dose to tissues beyond the air cavity is also increased because of additional electron scattering from surrounding tissues.[10] Changes in dose range from a 20% underdose behind bone to a 15% to 35% overdose behind air cavities.[10]

The situation for large tissue heterogeneities of uniform density differs from that of small heterogeneities.[10] The major factor responsible for changes in the dose distribution of large tissue heterogeneities of uniform density is absorption.[10] The determination of actual dose distribution resulting from a large heterogeneity depends on the complex interrelationships of several factors. However, the effect of large heterogeneities may be discussed in a general sense.[4]

At the boundary where the electron beam leaves the bone and enters tissue, there is a small increase in dose because of increased scattering of the electrons in the bone.[10] Tissues beyond the boundary of large high density heterogeneities such as bone receive a lower dose.[4] This results in the dose distribution being moved toward the surface.[4,10] Tissues beyond low density heterogeneities, such as lung, receive a greater dose because of the reduced absorption of the lung tissue. "This results in the dose distribution being moved toward greater depth.[10] In the lung, the range of the electrons is increased by a factor of 3, with an associated increase in dose to the lung and the tissue beyond the lung."[14] An additional concern with large heterogeneities involves areas of increased and decreased dose, or "hot and cold spots," which may appear at the lateral edges of the heterogeneity.[4]

Gaps in electron beam therapy

The use of combinations of two or more electron beams or electron beams and photon beams should be undertaken with great care. As previously stated, electron beam isodose curves have a characteristic shape (Fig. 13-2, *B*), which is described as a lateral bulge or ballooning of the isodose curves. Because of this characteristic shape, electron fields with adjacent treatment areas that abut each other on the surface will result in an overlap at depth.[8] Separating the treatment fields or placing a "gap" on the patient or phantom's surface results in an underdose or cold spot on the surface.[13] This is demonstrated in Fig. 13-5, which shows isodose distributions for adjacent electron fields. Note that the lowest dose to surface and superficial tissues results from the largest gap (1.5 cm). Similarly, the highest dose at depth results from the smallest

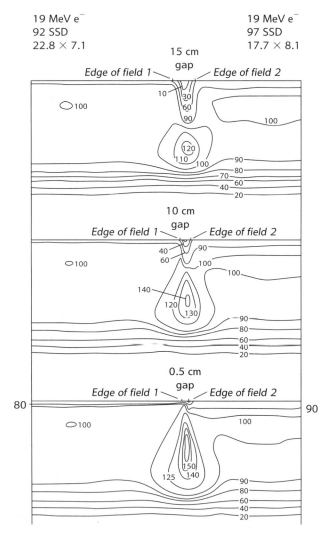

Fig. 13-5 Isodose distributions for adjoining fields with the same electron beam energy with different gap widths between fields. (From Tapley N, Almond PR, editors: *Clinical applications of the electron beam.* New York, 1976, Wiley.)

gap on the surface (0.5 cm). "In a clinical situation, the decision as to whether the fields should be abutted or separated should be based upon the uniformity of the combined dose distribution across the target volume."[9] To decrease the amount that the dose will vary to a particular anatomical location the abutment line may be moved two or three times during the patient's treatment course.[3] Treatments delivered in this fashion ensure that no one anatomical area will receive all of the increased or decreased dose.

A P P L I E D   T E C H N O L O G Y

Electron Beams in Radiation Therapy

In the next section, three cases are presented representing the clinical application of electron beams in radiation therapy. Various principles of treatment planning covered in the preceding portion of this chapter are demonstrated. The clinical cases are followed by a summary of the cases, which is meant to underscore the treatment planning principles outlined in each case.

Case studies

CASE I:

A 62-year-old woman with stage $T_2N_2M_O$ intraductal carcinoma of the left breast has had a left modified radical mastectomy and axillary lymph node dissection. The patient's past medical history is significant for hypertension, diabetes, asthma, and bronchitis. Family history is negative for malignancy.

Because the incidence of residual tumor after surgery is high for intraductal carcinoma, radiation therapy is used to treat the unresected microscopic involvement. After a mastectomy, the average thickness of the chest wall is 1.5 to 2.0 cm. The major characteristics of electron beam therapy are the rapid dose fall off, superficial dose distribution, and a skin dose of 80% to 100%, depending on the electron beam energy. With many critical structures such as lung, heart, and spinal cord underlying the chest wall, these beam characteristics make electron beam therapy an option for chest wall irradiation. Radiation therapy machines can produce a wide range of electron beam energies. The machine used for this particular treatment is a ScanditronixMM22-Microtron, which uses a dual scattering foil system to produce electron beam energies from 3 to 20 MeV. There are many considerations when determining which electron energy to use. For chest wall electron irradiation these may include the thickness of the chest wall, the surface skin dose needed, the use of tissue-equivalent material (bolus), and underlying critical structures. A 13 MeV electron beam is prescribed for a field 24 cm wide and 13 cm long (Fig. 13-6). A 1.0 cm thick bolus

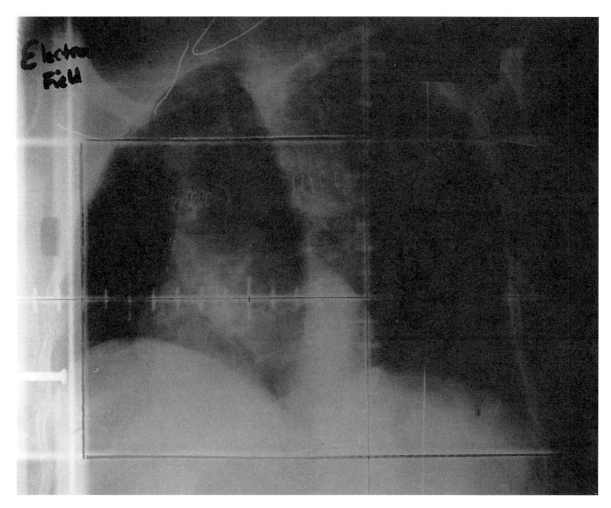

Fig. 13-6 Simulator verification film of the treatment volume for chest wall irradiation. The metal clips designate the mastectomy scar and the site of possible residual disease.

material is used to increase the surface skin dose. A dose of 5000 cGy will be delivered to the chest wall in 25 fractions, 200 cGy a day, to the 90% isodose line, which lies at a depth of 4.5 cm. The resulting dose to the skin surface is about 5222 cGy. A reduced area of the chest wall will be given anadditional 1000 cGy in 5 fractions, 200 cGy a day, to the 90% line with a 1.0 cm bolus.

The patient is set up and immobilized in a lateral oblique position with the left arm raised above the head (Fig. 13-7). Immobilization is achieved with the use of an alpha cradle. This position is accurately reproducible, allows the chest wall to be perpendicular to the central axis of the beam, and reduces the air gaps across the field. The central axis and borders of the electron field are located and marked in the simulator. Verification films and photographs are also taken at this time. In the treatment room a 100 cm SSD is set to the skin or to the top of the bolus material. The penumbra of the electron beam increases with an increase in distance between the patient skin surface and the electron cone. To avoid this problem, normal tissue and critical structures are spared by

the use of an electron cone with a Cerrobend (lead alloy) block placed close to the patient skin surface. The electron cone and Cerrobend block define the field to be treated.

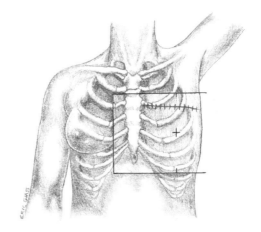

Fig. 13-7 Electron chest wall field that is to be treated.

CASE II:

A 50-year-old black woman had a mass in her left breast found on self-examination and confirmed by mammogram and biopsy. A modified radical mastectomy was performed with an axillary dissection. Postoperative workup and all 17 axillary lymph nodes removed were both negative for disease. She was diagnosed with a $T_1N_0M_0$ adenocarcinoma of the left breast. The patient was given tamoxifen and did well for approximately 1 year postoperatively.

After 16 months the patient noted some tenderness in the left chest wall, but presumed it resulted from arthritic changes. Because of progression of symptoms and the development of a sternal mass, a biopsy was performed 2 years after initial treatment. Histological examination confirmed locally recurrent breast cancer with metastatic disease in the sternum. She was referred to a radiation oncologist for consultation.

Examination revealed bilateral supraclavicular lymphadenopathy, which was believed to be malignant. Swelling in her upper medial left chest wall was consistent with internal mammary recurrence. CT scans were obtained to determine the dimensions of any residual masses as well as evaluate the possibility of subclinical disease, which would affect the approach for treatment. Planning was begun for a palliative course of radiation therapy. It was decided to use a combination of photons and electrons to treat all of the disease sites with an adequate and homogeneous dose while minimizing the dose to the lung. The dual-energy, dual-modality Siemens MD 6/15 unit was selected. This machine generates 6 and 15 MV photons and produces 5 to 14 MeV electrons with a single scattering foil. Electron and photon fields were treated on the same unit, which ensured accurate border matches. All ports were shaped with custom blocks.

Initially, 4000 cGy (200 cGy/fraction) was delivered by AP/PA fields with 15 MV photons used to treat the mediastinum, left internal mammary, and bilateral supraclavicular areas (Fig. 13-8, A). A 1.5 cm bolus was placed anteriorly to ensure adequate build-up due to superficial extension of disease. The disease in the inferolateral left thorax was limited to the chest wall only. To spare underlying lung tissue a 12 MeV electron field with a 0.5 cm bolus was delivered in an oblique direction and adjoined the photon fields at the medial and superior borders. The divergence from the PA port was calculated geometrically. Because of the difficulty in matching the exit point of the PA photon field with the entrance edge of the left anterior oblique (LAO) electron port (see Fig. 13-8, B) and the variance of the field size across the port, appropriate gaps were maintained between the AP and LAO ports at selected intervals. A final 1000 cGy was delivered to the sites of bulky disease using 10 MeV electrons with a 0.5 cm bolus to a total dose of 5000 cGy.

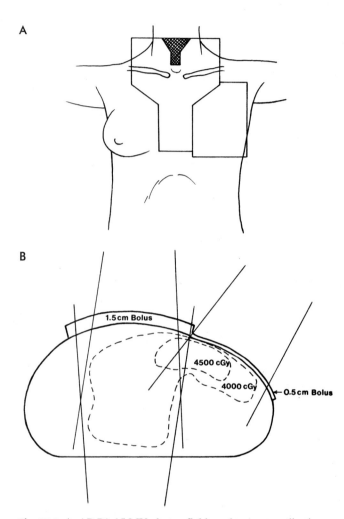

Fig. 13-8 **A**, AP-PA 15 MV photon field used to treat mediastinum, left internal mammary, and bilateral supraclavicular areas and the oblique 12 MeV electron beam used. **B**, Cross-sectional view showing orientation of the AP-PA photon fields, oblique electron field, and bolus materials.

CASE III:

A 52-year-old black man had a 1-month history of sore throat, hoarse voice, and hemoptysis. He was treated unsuccessfully with antibiotics. Triple endoscopy revealed prominent exophytic lesions involving the left false cord, extending to the epiglottis, and encroaching on the entire border of the left ventricular fold. CT scans were also obtained. He was diagnosed with a $T_3N_0M_0$ squamous cell carcinoma of the larynx.

The patient adamantly refused surgical treatment, but he agreed to a definitive course of radiation therapy. He was simulated supine with his arms in a reproducible position, and triangulation setup marks were tattooed. Measurements were taken from stable landmarks for each tattoo as well as the chin-to-suprasternal notch distance for proper head angulation. Isodistance photographs were taken for the construction of three-dimensional compensators to maximize the homogeneity of dose with the initial larger photon ports. All fields were shaped with custom Cerrobend blocks.

A hyperfractionated approach was used with a 100 cGy/fraction delivered twice per day and a 6- to 8-hour interval between fractions. Bilateral cobalt 60 ports (Fig. 13-9, *A*) were treated via a Theratron 780 so as to provide a homogeneous dose to the entire target volume, which included the primary tumor plus lymphatics. At 3960 cGy the photon ports were modified (Fig. 13-9, *B*) to exclude the dose-limiting spinal cord. Spinal cord tolerance is generally accepted as 4500 to 5000 cGy. This amount will vary with certain circumstances, such as the patient's overall condition, the length of the spinal cord irradiated, the dose per fraction, the number of fractions per day, and the use of chemotherapy. This patient was hyperfractionated and was tentatively scheduled to receive chemotherapy at the end of the radiation course. With this in mind, his spinal cord dose for the initial photon field was kept just below 4000 cGy.

The posterior neck nodes were matched to the off-cord photon fields and treatment continued twice per day at the same dose using 7 MeV electrons up to 5500 cGy. The dose was normalized to a depth of 1.6 cm, which was the maximum build-up for the energy. This energy was selected so as to provide an adequate dose to the nodes while delivering a minimal percentage to the spinal cord. A single-foil Siemens Mevatron XX was used. The primary site was central and anterior to the spinal cord (Fig. 13-9, *C*). It was boosted with bilateral cobalt 60 fields, which were also given at 100 cGy/fraction twice a day to a total dose of 6600 cGy delivered in 6 weeks.

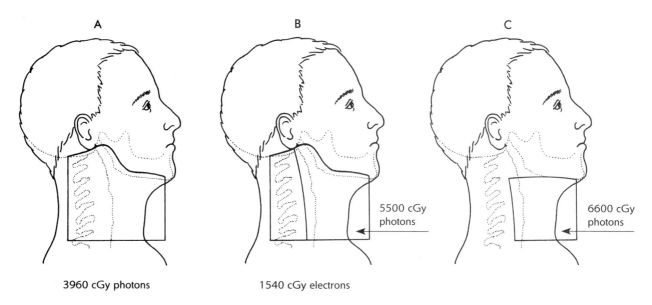

Fig. 13-9 A, Treatment port used to deliver 3960 cGy with cobalt 60 photons. **B**, Modified treatment ports. Anterior port treated to 5500 cGy with cobalt 60 photons; posterior port treated to 1540 cGy with 12 MeV electrons. **C**, Primary site boosted to 6600 cGy with cobalt 60 photons.

SUMMARY OF THE CLINICAL CASES

Case I details the use of an electron beam to treat a patient's chest wall after mastectomy. The goal of this treatment is to deliver a sufficient dose to the chest wall while preserving the lungs and pericardium, which are located just a few centimeters below the skin surface. A low energy electron beam that will spare the lungs and pericardium will also deliver a low dose to the superficial tissues and skin surface. The bolus in this treatment situation may be used to shape the dosage distribution to that of the patient as well as to increase the surface dose.[4]

Case II again deals with a postmastectomy breast cancer patient. The treatment goals are slightly different from those of the first case. The patient in case II has a parasternal mass and metastatic disease in the sternum. Treatment of these areas requires a homogeneous dose to the parasternal mass as well as the sternum. A megavoltage photon beam using parallel opposed fields was chosen to deliver

this homogeneous dose. A single direct electron beam with a rapid decrease in dose with increasing depth would not deliver a homogeneous dose to both parasternal mass and sternum. Additional, inhomogeneities could result from the scattering of electrons by the sternum near the parasternal mass. An adjacent area of the patient's chest wall was also involved. The chest wall was well suited to a single direct electron field, which allowed a dose to be delivered to the superficial tissues while preserving the lung directly beneath it. Abutting photon and electron fields are used to deliver a homogeneous dose to the anterior surface. The anterior megavoltage photon field is opposed by a posterior photon field. Other interesting features of this treatment include the use of bolus in both megavoltage electron and photon fields.

In case III, the goal of treatment was to deliver 5500 cGy to the lymph nodes of the patient's neck and 6600 cGy to the primary tumor. The parallel opposed cobalt 60 photons were used to provide a homogenous dose to the lymph nodes of the neck. If continued for the entire treatment course this would exceed the limit of spinal cord tolerance. A combination of electron and photon beams were used to overcome this problem. Cobalt 60 photons were used for the entire treatment course and electron beams were used at the end of the treatment course to treat the lymph nodes in the neck. This combination of cobalt 60 photons and electrons accom-

plished the goal of delivering 5500 cGy to the lymph nodes in the neck while limiting the dose to the spinal cord. In addition, the use of the cobalt 60 photons for the majority of the treatment course limited the dose to the patient's skin because of the skin-sparing effect of the megavoltage photon beam. To achieve the goal of delivering 6600 cGy to the primary tumor, the treatment field was reduced in size as treatment progressed.

Review Questions

Essay Questions

1. What is the predominate mode of electron beam interaction or scattering in the 1-20 MeV energy range used in radiation therapy?

2. List one advantage of the use of scattering foils in electron beam therapy.

3. A patient is to be treated with a 16 MeV electron beam. Calculate the depth of the 80% and 90% isodose lines.

4. A patient has a tumor at a depth of 4 cm. What energy of electron beam should be used so that the 80% isodose line encompasses the tumor?

5. What is the range in tissue of the electron beam used in question number four?

6. List two treatment planning considerations in the use of bolus in an electron beam used for radiation treatments.

7. Using the value of 2.4 for the constant C^4, determine the energy of an electron beam whose fifty percent isodose value is at a depth of 5 cm.

8. A patient is to be treated with a 7 MeV electron beam, how thick (in centimeters) should a lead shield be to reduce the dose to less than 5% of the useful beam?

9. Two electron beams adjoin or abut each other on the patient's skin surface. How does this affect the dose to the patient at depth below the point where the fields abut?

10. A 12 MeV electron beam is used to deliver a dose to a 4 cm by 4 cm field size. What should be considered for this particular treatment?

11. A patient is to be treated with a 15 MeV electron beam to a treatment volume which measures 5 centimeters in width and length at depth. Discuss the selection of field size for treatment?

Questions to Ponder

1. Compare and contrast the of the use of 1-20 MeV electron beams with that of photon beams in radiation therapy?

2. Discuss the situations in which a special calibration of an electron beam may be required.

3. Describe two specific clinical situations in which electron beam therapy is useful.

4. Compare and contrast the relationship between electron beam energy and the depth of maximum dose with that of photon beams?

REFERENCES

1. Cunningham R, Johns HE: *The physics of radiobiology*, ed 4. Springfield, IL, 1983, Charles C Thomas.

2. Grimm DF, et al: Electron beam port films. *Med Dosim* 14:31-33, 1989.

3. Hogstrom KR: Treatment planning in electron beam therapy. In Vaeth JB, Meyer JL, editors: *Frontiers of radiation therapy and oncology*, Vol 25. *The role of high energy electrons in the treatment of cancer*. New York, 1991, Karger.

4. ICRU Radiation Dosimetry: *Electrons with initial energies between 1 and 50 MeV*, report No. 21. Washington, DC, 1972, International Commission on Radiation Units and Measurements.

5. Karzmark CJ, Nunan CS, Tanabe E: *Medical electron accelerators*. New York, 1993, McGraw-Hill.

6. Khan FM: Basic physics of electron beam therapy. In Vaeth JB, Meyer JL, editors: *Frontiers of radiation therapy and oncology*, Vol 25. *The role of high energy electrons in the treatment of cancer*. New York, 1991, Karger.

7. Khan FM, et al: Clinical electron-beam dosimetry. Report of AAPM Radiation Therapy Committee Task Group No. 25. American Association of Physicists in Medicine (AAPM) *Med Physics* 18:73, 1991.

8. Khan FM: *The physics of radiation therapy*. Baltimore, 1984, Williams & Wilkins.

9. Khan FM: *The physics of radiation therapy*, ed 2. Baltimore, 1994, Williams & Wilkins.

10. Klevenhagen SC: *Physics of electron beam therapy, Medical Physics Handbooks* Bristol, Great Britain, 1985, Adam Hilger.

11. McPharland BJ: *Med Dosimetry* 14:17, 1989.

12. Mould RF: *Radiotherapy treatment planning*. Great Britain, 1981, Adam Hilger.

13. Olch A, et al: External beam electron therapy: pitfalls in treatment planning and deliverance. In Vaeth JB, Meyer JL, editors: *Frontiers of radiation therapy and oncology*, Vol 25. *The role of high energy electrons in the treatment of cancer*. New York, 1991, Karger.

14. Perez CA, Brady LW: *Principles and practice of radiation oncology*, Philadelphia, 1992, Lippincott.

15. Rustgi SN, Working KR: Dosimetry of small field electron beams. *Med Dosim* 17:108, 1992.

16. Tapley N duV: *Clinical applications for the electron beam*. New York, 1976, Wiley.

Glossary

absorbed dose Energy absorbed per unit mass of any material; units are the rad (100 ergs per gram) or gray (1 Gy = 1 joule per kilogram). 1 Gy = 100 rad.

activity Rate at which a radioactive isotope undergoes nuclear decay; units are the Curie (Ci) or becquerel (Bq = 1 disintegration per second). 1 Ci = 3.7 × 10^{10} Bq.

advisory agency An organization that collects and analyzes data and information and makes recommendations.

afferent lymphatic vessel Lymphatic vessels that flow into a lymph node. There are more afferent vessels than efferent vessels associated with each lymph node.

afterloading A system that was developed to allow devices known as applicators to be inserted into the treatment area first, then loaded with radioactivity quickly and safely. In this way, dose to personnel is kept to a minimum.

ALARA As Low As Reasonably Achievable; regulatory concept which stresses that radiation exposures to personnel and the public should be kept to a minimum.

algebraic equation A mathematical formula that describes a physical phenomenon based on the interaction of several factors or variables. Algebraic equations are typically used to find an unknown value when related factor values are known.

Alpha Cradle Trade name for an immobilization device created from a Styrofoam shell and foaming agents.

alpha particle Particulate radiation, positively charged, which consists of two protons and two neutrons; emitted during nuclear decay.

anatomical position Position in which the subject stands upright, with feet together flat on the floor, toes pointed forward, eyes looking forward, arms straight down by the sides of the body with palms facing forward, fingers extended and thumbs pointing away from the body.

anterior Relates to anatomy nearer to the front of the body.

applied dose The applied dose is the dose delivered at the depth of D_{max} for a single treatment field. Sometimes referred to as *given dose*.

Aquaplast Trade name for a thermoplastic that is frequently used as an immobilization device.

aspect of care Those activities considered to be of the most importance in providing health care services.

atlas First cervical vertebral body with the specialized function of supporting the skull and allowing it to turn.

attenuation The removal of photons and electrons from a radiation beam by scatter or absorption as it travels through a medium, typically tissue or tissue equivalent materials.

autoradiograph A signature exposure of a radioactive source obtained by placing the source on an unexposed x-ray film for a period of time long enough to darken the film. The film may be scanned to check for dose uniformity.

backscatter factor The ratio of the dose rate with a scattering medium (water or phantom) to the dose rate at the same point without a scattering medium (air).

backup timer setting The backup timer device refers to a safety device that will stop the treatment if the primary timer device fails.

beam restricting diaphragms Made of 2 mm to 3 mm of lead, the diaphragms (also called x-ray shutters, blades, or collimators) define both the size and the axis of the x-ray beam.

beta particle Electrons (B⁻, negatively charged) or positrons (B⁺, positively charged) emitted during nuclear decay.

bite block An object placed between the patient's teeth to assist in immobilization and to position the tongue.

blocked field size The equivalent rectangular field dimensions of the open treated area within the collimator field dimensions. The blocked field size is the actual area treated. Therefore, the blocked field size is normally smaller than the collimator field size.

body cavities The spaces within the body that contain internal organs.

body habitus The physique of the human body. The internal anatomy of a person varies with the physique. The four standard body habiti are hypersthenic, sthenic, hyposthenic, and asthenic.

bolus Tissue equivalent material that is usually placed on the patient to increase the skin dose and/or even out irregular contours in the patient. When bolus is placed on the skin surface for megavoltage irradiation, skin sparing is lost.

brachytherapy Radiation therapy technique that involves the application of radioactive material directly into or immediately adjacent to the tumor, rather than through external beams. The advantage of brachytherapy is that it delivers a large amount of dose directly into the area to which it was administered and rapidly falls off as distance increases from the sources.

build-up region The region between the skin surface and the depth of D_{max}. A build-up region is a characteristic of megavoltage irradiation. In this region the dose increases with depth until it reaches a maximum at the depth of D_{max}.

calvaria The part of the skull that protects the brain.

central axis It is the central portion of the beam emanating from the target; the only part of the beam that is not divergent.

chin to SSN measurement A measurement taken between the anatomical landmarks of the tip of chin and the suprasternal notch (SSN).

Clarkson integration or Clarkson technique is a method used to calculate the dose in an irregularly shaped field.

collimation Restricting the simulator's x-ray beam using the lead diaphragms.

collimator An arrangement of shielding material designed to define the dimensions of the beam of radiation. The collimators are located in the treatment head. The secondary collimators are used to set the field size.

collimator assembly The collimator assembly provides support for the x-ray tube aperture, field defining wires, light field indicator, beam limiting diaphragms, an accessory holder, and other essential equipment within the head of the gantry.

collimator field size The unblocked or open field size as defined by the collimator setting and projected at the reference distance, usually the isocenter of the machine.

common iliac nodes Lie at the bifurcation of the abdominal aorta at the level of L4.

These nodes directly drain the urinary bladder, prostate, cervix, and vagina.

compensatory curves Specific sections of the curvature of the vertebral column that form after birth due to the development of muscles as an infant grows. The cervical and lumbar curves are compensatory curves.

complex immobilization devices Individualized devices that restrict patient movement and ensure reproducibility in positioning.

continuous quality improvement (CQI) Same as for quality improvement; it is an ongoing improvement of health care services through the systematic evaluation of processes.

contralateral The opposite side of the body.

coronal plane Perpendicular (at right angles) to the sagittal plane and vertically divides the body into anterior and posterior sections.

CT simulation/virtual simulation A type of simulation that operates along with a 3D geometric planning computer. The extension of a CT system (usually a high performance spiral CT acquisition system) allows the single acquisition of many thin slices over a required treatment area. Virtual simulation is a geometrical planning function. It is not a 3D radiation treatment planning function, as it does not include or require dose computation. To complete the process of simulation, true virtual simulation systems allow the generation of DRR on the interactive basis.

decay constant The total number of atoms that decay per unit time.

depth The distance beneath the patient's skin to the point of calculation.

dimensional analysis A process that involves assessment of units of measure used in calculating some scientific quantity. This practice involves canceling of common units in an effort to leave the specified unit.

direct proportionality Relationship between measurable quantities/factors; as one increases, the other increases and vice versa.

divergence Divergence is the spreading out of the beam of radiation. The farther

from the source, the more the beam has spread. We need to be aware of beam divergence when setting up adjacent fields or where field edges are near critical structures. The divergence of the beam is taken into account when performing field size calculations and many dose calculations.

D_{max} The depth at which electronic equilibrium occurs for photon beams. This is also the depth of maximum absorbed dose and ionization, for photons, from a single treatment field. The depth of maximum ionization and maximum absorbed dose are usually not the same depth for electrons.

dose equivalent Product of the absorbed dose and a quality factor (QF), which takes into account the biological effects of different types of radiation on humans; units are the rem (1 rem = 1 rad × QF) or sievert (1 Sv = 1 Gy × QF). 1 Sv = 100 rem.

dose rate Also known as output, the dose rate of a treatment machine is the amount of radiation exposure produced by a treatment machine or source as specified at a reference field size and at a specified reference distance.

edema Excessive accumulation of fluid in a tissue, producing swelling.

effective dose equivalent The dose equivalent weighted by the proportionate risk for various tissues. That is, it is the sum over specified tissues of the products of the dose equivalent in a tissue and the weighting factor for that tissue.

effective field size (EFS) Another term for blocked field size (BFS). The effective field size (EFS) is the equivalent rectangular field dimensions of the open or treated area within the collimator field dimensions. The effective field size is the actual area treated.

efferent lymphatic vessels Lymphatic vessels that flow out of the hilum of a lymph node.

exposure Amount of ionization produced by photons in air per unit mass of air; units are the roentgen (R) or Coulomb per kilogram (C/kg). 1 R = 2.58 × 10⁻⁴ C/kg.

equivalent square The square field that has the same percentage depth dose and output of a rectangular field.

exit dose
The term exit dose is used for the dose at the exit surface of the patient or to a depth that is the equivalent of the depth of D_{max}.

extended distance setup An extended distance set up occurs when the set up SSD is greater than the reference SSD. The reference SSD is normally 80 cm for cobalt 60 treatment machines and 100 cm for linear accelerators.

fiducial plate Plastic trays imbedded with lead markers at regular intervals. These trays, sometimes referred to as a reticule or beaded trays, are positioned in the head of the gantry between the field defining wires and accessory holder.

field defining wires They are small tungsten wires (also called delineators), located in the collimator assembly, that represent the edge of the treatment field.

field size The dimension of a treatment field at the isocenter, represented by width × length.

film badge A device for measuring dose. It utilizes the phenomenon that when film is exposed to radiation and subsequently developed, the amount of blackening is proportional to the dose delivered to the film. Metal filters in the film badge holder are used to allow discrimination of the energy levels of the radiation.

flow chart A diagram illustrating a sequence of steps to be utilized in the completion of a process.

free space Term used for dosimetry measurements using a build-up cap or miniphantom.

gamma rays High energy electromagnetic radiation of no mass and no charge emitted during nuclear decay.

gantry On a simulator, it is a mechanical C-shaped device that supports the x-ray tube and collimator device at one end and an image system at the other and allows the duplication of treatment unit motions.

gap The distance between the borders of two adjacent fields. The gap is usually measured on the patient's skin. The skin gap is usually calculated to verify the depth at which the two adjacent fields abut.

genetically significant dose The dose equivalent to the gonads weighted for the age and sex distribution in those members of the irradiated population expected to have offspring; units are the rem or sievert.

given dose The given dose (GD) is the dose delivered at the depth of D_{max} through a single treatment field. Also known as *applied dose* or D_{max} dose.

grid A device constructed with thin lead foil strips and plastic spacers. It should be employed during simulation both to absorb the scattered radiation emitted from the thicker body parts, and to allow the use of beam energies needed to maximize differential absorption between similar tissues.

half-life The time period in which the activity decays to one-half the original value. It is the essential value to employ the decay formula for a particular isotope.

health care organization A generic term used to describe all types of groups that provide health care services.

image intensifier It is a useful tool during fluoroscopy, as it converts an x-ray image into a light image.

immobilization The process of ensuring that a patient does not move out of treatment position, thus allowing for reproducibility and accuracy in treatment.

immunity The ability of the body to defend itself against infectious organisms, foreign bodies, and cancer cells.

inferior Toward the feet.

internal mammary lymphatic pathway Lymphatic chain that runs toward the midline and passes through the pectoralis major and intercostal muscles close to the body of the sternum (T4-T9).

interpolation To estimate values between two measured, known values. A mathematical process used in radiation therapy in which unlisted values in tables can be derived.

interstitial brachytherapy Treatment technique that is characterized by the placement of radioactive sources directly into a tumor or tumor bed. Interstitial implants can be either permanent or temporary.

intracavitary brachytherapy In this aspect of brachytherapy, radioactive

sources are placed within a body cavity for treatment. This type of brachytherapy has been the mainstay in treatment of cervical cancer for over 50 years.

intraluminal brachytherapy Closely associated with interstitial brachytherapy, intraluminal brachytherapy place sources of radiation within body tubes such as the esophagus, uterus, trachea, bronchus, and rectum. Many high dose rate applications are performed for intraluminal applications.

inverse proportionality Relationship between measurable quantities/factors, in that as one increases, the other decreases, and vice versa.

inverse square law A mathematical relationship that describes the change in beam intensity as the distance from the source changes. The change in intensity is primarily due to the divergence of the beam.

ionizing radiation Radiation with sufficient energy to separate an electron from its atom.

ipsilateral Refers to a body component on the same side of the body.

irradiated volume The volume of tissue receiving a significant dose (e.g., >50%) of the specified target dose.

isocenter The gantry of both the simulator and treatment unit rotates around a fixed point in space, called the isocenter. It is a reference point, located at a fixed distance (80 cm to 100 cm) from the target.

Joint Commission on the Accreditation of Healthcare Organizations An independent, not-for-profit organization dedicated to improving quality of care in organized health care settings. It is the accrediting body for health care organizations.

kyphosis An excessive curvature of the vertebral column that is convex posteriorly.

lasers Each positional laser projects a small red beam of light toward the patient during the simulation or treatment process. This provides the therapist several external reference points in relationship to the position of the isocenter.

lateral Toward one side or the other.

LET Linear energy transfer; the average energy deposited per unit path length to a medium by ionizing radiation as it passes through that medium.

light cast A fiberglass tape that contains resin, which can be molded around a patient. When exposed to ultraviolet light, it hardens, creating a rigid immobilization device.

localization The geometrical definition of the tumor and anatomical structures using reference of surface marks.

logarithm The inverse or exponential notation. The exponent that indicated the power to which a number is raised to produce a given number.

lymph Excessive tissue fluid consisting mostly of water and plasma proteins from capillaries.

lymphangiography A radiographic study that uses special injected dyes that aid in visualizing the lymphatic system on x-ray.

magnetic resonance imaging (MRI) A diagnostic, nonionizing means of visualizing internal anatomy through noninvasive means. Imaging is based on the magnetic properties of the hydrogen nuclei.

mastoid process An extension of the mastoid temporal bone at the level of the ear lobe.

Mayneord's factor Used to convert the percentage depth dose at the reference distance to the percentage depth dose at a nonreference distance. This would occur at extended distance setups.

mean life The average lifetime for the decay of radioactive atoms. It is the time period for a hypothetical source that decays at a constant rate equal to its initial activity to produce the same number of disintegrations as the exponentially decaying source that decays for an infinite period of time. It is primarily applicable to dose calculations in permanent implants, typically gold-198 (198Au) and iodine-125 (125I).

medial Toward the midline of the body.

median sagittal plane Also called the midsagittal plane, divides the body into two symmetric right and left sides. There is only one median sagittal plane.

meter setting Used for the monitor unit setting for linear accelerators and the minute setting for cobalt 60 treatment machines.

monitor unit A unit of output measure used for linear accelerators. The accelerators are calibrated so that one MU delivers 1 cGy for a standard, reference field size at a standard reference depth at a standard source-to-calibration point.

nasion The center depression at the base of the nose.

natural background radiation Ionizing radiation from natural sources including cosmic rays from outer space and our sun, terrestrial radiation from radioactive materials in the earth, and internal radiation from radioactive materials normally present in the body.

nuclear medicine The branch of medicine that uses radioisotopes in the diagnosis and treatment of disease.

occupancy factor (T) The fraction of time that an area adjacent to a source of radiation is occupied.

optical distance indicator (ODI) Sometimes called a rangefinder, it projects a scale onto the patients' skin, which corresponds to the SSD used during the simulation or treatment process.

outcomes The result of the performance, or lack of performance, of a process.

output Referred to as the dose rate of the machine. Dose rate should be specified for field size, distance, and medium.

output factor The ratio of the dose rate of a given field size to the dose rate of the reference field size.

ovoid Also called colpostats, these applicators are oval-shaped and insert into the lateral fornices of the vagina. They can hold radioactive sources and shielding material and are used in the treatment of gynecological tumors.

para-aortic nodes Efferent to the cisterna chyli, which is the beginning of the thoracic duct. These nodes run adjacent to the abdominal aorta from T12 to L4. This major section of the lymphatic system eventually receives lymph from most of the lower regions of the body.

paranasal sinuses Air spaces in the skull, lined by mucous membranes, that reduce the weight of the skull and give the voice resonance. The four paranasal sinuses are the ethmoid, maxillary, sphenoid, and frontal.

patient positioning aids Devices that place the patient in a particular position for treatment, but do not ensure that the patient does not move.

patient support assembly (PSA) Also called a "couch" or "table," it allows the table top its mobility, permitting the precise and exact positioning of the isocenter during simulation or treatment. A standard feature allows the table top to mechanically move vertically, radially, horizontally, and in a lengthwise direction.

peak scatter factor The peak scatter factor is a backscatter factor sometimes normalized to a reference field size, usually $10 \, cm \times 10 \, cm$, for energies of 4 MV and above.

peer review An evaluation by health care professionals of the same credentials in which standards of practice are applied to evaluate professional performance and processes. This evaluation may be conducted by health care professionals within the same organization or from another health care organization.

pendant A set of hand-held local controls suspended from the ceiling or attached to the treatment couch that mimic those of the treatment unit.

percentage depth dose (PDD) The ratio, expressed as a percentage, of the absorbed dose at a given depth to the absorbed dose at a fixed reference depth, usually D_{max}.

pharynx A membranous tube that extends from the base of skull to the esophagus and connects the oral and nasal cavities with the larynx and esophagus.

photon Small packet of electromagnetic energy, e.g., radiowaves, visible light, and x-rays and gamma rays.

pocket ionization chamber (pocket dosimeter) A device for measuring exposure. It utilizes the phenomenon that when air is irradiated, the ions formed partially discharge the static electricity on a fine filament, allowing it to move across a scale. The filament and scale can be visualized by holding the cylindrical device up to a light and looking through one end.

positrons Positively charged electrons.

quality assessment The systematic quality analysis and review of patient care data.

quality assurance (QA) A systematic monitoring of the quality and appropriateness of patient care with an emphasis on performance levels.

quality control (QC) A component of quality assurance used in reference to the mechanical and geometrical tests of the radiation therapy equipment.

quality improvement (QI) The continuous improvement of health care services through the systematic evaluation of processes.

quality indicator A measurement tool used to evaluate an organization's performance.

radiation oncology team A group consisting of all staff employees in radiation oncology who come in contact with the patient and/or family members throughout the course of radiation treatments.

radiation therapy prescription A legal document written by a radiation oncologist that provides the therapist with the information required to deliver the appropriate radiation treatment. It defines the treatment volume, intended tumor dose, number of treatments, dose per treatment, and frequency of treatment.

radiopaque marker A material with a high atomic number used to document structures radiographically.

radium substitute Any isotope used for brachytherapy whose dosimetry is based on the original radium work.

ratio A mathematical comparison of two numbers, values, or terms that denotes a relationship between the two.

regulatory agency An organization that may promulgate rules and regulations which have the force of law; license users; and provide inspection and enforcement actions.

scatter Radiation that changes direction.

scatter air ratio (SAR) The ratio of the scattered dose at a given point to the dose in free space at the same point. The scatter air ratio is the difference between the tissue air ratio for a given field size and the tissue air ratio for a zero field size. An equation can be written for the SAR: SAR = TAR(d,r1) - TAR(d,0); where d is the depth of calculation and r1 is the field size at the depth. TAR(d,0) represents the primary component of the beam. There is no dose from the scatter components in TAR(d,0).

separation The measurement of the thickness of a patient along the central axis or at any other specified point within the irradiated volume, also referred to as IFD.

sim CT/simulated CT The extension and adaption of a conventional simulator to allow the acquisition of axial "slices". They simulate CT slices. Usually these are limited to a small number of thick slices and are adequate for localization and 2D treatment planning, but generate poor quality DRR images.

simple immobilization devices Devices which restrict movement but require a patient's voluntary cooperation.

simulation Can be a process carried out by the radiation therapist under the supervision of the radiation oncologist. It is the mockup procedure of a patient treatment with radiographic documentation of the treatment portals.

simulator A specialized x-ray machine that imitates the mechanical and geometrical features of several different treatment units.

skin sparing A property of megavoltage irradiation where the maximum dose occurs at some depth beneath the skin surface.

source axis distance (SAD) The distance from the source of radiation to the axis of rotation of the treatment unit.

source skin distance (SSD) The distance from the source of radiation to the patient's skin.

specific activity The activity per unit mass of a radioactive material (Ci/g). The specific activity dictates the total activity that a small source can have.

table top That part of the patient support assembly (PSA) on which a patient is positioned during treatment or simulation; may be called a treatment couch or patient table top.

tandem A long narrow tube that inserts into the opening of the cervix (cervical os) into the uterus. They can hold radioactive sources and are used in the treatment of gynecological tumors.

target volume Consists of the tumor, if present, and any other tissue with presumed tumor.

"tennis racket" This may be a square or rectangular section of the table top, similar to a tennis or racquetball racquet

woven tightly together. After extended use, the "tennis racquet" section should be re-strung to provide more patient support and reduce the amount of "sag" during simulation.

thermoluminescent dosimeter (TLD) A device for measuring dose. It utilizes the phenomenon that some solid materials, when irradiated, will subsequently give off light when heated. The amount of light emitted is proportional to the dose delivered to the crystal.

tissue air ratio The ratio of the absorbed dose at a given depth in phantom to the absorbed dose at the same point in free space.

tissue absorption factor The beam of radiation gives up energy as it travels through the body. The more tissue the beam traverses, the more it is attenuated. There are a number of different methods for measuring the attenuation of the beam as it travels through tissue. These are *percentage depth dose, tissue air ratio, tissue phantom ratio,* and *tissue maximum ratio*. The first method used was *percentage depth dose*.

tissue maximum ratio The ratio of the absorbed dose at a given depth in phantom to the absorbed dose at the same point at the level of D_{max} in phantom.

tissue phantom ratio The ratio of the absorbed dose at a given depth in phantom to the absorbed dose at the same point at a reference depth in phantom. If the reference depth is chosen to be the depth of D_{max}, then the tissue phantom ratio is called the *tissue maximum ratio*.

topical brachytherapy Radioactive sources are placed on top of the area to be treated. Molds of the body part to be treated may be taken and prepared to place the sources in definite arrangements to deliver the prescribed dose.

total quality management (TQM) Synonymous to CQI. An organization-wide systematic approach designed to improve services and reduce costs by concentrating on processes.

transmission factor Any device placed in the path of the radiation beam will attenuate the beam. The transmission factor is the ratio of the radiation dose with the device to the radiation dose without the device. Examples of commonly used devices in radiation therapy are blocking trays, wedges, and compensators.

treatment time   The amount of time required to deliver a prescribed dose of radiation, taking all pertinent treatment factors such as field size, energy, depth, etc. into account. Treatment time is used in treatment with Cobalt 60.

treatment verification   A process using diagnostic quality radiographs of each treatment field from the initial simulation procedure to determine the accuracy of the treatment plan.

treatment volume   Generally larger than the target volume, and encompasses the additional margins around the target volume to allow for limitations of the treatment technique.

tumor localization   This may involve the use of a simulator in determining the extent of the tumor and location of critical structures.

use factor (U)   The fraction of time that the radiation beam is directed at a barrier; the use factor for scatter and leakage radiation is always 1.

Vac-lok   Trade name for an immobilization device that consists of a cushion and a vacuum compression pump.

vacuum-formed shell   An immobilization device that is formed when a piece of plastic is molded over a plaster cast of a patient's anatomy.

verification   A final check that each of the planned treatment beams does cover the tumor or target volume and does not irradiate normal tissue structures.

wedge filter   A tool that modifies the isodose distribution of a beam to correct for oblique incidence or tissue inhomogeneities by progressively decreasing beam intensity across the field irradiated.

workload (W)   For superficial and orthovoltage units, the milliamperage (mA) used and beam on time per week; for high energy units, the Gy (rad) per week at isocenter.

x-ray generator   It provides radiographic and fluoroscopic control of the simulator through the selection of various exposure factors, which include: focal spot, mAs, kVp, and time.

x-rays   High energy electromagnetic radiation of no mass and no charge resulting from the rearrangement of electrons in the electron shells or from the process of bremsstrahlung.

Answers to Review Questions

CHAPTER 1

1. c
2. a
3. a
4. a
5. b
6. True
7. False

CHAPTER 2

1. c
2. d
3. c
4. e
5. c
6. b
7. a
8. d
9. e
10. e

CHAPTER 3

1. d
2. c
3. b
4. a
5. c
6. b
7. c
8. c

9. d
10. a
11. c
12. c
13. b
14. d
15. a

CHAPTER 4

1.
Term	Answer
Exposure	g
Activity	f
Absorbed dose	g
Dose equivalent	e
Gamma ray	b
X-ray	a
Positron	d
Alpha particle	c

2. c
3. b
4. b
5. c
6. c
7. c

CHAPTER 5

1. According to JCAHO, the departmental medical director is responsible for the establishment and continuation of a quality improvement program. However, the responsibility may be met by appointing a Quality Improvement Committee.

2. Quality improvement programs are important in radiation oncology because they are directly correlated to an increase in quality of service and cost reduction. It is a way or ensuring a consistent and safe delivery of radiation to all patients at all times.
3. The radiation therapist has an integral role in the quality improvement process. He is not only involved with patient care and treatment delivery activities, but also equipment performance and documentation.
4. Quality assurance is department specific and emphasizes the level of performance. Whereas, quality improvement emphasizes total involvement of all staff members, is organization-wide, and focuses on customer satisfaction. It is based on the premise that even the best process can be improved.
5. The data collected in a quality improvement plan should be systematically analyzed against customer satisfaction and put into meaningful form. Solutions for improvement should be based on the results of the data analysis. The results should be distributed to all staff employees.

PONDER QUESTION RESPONSES

1. The phrase, "If it ain't broke, don't fix it," cannot be applied in a quality improvement plan. The phrase assumes that if something works, then there is nothing wrong with it and therefore needs no attention. The basic concept in a quality improvement plan involves continually refining a process or processes perpetually, because it is believed that even the best process can be improved.
2. Development of port film example (flow chart):

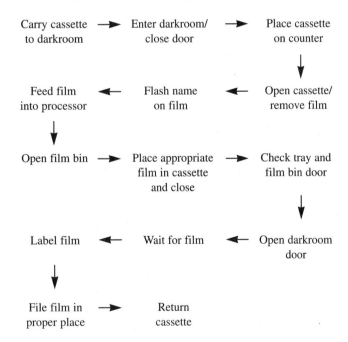

3. According to CQI and Deming's principles of management, the power to improve the process rests specifically with the employees. I would recommend that the coworker, in cooperation with management, make a flow chart defining the activities surrounding the process. If it involves the responsibility of more than one staff employee, then a team should be formed to study the process and how it can be improved.

CHAPTER 6

1. c
2. d
3. a
4. a
5. d
6. b

CHAPTER 7

1. b
2. b
3. e
4. True
5. False
6. True
7. True
8. True
9. False
10. False

CHAPTER 8

1. Median or midsaggital
2. Diaphram
3. Thoracic duct
4. C-2
5. Ureters
6. d
7. b
8. b
9. c
10. c

CHAPTER 9

1. False
2. True
3. d
4. c
5. d
6. b
7. b
8. b
9. a
10. d

CHAPTER 10

1. a
2. d
3. a
4. c
5. d
6. a
7. d
8. True
9. False

CHAPTER 11

1. b
2. a
3. b
4. c
5. c
6. c
7. b
8. a
9. True

CHAPTER 12

1. d
2. b
3. d
4. c
5. d
6. d
7. d
8. True
9. False
10. True

CHAPTER 13

1. The predominate mechanism of the interaction of electron beams in the 1-20 MeV energy range used in radiation therapy is collisional interactions. This is due to the low Z number of tissue that interacts with the electron beam.
2. Scattering foils are a relatively simple and reliable method of producing a clinically useful electron beam (when compared to the scanning beam method).
3. The depth of the 80% isodose line = MeV/3
   by substitution 16 MeV/3 = 5.3 cm
   The depth of the 90% isodose line = MeV/4
   by substitution, 16 MeV/4 = 4.0 cm
4. The depth of the 80% isodose line = MeV/3
   solving for the energy, MeV/3 = 4.0 cm, 3 × 4.0 = 12 MeV
5. E_r = MeV/2, range of an electron beam in tissue,
   by substitution 12 MeV/2 = 6
6. 1) A partial bolus should never be used with electron beams.
   2) The "edge effect" (areas of increased and decreased dose) produced by a large bolus with an edge perpendicular to the surface.
   3) Electron beams less than 12 MeV may require a bolus to increase surface dose.
   4) Bolus may also be used to shape isodose distributions to conform to the treatment volume or as a tissue compensator.
7. $E_o = C_4R_{50}$, By substitution, E_o = 2.4 × 5.0 cm = 12 MeV.
8. Shield thickness in millimeters of lead = MeV/2
   By substitution, 7/2 = 3.5 mm
   NOTE: Khan suggests that an additional millimeter of lead should be added to the amount indicated by the rule of thumb as follows:
   7/2 = 3.5 + 1.0 = 4.5 mm
9. This would result in an area of increased dose below the location where the two treatment fields adjoin or abut.
10. The output of this treatment field may require a calibration measurement due to the diameter of the treatment field being less than the practical range (E_r = MeV/2) of the treatment beam.
11. Due to lateral constriction of the higher isodose lines at 15 MeV a larger area on the surface must be irradiated to cover a given area at depth. A margin of 1 cm is recommended between the lateral edge of the target volume and the edge of the collimator.

Index